Contemplative Practices for Sustaining Wellness

Bold Visions in Educational Research

VOLUME 78

The titles published in this series are listed at *brill.com/bver*

Contemplative Practices for Sustaining Wellness

Priorities for Research and Education

Edited by

Kenneth Tobin and Konstantinos Alexakos

BRILL

LEIDEN | BOSTON

Cover illustration: Photograph by Konstantinos Alexakos

All chapters in this book have undergone peer review.

Library of Congress Cataloging-in-Publication Data

Names: Tobin, Kenneth George, 1944- editor. | Alexakos, Konstantinos, editor.
Title: Contemplative practices for sustaining wellness : priorities for research and education / edited by Kenneth Tobin and Konstantinos Alexakos.
Description: Leiden ; Boston : Brill, [2022] | Series: Bold visions in educational research, 1879-4262 ; volume 78 | Includes bibliographical references and index.
Identifiers: LCCN 2022034742 (print) | LCCN 2022034743 (ebook) | ISBN 9789004527324 (paperback) | ISBN 9789004527331 (hardback) | ISBN 9789004527348 (ebook)
Subjects: LCSH: Health. | Health promotion. | Self-care, Health.
Classification: LCC RA776 .C759 2022 (print) | LCC RA776 (ebook) | DDC 613--dc23/eng/20220802
LC record available at https://lccn.loc.gov/2022034742
LC ebook record available at https://lccn.loc.gov/2022034743

Typeface for the Latin, Greek, and Cyrillic scripts: "Brill". See and download: brill.com/brill-typeface.

ISSN 1879-4262
ISBN 978-90-04-52732-4 (paperback)
ISBN 978-90-04-52733-1 (hardback)
ISBN 978-90-04-52734-8 (e-book)

This book is printed on acid-free paper and produced in a sustainable manner.

Contents

PREFACE

Our Research on Emotion and Wellness

In this preface we provide a context for authentic inquiry, an important component of the approach we adopt in our research. We address the salience of theoretical frameworks, emphasizing that we do not regard them as pathways toward truths, but as ways to illuminate lived experiences. We provide context for our multilogical approach with introductory reviews of the sociocultural and interpretive methodologies that are emergent and contingent. In so doing, we are mindful of limitations due to a crisis of representation. Our research designs acknowledge that there always will be more than we can illuminate with research. We can always do and learn more. Because all authors/researchers who contributed to the book use narrative in their chapters, we present an overview of the importance of narrative in our research.

Our prior research on emotions connects with changes in physiology and associated health issues. Accordingly, we provide brief insights into our research on emotion, its association with wellness projects, and healing dis-ease.[1] Because emotions and dis-ease are pervasive across the lifespan and encompass the entire world, we conclude with an exhortation to expand foci for research to embrace the life spectrum from pre-birth through death, and to expand the places in which research is undertaken. That is, global perspectives are a priority and foci also should include aspects of the entire spectrum of everyday life. There is a priority for research in wellness that goes beyond just formal schools, to include places like hospitals, home, and even our own bodies.

Our Methodologies

The 31 authors of the 19 chapters that comprise this book embrace a goal that the research in which they engage can and should catalyze positive changes in social life, while also contributing to the knowledge system we label as education. In our ongoing research we have employed authentic inquiry, seeking to ensure that we learn from the research we undertake (Tobin & Alexakos, 2021a). Also, we endeavor to educate participants in our research about what we learn, ensuring that they understand the diversity of perspectives extant within different clusters of participants. Importantly, others' perspectives are to be valued, respected, and considered as resources from which to learn. We regard authentic inquiry as a catalyst for change and to assist all participants to benefit from what we have learned in research by changing their practices if and when it is appropriate to do so. We recognize that some participants are better placed than others to benefit from what we have learned in our research. Accordingly, we plan and enact to ensure that beneficence is equitable for everyone involved in regards to improving the quality of social practices that are enhanced from understandings of what we are learning from ongoing authentic inquiry.

Illuminating Pathways for High Priority Research

Our approach to research has been to recognize that the answers to questions like: What is happening? Why is it happening? and What more can be learned? depend on the theories we use to frame our research experiences. What we see as we undertake research depends on what we are aware of – so that when it happens we take note because of its salience to the research. We know full well that theory illuminates, as it obscures. For example, consider the research we were undertaking in Australia – collaborating with Steve Ritchie, Donna King, and colleagues (Tobin et al., 2016). As we were in the process of analyzing expressed emotions and associated physiological responses, we were aware that when Donna addressed her science education class, there were times when students found her voice annoying (Tobin, 2018). As we studied the prosody of her utterances we noticed that when she was teaching with low levels of blood oxygenation, some vowels had high-frequency components that were uttered with high intensity. We heard this as a twang, and re-searched our database to find as many occurrences of twangs as we could.

At the time we were doing these analyses, Maria Miniello, a colleague who was involved in complementary medicine, introduced us to The Polyvagal Theory (PVT; Porges, 2011). Maria felt PVT might apply to our ongoing work on using healing practices to treat everyday health issues such as seasonal allergies, headache, skin rashes and dermatitis, and injuries to muscles and connective tissue.

After a relatively short time we saw the relevance of PVT to healing work and also noted its potential applicability to our studies of physiological responses to expressed emotions. Also, based on our emerging understandings of PVT, through the theoretical lights of Stephen Porges' publications and videos, we began to view oximetry data in terms of autonomic functioning of the nervous system (ANS) – especially the role of the vagus nerve. PVT allowed us to interrelate states of the ANS with breathing patterns, expressed emotions, and physiological changes. From the perspective of PVT, a relatively low blood oxygenation might be regarded by Donna's monitoring system as a threat to the wellbeing of her body.

Without consciously trying to do so, Donna's body's nervous system might favor sympathetic innervation, which is frequently described as a fight-flight mode of functioning (Dana, 2018). Of salience to our study of prosody, when the ANS functioning is primarily sympathetic, the prosody of the voice is constrained to express orally in ways that are suited to situations of physical and social risk – such as being able to express fear and anger. Hence, to the extent that Donna's ANS functioning is sympathetic, her voice would show less variation – possibly permitting high and low intensity and features that might frighten away attackers and alert caregivers, if and when necessary. In contrast, when parasympathetic functioning of the ANS is favored, the muscles attached to the tongue receive the energy necessary to create a wider range of prosodic functions that can enhance social communication.

With insights like these we re-examined prosodic trends and video images coordinated with oximetry data that allowed us to compare at rest oximetry measures with prosody in an environment in which pulse rate, blood pressure, and blood oxygenation varied from normal (e.g., getting ready to teach).

Once we envisioned the benefits of including PVT in a multilogical framework, we began to use it to deepen and expand the understanding and scope of our research. Importantly, PVT illuminated the importance of nasal breathing, its association with nitric oxide, and functioning of the ANS. For example, in our program of research on contemplative practices, emotions, and wellness, we ensured that in designing meditation protocols we emphasized the value of breathing in and out through the nose, and of humming audibly on the outbreath (Tobin & Alexakos, 2022).

Several authors in this volume specifically mention PVT as one of the theoretical frames they use in their research. For the most part, our research incorporates multilogicality, whereby each study uses complementary frameworks for purposes associated with authentic inquiry (i.e., learning from research, transforming practice, and using research to attain and maintain equity). We stress that the bricolage of frameworks changes continuously because of the emergent and contingent nature of our research. Also, the constituent theories themselves change as we learn more about them and the nuances they entail. We do not see our bricolage as truths (Kincheloe, 2005). Instead, we see our frameworks as lights that illuminate salient practices and events while obscuring others. Ken wrote about this stance in an editorial published in *Cultural Studies of Science Education* (CSSE) in 2008:

> In creating CSSE we sought to provide a forum for social and cultural theories to inform scholarship in science education. In so doing we did not seek to extinguish psychological models from being employed in research and scholarship in science education, nor do we seek to represent sociocultural frameworks as viable master narratives. Hence, in laying out theories, associated critical reviews, and forum discussions we hope to provide the kernels for fresh conversations and the hoisting of lamplights to illuminate fresh fields for the conduct of research in science education. In so doing, it is important to acknowledge that the theories used to give meaning to social life, while informative, are neither complete nor unique. Through the use of multiple frameworks, different events and phenomena may become salient as objects for research. (Tobin 2008, p. 229)

For this reason, it is important to be specific about our frameworks and open to research grounded in different theoretical frames. We suggest that in our work we seek to learn through the use of practices that are intensive and extensive, ensuring that what we learn is explicitly linked to the theories we appropriate. Consistent with William Sewell Jr's theory of culture, we not only learn from patterns of coherence in participants' practices, but also from dialectically related contradictions (i.e., patterns of coherence | contradictions) so that nuance is attained in what we learn from research (Sewell, 2005).

In a long journey that began with Fred Erickson's Interpretive Research (Erickson, 1986), in the mid-1980s, we developed authentic inquiry to address what is happening and why it is happening (Tobin & Alexakos, 2021a). Also, we embrace a mantra "what more is there?" – because there always will be more than can be spoken and written (Greene, 1994). Also, as ethnomethodologists made clear (Garfinkel, 1967), culture reveals itself in unsettled times (Swidler, 1986). When perturbations occur, previously hidden forms of culture can emerge and be seen. For this reason, we view the three broad questions of what, why, and what more as constituents of participatory inquiry that includes authentic inquiry, event-oriented inquiry, and an array of methods | methodologies that we employ if, when, and as needed (Tobin, 2021).

The theories we employ in our multilogical approach are not as others – such as Porges, Sewell, and Bourdieu might understand their own work. Citations signify our appropriation of others' work. We build understandings of their research and then adapt and apply what we have learned, and value, in ways that are consistent with overarching schemas of emergence and contingence. We read others' work from a context of lived experiences and expectations that we may appropriate from what we learn for the purpose of enhancing our research. In citing research, we acknowledge the roots of our appropriations, and do not imply that those cited would necessarily see the affordances of their work in our contexts and associated research goals.

As our frameworks evolve it is often possible to re-analyze data sets to obtain deeper and complementary insights. In the case of Donna's teaching of science education, we did not only learn about mouth and nose breathing, nitric oxide, modes of autonomic functioning, prosody, blood oxygenation, and pulse rate (Tobin, 2018). We also learned that our initial understandings of PVT were even more appropriate and powerful when we considered the modes of autonomic functioning as dialectically related. For example, instead of seeing sympathetic and parasympathetic functioning as binary states, we view social systems as dynamically shifting with different states of equilibria being dependent on context. The relationship we found most useful was sympathetic | parasympathetic. This was specifically important in our studies of healing, using soft touch healing and other contemplative practices (Tobin & Alexakos, 2022).

When we speak and write about frameworks, our purpose in so doing is to communicate with those who seek to learn about our work. Accordingly, we try to write plainly so that it is not necessary to be checking back and forth with dictionaries, other articles, and books. The dissemination of our research is part of our adherence to authentic inquiry. Our efforts to disseminate are not constrained to only one article or to just one book. To capture the nuances and extent of what we have done and learned, we invite readers of this volume to also read others in our recently published set of four books (Tobin & Alexakos, 2021a, 2022, forthcoming), and then to look beyond to access websites,[2] videos, courses, and other prior and subsequent publications.

The Place of Narrative

Narrative inquiry is an integral component of our methodology. We see narrative as an extension of lived experience – one way to represent what happened, why it happened, and aspects of life that are "beneath the surface." Narrative is a complement to other modes of representation, including but not limited to photography, painting, sketching, poetry, summarizing key points, and statistical modeling. As is the case with all modes of representation, narrative, no matter how polished and detailed, falls short of communicating all that could be told. Re-viewing, revising and adding post-scripts may increase the fidelity of narrative, but the final completed and polished project will be an underrepresentation of an experience (Greene, 1994).

An author can use narrative to represent what is being learned from research. In writing a narrative there usually will be other frames that shape the text. For example, since we emphasize nuance and a dialectical relationship between patterns of coherence and contradictions, we will have this in mind when we make claims within a narrative. Also, because event-oriented inquiry is salient to most of our studies, we frequently storyboard a narrative around selected events that characterize the aspects of lived experiences being described. Since an event is a spike upward in the curve of what is happening, or a spike downward, it is a potential game changer (Tobin, 2021). Accordingly, we are aware of the importance in preparing a narrative of the events that transformed an aspect of social life. In telling about the changes that occurred, we take care to be nuanced so that it is clear to readers that, for all patterns of coherence there are contradictions i.e., for any descriptions in a narrative there are exceptions. In this sense, a narrative is like an impressionistic tale (Geelan, 2007; Van Maanen, 2011).

Readers of a manuscript make sense of what they read in terms of their personal lived experience, which incorporates a knowledge base they hold to be viable for the many aspects of their lives. This knowledge base includes values and expectations. As a reader makes sense of text, they do so by giving heft to parts of a narrative that connect with their expectations and values. After reading a section of text, a reader can decide whether any, all, or none of what has been read applies to their own practices and lifeworlds. For example, a person may highlight what they consider to be important in a text. Then, after completing their reading, they may review what they have highlighted and, almost immediately, change aspects of their conduct. That is, they appropriate selected parts of the narrative for the purposes of changing personal conduct in a particular field. As they enact changed practices, others in the field experience a stream of actions that have appropriated aspects of the narrative that was read and highlighted. We name this process as ripple effects and consider it to be a prevalent mode of generalizing from narrative – that is, what was learned from research in a particular setting is then appropriated for use when, where, and how a person chooses to adopt specific culture (Tobin, 2009). Having read a text, appropriation can be passive (Roth, 2007), in which case a stream of actions that includes appropriations from the narrative also is enacted without awareness. Subsequently, others in a field experience this practice as a resource, which can be appropriated according to an agency | passivity relationship (Tobin & Alexakos, 2021a).

Emotions and Teaching

Because of the historical constitution of lived experience, we briefly examine the grounding of our current research on wellness, its relationship to research on emotions, and our present interests in contemplative practices, healing, and applications of complementary healing practices to our ongoing work.

Emotions and Metaphors

Emotional aspects of teaching have been apparent in our research for many decades. For example, in Tobin, Kahle, and Fraser's *Windows into Science Classrooms,* Peter's projected emotions while teaching appeared to be related to the metaphors he used to frame segments of his teaching (Tobin, Kahle, & Fraser, 1990). When Peter taught as *the entertainer,* he was happy, playful, and humorous. At times, he was flirtatious, thereby situating female students in particular, in awkward environments. In contrast, when Peter framed his teaching as *captain of the ship,* he projected sternness. He was clearly in charge of his crew and any transgressions were dealt with using an angry demeanor.

Emotions associated with Peter's imagery of teaching were expressed overtly in his teaching practices, including interactions with students and physical resources in the classroom. Accordingly, emotions were visible to students and, consistent with research on emotion, students resonated with the expressed emotions (Collins, 2004) and often produced similar emotions or emotions that were reactions to Peter's package of emotions and interrelated actions. For example, if Peter was angry, students may have expressed fear or sadness. In some circumstances, anger may have triggered anger for some of the students. Similarly, as an entertainer, Peter may have triggered students' emotions such as happiness, amusement, sarcasm, and less frequently, annoyance (Goleman, 1998). Not all students enjoyed Peter as an entertainer.

Modifying Metaphors to Change Teaching

In follow-up studies in which Sarah Ulerick was the teacher | researcher, the broad questions studied by Sarah, Ken, and several colleagues was, "why can't Sarah teach the way she wants to?" Sarah struggled to produce and sustain learning environments that reflected order, cooperation, collaboration, and courtesy. Accordingly, teaching was highly stressful for her and frequently she was tearful, and expressed sadness (Tobin & Lamaster, 1995). Like Peter, Sarah tended to frame her teaching metaphorically and her initial approach was aligned with the metaphor of *teacher as performer*. Based on her lack of success in subsequent reflections, Sarah created a metaphor as *social director,* which took account of her beliefs about constructivism and collaborative learning. Although the learning environments improved, some students refused to cooperate with her. Ongoing research in her classroom pointed to students being dissatisfied with their grades. Even though Sarah considered herself to be a fair judge, a demonstrative minority of the students were angered by the grades they received. The students frequently were disruptive as they expressed their anger in ways that diminished opportunities for others to learn and for Sarah to teach as effectively as she liked. Sarah decided to alter her metaphor for assessment from fair judge to "looking through a window into the students' minds – opportunities for students to show what they know." When this metaphor was enacted, the classroom environment improved substantially, and Sarah and students expressed emotions consistent with productive social communication.

Although emotions were not the primary focus of the research with Sarah, the research on metaphors and teaching provided a foundation for ongoing research on emotions, situated in urban science classrooms.

Emotions and Learning Environments

Two theoretical sociologists from the University of Pennsylvania catalyzed perspectives that placed emotions at the center of learning in urban schools. Elijah Anderson (1999) addressed the issue of culture having no boundaries, raising the probability that the culture needed to survive and thrive on the streets of inner-city Philadelphia would not be checked at the door when urban youth attended school. Accordingly, respect, which was the currency of the streets, was bound to be highly valued throughout a school. Since respect is transactional, it would be necessary for all participants to earn respect. Furthermore, an important way to earn respect would likely involve showing disrespect to others. This framework was highly influential in making sense of our research on teaching, learning, and learning to teach. Studies of respect and trust led us to look for evidence of fear, anger, and sadness, as well as happiness and joy.

Randall Collins' research on interaction ritual chains also altered the way we examined social interactions in classrooms (Collins, 2004). We examined verbal and nonverbal conduct for evidence of synchrony, and when we observed synchrony among participants we watched for entrainment (i.e., social resonance) as a precursor to the emergence of a shared mood – a form of social contagion (Goleman, 1998). We regarded shared mood as emotional energy, which had a role in the spread of emotions throughout a social field (i.e., a community). Shared, intense emotions have tremendous impact on participants' solidarity, social bonds, coping, perseverance and success (Alexakos, Jones, & Rodriguez, 2011; Tobin, 2005).

Connecting Emotions and Wellness

Connection between emotion and wellness became a primary focus of our research that was situated in Bronx, New York City, science classes in which Rey Llena was a teacher | researcher (Tobin & Llena, 2012). Classroom environments were characterized by noise, obstruction of teaching, anger, fear, and sadness. Rey admitted that he often feigned anger, and within our research squad, we frequently ask Rey whether his body knew the difference between real anger and feigned anger. As far as the classroom environments were concerned, there were continuous efforts by students to disrupt, loud conversations between students, and shouting from the teacher as he sought to teach science.

We were shocked when one day after school Rey experienced heart problems and was rushed to a hospital. Rey considered that "teaching makes me sick" and his physician concurred, advising Rey to discontinue his teaching career because it impacted his heart, a stress inducing activity that triggered cardiac problems, leading to Rey's premature retirement.

Our research with Rey set the stage for our use of finger pulse oximeters so that we could study physiological expression of emotions while teaching. Accordingly, we examined blood oxygenation and pulse rate in research undertaken in Brooklyn (Alexakos, 2015) and Australia (Tobin et al., 2016). Although the oximeters provided data on the plethysmograph, a proxy for blood pressure, we have not examined the various representations of these data in detail (Amat et al., 2016). Suffice to say, we noticed that intense expressions of emotion are evident as pounding of the heart in the visual display of the plethysmograph. However, plethysmographs are related to pressure applied in arterial pulses. Accordingly, these are data that can be explored in conjunction with blood oxygenation and heart rate to directly address cardiological data and their relations to facial and other bodily expressions of emotion – including gestures, proxemics, and prosody.

As is always the case in education research, there is more to be done and advances in technology create possibilities that important follow up work will occur, including interventions to minimize health hazards that might be associated with teaching and learning.

Enhancing Participants' Lifeworlds

Health literacy must be a priority at this moment in time. Importantly, most individuals will have wellness projects that can be addressed through self-care if they have been appropriately educated early in life. Know myself can be a mantra for educating the world's citizens so that they have options when it comes to dis-ease and disease. Lifestyles can be explored in relation to wellness and changes can be made to lifestyle if and as necessary. What we allow into our body can promote good health and/or contribute to disharmonies that trigger disease. If a disease goes untreated or is mistreated, it can become chronic and/or acute. Foci for ongoing authentic studies are: the air we breathe, the water we use, and the food we eat as well as how we do these. Similarly, issues concerning exercise also can catalyze health projects and it is for individuals to learn to notice disharmonies where and when they occur.

Typically, schools, homes, and institutions like places of worship, have had the responsibility to educate the mind for wholesome living, not as a hermit on a mountain and not solely focused on ego (i.e., the conscious mind), but also as a member of a community. Saul McLeod (2018) explained that Carl Jung regarded ego as the conscious mind, which coexisted with personal unconscious knowledge (forgotten and repressed knowledge) and collective unconscious (transpersonal memory traces shared with other humans). Consistent with Heesoon Bai and Avraham Cohen (2014), we assign priority, as teachers, to providing students with activities in which they build understandings of interbeing, seeing their co-relations with resources – living and nonliving and also human and non-human. As Thich Nhat Hanh (2020) noted, it is desirable to learn about interbeing in ways that transcend words and images to include enacting everyday life. This involves understanding self as part of a dynamic ecosystem and realizing there is no self that is separate from other living/non-living things.

We regard it as essential for our ongoing work, including chapters published in this volume, to always probe for more than can be represented during person-person communication. We consider each person's knowledge as a dialectical relationship between conscious (i.e., ego) and unconscious knowledge (personal and collective). Building on Jung's work we consider ego as dialectically related to two interconnected components of unconscious knowledge (Ruf, 1999) – personal (forgotten and repressed knowledge) and collective (transpersonal memory traces shared with other humans). Thus, we believe, it is important, in addition to learning about self (i.e., know myself) and self-care, to actively care and work for the benefit of all on our planet, living and non-living (i.e., to adopt an ecological approach).

Having set the stage for the research that is presented in *Contemplative Practices for Sustaining Wellness*, we provide insights in chapter 1 into what is to follow. The research involves emotions, illness and wellness, educating self and others, contemplative practices, and complementary approaches to healing so as to attain and sustain wellness. We anticipate that readers will deepen their understandings of each of the categories mentioned above, while considering the wellness of self and others within a context of engaging in projects related to furthering our understandings of self and questions of who am I, self-help, and helping others. Also, we anticipate that many readers will undertake research that orientates toward foci such as enlightenment, transcendence, liberation, and equanimity.

Educating to Stay Connected with Life

As we finish *Contemplative Practices for Sustaining Wellness: Priorities for Research and Education,* we move forward with the completion of *Educating for Wellness and Sustainability from Pre-birth through Death,* the final book in a series of four. We would be remiss not to address key aspects of a world that is topsy turvy, seemingly in a state of disarray. The current context is one in which a large majority of people are not well placed to benefit from our research, and other studies like it, because of a tsunami of interests that greatly disadvantage many, in favor of benefiting a small number of people with power, influence and wealth. We conclude by addressing this problem, which we regard as a misalignment between education and a necessity for citizens to attain and sustain lifestyles that afford wellbeing. Turbulent times provide a context that will permeate the pages of *Educating for Wellness and Sustainability from Pre-birth through Death.*

It is a concern that much of the knowledge discussed in *Contemplative Practices for Sustaining Wellness: Priorities for Research and Education* is not widely available to the public (at least in the West) and so we are conscious of our intentions to make this information available by spreading what we know from the research and what readers learn from the book. We acknowledge that right now it is not only knowledge to keep ourselves healthy that people have difficulty finding. Political tendencies and practices, together with economic tides, combine to restrict, alter, and pervert knowledge that would otherwise expand wellness and harmony.

Knowledge alone is not sufficient for success in a contemporary society like we have in the West, where intentional acts create a scarcity of resources related to nutrition because price fixing practices and self-interest exploit vast numbers of people, not only in the United States, but worldwide. Throughout the world there are incredible rises in food and housing prices, pressing untold millions further into poverty and famine. Meanwhile the savage exploitation of our planet and its resources (Tollefson, 2019), further contributes to disharmony of the Earth's ecosystems and of humanity. It is estimated (Patel, 2022) that 1 in 6 deaths worldwide stem from air and water pollution and from lead poisoning and other chemical toxins – the great majority of these deaths were in low- and middle-income countries. Furthermore, millions have died in the COVID 19 pandemic and more are continuing to die. Just as staggering, over 100,000 died in 2021 from drug overdose in the USA alone (Kornfield, 2022).

Rights pertaining to our own bodies face legal and extra-legal attacks, especially for people of color, women, and gender non-conforming and transgender people. How much can we do for personal improvements when many go to sleep hungry, are confined to concentration camps, and are denied basic human recognition? For example, in the USA rights to our bodies conflict with political agendas prescribed in the legal and health system.

Knowing thyself and living in harmony with those around us require advocacy and calls to action for personal and global wellness and sustainability. We regard the grand challenges to wellness and sustainability mentioned above as examples of a plethora of high priority foci for research (Tobin & Alexakos, 2021b), especially studies that incorporate authentic inquiry with an emphasis on self-help, caring for others, inclusiveness, compassion and expanding human agency to attain and sustain wellbeing (Tobin & Alexakos, 2021a).

The authors | researchers who contributed to this volume share their personal stories and narratives of their paths, struggles and challenges to wellness as they live their lives in the complexity of being of and in this world. In so doing, authors courageously address a diverse set of critical issues, including education, resilience, vulnerability, racism, misogyny, bigotry, and poverty. It is our hope that the knowledge produced by reading this book contributes to understanding, wellness, and healing of us all.

Notes

1 Dis-ease conveys a lack of feeling at ease. We are not speaking of a diagnosis of a disease, which often accompanies a label and an associated prescription. In general, as practitioners of complementary healing practices, we are interested in identifying disharmonies in the functioning of an individual and using practices to restore harmony and a feeling of ease.
2 https://cinquiry.com/; kennethtobin.com

References

Alexakos, K. (2015). *Being a teacher | researcher: A primer on doing authentic inquiry research on teaoching and learning.* Sense Publishers. https://doi.org/10.1007/978-94-6300-295-0

Alexakos, K., Jones, J., & Rodriguez, V. (2011). Fictive kinship as it mediates learning, resiliency, perseverance, and social learning of inner-city high school students of color in a college physics class. *Cultural Studies of Science Education, 6*(4), 847–870. https://doi.org/10.1007/s11422-011-9317-7

Amat, A., Zapata, C., Alexakos, K., Pride, L. D., Paylor-Smith, C., & Hernandez, M. (2016). Incorporating oximeter analyses to investigate synchronies in heart rate while teaching and learning about race. *Cultural Studies of Science Education, 11*(3), 785–801. https://doi.org/10.1007/s11422-016-9767-z

Anderson, E. (1999). *Code of the street: Decency, violence, and the moral life of the inner city*. W. W. Norton & Company.
Bai, H., & Cohen, A. (2014). Zen and the art of storytelling. *Studies in Philosophy and Education, 33*(6), 597–608.
Collins, R. (2004). *Interaction ritual chains*. Princeton University Press. https://doi.org/10.1515/9781400851744
Dana, D. (2018). *The polyvagal theory in therapy: Engaging the rhythm of regulation*. W. W. Norton & Company.
Erickson, F. (1986). Qualitative research on teaching. In M. C. Wittrock (Ed.), *Handbook of research on teaching* (3rd ed., pp. 119–161). MacMillan.
Garfinkel, H. (1967). *Studies in ethnomethodology*. Prentice Hall.
Geelan, D. (2007). Songs of innocence and of experience: Impressionist tales and secret stories of life in classrooms. In P. C. Taylor & J. Wallace (Eds.), *Contemporary qualitative research: Exemplars for science and mathematics educators* (pp. 139–148). Springer. https://doi.org/10.1007/978-1-4020-5920-9_13
Goleman, D. (1998, November–December). What makes a leader? *Harvard Business Review*, 93. https://doi.org/10.1002/ltl.40619981008
Greene, M. (1994). Postmodernism and the crisis of representation. *English Education, 26*, 206–219.
Hahn, T. N. (2020). *Interbeing: The 14 mindfulness trainings of engaged Buddhism* (4th ed.). Parallax Press.
Kincheloe, J. L. (2005). On to the next level: Continuing the conceptualization of the bricolage. *Qualitative Inquiry, 11*(3), 323–350. https://doi.org/10.1177/1077800405275056
Kornfield, M. (2022, May 11). U.S. surpasses record 100,000 overdose deaths in 2021. *The Washington Post*. https://www.washingtonpost.com/health/2022/05/11/drug-overdose-deaths-cdc-numbers/
McLeod, S. A. (2018). *Carl Jung*. Retrieved May 8, 2022, from https://www.simplypsychology.org/carl-jung.html
Patel, K. (2022, May 17). Pollution caused 1 in 6 deaths globally for five years, study says. *The Washington Post*. https://www.washingtonpost.com/climate-environment/2022/05/17/pollution-caused-1-6-deaths-globally-five-straight-years-study-says/
Porges, S. (2011). *The polyvagal theory: Neurophysiological foundations of emotions, attachment, communication and self-regulation*. W.W. Norton & Company.
Roth, W.-M. (2007). Theorizing passivity. *Cultural Studies of Science Education, 2*(1), 1–8. https://doi.org/10.1007/s11422-006-9045-6
Sewell, W. H. Jr. (2005). *Logics of history: Social theory and social transformation*. University of Chicago Press. https://doi.org/10.7208/chicago/9780226749198.001.0001
Swidler, A. (1986). Culture in action: Symbols and strategies. *American Sociological Review, 51*, 273–286. https://doi.org/10.2307/2095521

Tobin, K. (2005). Teaching urban science as culturally and socially adaptive practice. In K. Tobin, R. Elmesky, & G. Seiler (Eds.), *Improving urban science education: New roles for teachers, students and researchers.* Rowman & Littlefield.

Tobin, K. (2008). In search of new lights: Getting the most from competing perspectives. *Cultural Studies of Science Education, 3*, 227–230. https://doi.org/10.1007/s11422-008-9109-x

Tobin, K. (2009). Repetition, difference and rising up with research in education. In K. Ercikan & W.-M. Roth (Eds.), *Generalizing from educational research* (pp. 149–172). Routledge.

Tobin, K. (2018). Methodological bricolage. In S. M. Ritchie & K. Tobin (Eds), *Eventful learning: Learner emotions* (pp. 31–55). Brill. https://doi.org/10.1163/9789004377912_003

Tobin, K. (2021). The spike in the curve. In K. Tobin, & K. Alexakos (Eds.), *Doing authentic inquiry to improve learning and teaching* (pp. 43–58). Brill. https://doi.org/10.1163/9789004446885_003

Tobin, K., & Alexakos, K. (Eds.). (2021a). *Doing authentic inquiry to improve learning and teaching.* Brill. https://doi.org/10.1163/9789004446885

Tobin, K., & Alexakos, K. (2021b). Global challenges need attention now: Educating humanity for wellness and sustainability. *Cultural Studies of Science Education, 16*(3), 651–673. https://doi.org/10.1007/s11422-021-10080-6

Tobin, K., & Alexakos, K. (Eds.). (2022). *Transforming learning and teaching: Heuristics for educative and responsible practices.* Brill. https://doi.org/10.1163/9789004507609

Tobin, K., & Alexakos, K. (Eds.). (forthcoming). *Educating for wellness and sustainability from pre-birth through death.* Brill.

Tobin, K., Kahle, J. B., & Fraser, B. J. (Eds.). (1990). *Windows into science classrooms: Problems associated with higher-level learning.* Falmer Press.

Tobin, K., King, D., Henderson, S., Bellocchi, A., & Ritchie, S. M. (2016). Expression of emotions and physiological changes during teaching. *Cultural Studies of Science Education, 11*, 669–692. https://doi.org/10.1007/s11422-016-9778-9

Tobin, K., & Lamaster, S. (1995). Relationships between metaphors, beliefs and actions in a context of science curriculum change. *Journal of Research in Science Teaching 32*(3), 225–242. https://doi.org/10.1002/tea.3660320304

Tobin, K., & Llena, R. (2012). Colliding identities, emotional roller coasters, and contradictions of urban science education. In M. Varelas (Ed.), *Identity construction and science education research: Learning, teaching, and being in multiple contexts* (pp. 141–156). Sense.

Tollefson, J. (2019). Humans are driving one million species to extinction. *Nature, 569*(7755), 171.

Van Maanen, J. (2011). *Tales of the field: On writing ethnography* (2nd ed.). University of Chicago Press.

Figures and Tables

Figures

Tables

Notes on Contributors

Konstantinos Alexakos
is Professor and program coordinator for Adolescence Science Education at the School of Education, Brooklyn College, CUNY as well as a professor in the PhD Program in Urban Education, at The Graduate Center, CUNY. His research focuses on teaching and learning, emotions, wellness and critical social issues such as race, gender, and sexuality with the goals of improving personal and global well-being, sustainability and education.

Fatima Alexander
has been an early childhood educator for 14 years. She holds a master's degree in early childhood. She started her teaching journey after the birth of her first son who is now 17 years old. She is a mother of 3 boys. Fatima enjoys teaching 3-year-olds. She has taught this age group for the past 9 years. Early childhood is a rewarding career for Fatima, and she enjoys teaching young children very much.

Carolyne Ali-Khan
is Associate Professor and the Graduate Program Coordinator for the MEd Program in the Department of Teaching Learning and Curriculum at the University of North Florida. She obtained her PhD in Urban Education in 2011, and before this was a high school teacher in New York for 20 years. She is interested in the complexities of what it means to engage in transformative, critical, creative and joyful education.

Corinna Brathwaite
completed her doctoral degree in the Urban Education Department of The Graduate Center, CUNY, in the Spring of 2019. She works at St Hope Leadership Academy in New York City teaching mathematics to middle schoolers and co-leading The Natural Hair Club. She also is an adjunct at the City College of New York teaching Elementary Math Methods to pre-service and in-service teachers.

Mary Bullen
is interested in teaching, which is not surprising since her parents and four siblings were/are educators in the Caribbean. Mary is an immigrant and her first job in the United States was caring for young children as a nanny. When

Mary became a mother to two daughters, her children attended public school and she saw the support, dedication, and passion in her children's elementary school teachers. Her children's success inspired her to give back to the public school system and pursued her master's degree in early childhood education. She currently works for a city agency but is in the process of changing her career to be in a classroom. Mary's journey to be in a classroom has been long and difficult but she is determined to see her passion become a reality.

Maria Cadme
has been an early childhood educator for 7 years. She holds a master's degree in early childhood general and special education. Maria discovered her love for teaching with her first-born son, Anthony, who is now 12 years old. Through her education career she saw first-hand the findings of all theorists and understood even more when her daughter, Anahi, was born in 2013. She currently works as a Universal Pre-Kindergarten teacher. Maria enjoys teaching all age groups paying close attention to social and emotional development through music.

Piyanate Chuychai
is currently an independent researcher and part-time teacher in physics and mathematics. She received her PhD in physics in 2004. After graduation, she worked as a postdoctoral researcher in space physics for almost 3 years, a university lecturer for 7 years, and a volunteer teacher in Agri-nature Foundation for 1 year. In her life, she experienced depression at various levels. Suffering and pain from the illness motivated her to be a lifelong learner. To live with depression, she learned to change her lifestyle, such as doing exercise, dieting, and practicing mindfulness for over 10 years.

Hema Daswani
is a graphic design consultant and works 2 days a week for a medical device company. The remaining three days, she treats patients in the NY/NJ area using JSJ, acupuncture and nutrition. Both graphic design and the human body share this fundamental principle: form follows function. There is a certain satisfaction in creating print collateral and packaging that is both esthetically pleasing, compelling, and where every element has a reason for being. Within the human body, every cell, tissue and organ follow the same principle. Having been a witness to the body's regenerative powers, her thrust and mission today is to share her knowledge with those interested in empowering themselves through simple self-help techniques. It is nothing short of pure joy watching

this transformation. A resident of northern New Jersey, and in close proximity to the mountains, she finds her heart most open when she's in nature. She sees herself as an eternal student and a seeker of the Truth.

Suskya Goodall
is a doctoral candidate in the Faculty of Education at Victoria University of Wellington with a research focus on actively enhancing wellbeing in centers, kura and schools of Aotearoa New Zealand. She is involved with initial teacher education, research fellow work, various committees and leads a project for doctoral students. Her work with schools, clusters, Ministry of Education projects centers around her passion for wellbeing at individual, organizational and sector wide levels with theoretical influences of strengths-based and authentic leadership, ecological systems, appreciative inquiry and positive psychology.

Xiao Ling He
holds a master's degree in early childhood education and has been teaching children between the ages of 3 and 4 for the last 4 years. Before Xiao Ling decided to become an educator, she realized the importance of early childhood education and pursued her career in the field. She loves being around children and enjoys teaching and finds it meaningful to learn from each individual child. Teaching has been a gift to Xiao Ling and her goal is to create an inclusive classroom that supports all children.

Joanna Higgins
is an associate professor at the Faculty of Education, Victoria University of Wellington, New Zealand where she teaches in initial teacher education, masters and doctoral programs. She supervises masters and doctoral projects that focus on policy implementation, professional learning and development, leadership and wellbeing initiatives in schools and universities. Joanna's research focuses on learning environments and policy implementation. Her work from sociocultural perspectives includes instructional reform in mathematics education, professional inquiry of teachers and teacher educators, and analyses of wellbeing policy and practice.

Francie Johnson
is a passionate educator with over 20 years of dance teaching experience in K-12 and studio settings. She also is a curriculum writer and facilitator for the Professional Development Office of Arts for New York City dance teachers. Francie is a PhD candidate in the Urban Education program at CUNY Graduate

Center with interests including cultural identity, dance as an agent of transformation, art-based research, and K-12 public education.

Sara E. Johnson
has a passion for the performing arts, ultimately leading her to pursue a Master of Science in Early Childhood General and Special Education in order to share her enthusiasm for the arts and play with the next generation. She also holds a Bachelor of Music (Classical Vocal Performance) and a Professional Studies certification (Meisner Technique).

Anna Malyukova
is a lecturer in the Early Childhood department at Queen's College (CUNY). She has a PhD in Urban Education earned at the Graduate Center, CUNY. Anna is very passionate about mindfulness and emotions in the process of learning on the birth-death continuum. She began her education in Russia in 1997 pursuing her degree in engineering, but has since become interested in education and received an AS in Early Childhood Education from BMCC, CUNY, a BA in Liberal Arts from City College, CUNY, and a Master's degree in Liberal Arts from The Graduate Center, CUNY. In her collaboration with Kenneth Tobin and Konstantinos Alexakos, she became very interested in mindfulness and wellness in learning and has published several works on these topics.

Corie A. McCallum
completed her doctoral degree in Urban Education at The Graduate Center, CUNY, in Summer of 2021. While completing her chapter, she was a Student Conduct Officer at New York City College of Technology, CUNY. Recently, she accepted a position as Assistant Dean for Community Standards and Student Well-being at Fashion Institute of Technology, SUNY. Her interests lie in emotions in teaching and learning and the experiences of student affairs administrators in higher education. Prior work experience includes residence life, event management, student conduct, and diversity initiatives.

Tabitha McKenzie
(Ngāti Hinerangi, Ngāi Te Rangi, Ngāti Ranginui) is a staff member within Te Kura Māori at the Faculty of Education, Victoria University of Wellington. She has taught across a range of programs and has worked on numerous Ministry of Education projects, both focused particularly around Māori education and Māori language. Overall Tabitha's work and research interests are concerned with the wellbeing of Māori students, education and language as well as digital technologies. She has also been an IronMāori participant.

Eleanor A. Miele
is Chair of Secondary Education and Coordinator of General Science at Brooklyn College of the City University of New York where she has been on the faculty since 1998. After leaving research in molecular biology, Miele taught courses in human genetics and molecular biology to high school students in the Science Honors Program of Columbia University for 16 years. Since first assuming a faculty position as a teacher educator, Miele has focused on holistic approaches to science teaching, including integration of choice in learning, informal and place-based science learning and reducing stress in the science classroom.

Beatriz Verónica Panduro Espinoza
has a doctorate in education research and is a pediatrician certified in Pediatric Nephrology. For 14 years she has been working in a third level hospital, that is to say that in addition to the basic services it offers specialties and subspecialties to multi infringed populations, where she has developed education projects for improving a patient's health and quality of life.

Andre Poole
is a STEM teacher with the NYC Department of Education by day and an adjunct assistant professor with the Brooklyn College, CUNY. His teaching | learning interests are centered on STEM education and the health, wellness, and longevity of teachers. Andre earned his PhD from the Graduate Center, CUNY. As a STEM educator his goal is to develop science and instructional technology literacy with teachers, teacher educators, and elementary school students.

S. Lizette Ramos de Robles
is a professor and coordinator of the Environmental Health Master program in the Department of Environmental Sciences at the University of Guadalajara. Her research focuses on sociological and cultural aspects of discourse in the teaching and learning of science. In order to understand more deeply scientific literacy, she uses sociocultural and sociolinguistic perspectives. In addition, her research also focuses on socio-environmental aspects related to Environmental Health and Health Education.

Wolff-Michael Roth
is Lansdowne Professor of Applied Cognitive Science at the University of Victoria (since 1997). He taught high school science, mathematics, and computer science for much of the period from 1980 to 1992 after which he began

a university career teaching quantitative and qualitative research methods (Simon Fraser University). He has been investigating knowing and learning across the lifespan in formal educational, workplace, and leisure settings.

Jenna Sclafani
has been an early childhood educator since 2016. A lover of all creatures big and small makes celebrating nature with children a very joyful experience. She received her master's in early childhood education and is certified in general and special education. Currently, she works as a teacher and education director at a nature preschool.

Theila Smith
is currently pursuing a PhD at the University of Groningen in the Netherlands. Her research interests lie in the areas of science identity and informal science education. Previously, she was a science teacher in the NYC DOE school system. Theila adjuncts at Brooklyn College during the summers since 2018. Where she teaches an Urban Ecology and Eco-justice course through the school-to-university partnership program, College Now.

Suellen Taragano
has been involved in Early Childhood Education for twenty-seven years. She was in the classroom for many years when she got an opportunity to become the Early Childhood Director of the same school. Next, she became the Educational Director for a school. She made the transition back to the classroom teaching Universal Pre-Kindergarten and decided this was where she truly belonged. She holds a master's degree in Early Childhood Education. She is a mother of two daughters and a grandmother of two. She had found the joy of teaching many years ago and continues to have the same joy watching children blossom each year in her classes.

Sister Tibebwa
is a citizen of the world, having grown up in Europe and lived in Ethiopia for many years, now settled on the island of Lamu in Kenya, Sister Tibebwa is mother to many children and has a background as a healer, tree planter and as an environmental and permaculture activist. She is a certified Ipsalu Tantra KriyaYoga (Level 1) instructor, a teacher of both Afrikan and Kemetic Yoga, as well as a co-founder of the Ta-Nut-Ra Afrikan Tantra. She is also a Sister Goddess graduate from Mama Gena's School of Womanly Arts and a Priestess of the Divine Feminine. Tibebwa's foundation is a devout Rastafarian and member of

the Ethiopian Orthodox Tewahedo Church. She has journeyed through many practices and disciplines over the past 20 years, yet finding herself drawn to the activation of her own sacred sexual energy as a mode of consciousness expansion and rising Kundalini life force.

Kenneth Tobin
is Presidential Professor Emeritus in the Urban Education program at the Graduate Center of CUNY (2003–2019). Prior to becoming a university science educator in Australia in 1974, Tobin taught high school physics, chemistry, biology, general science, and mathematics for 10 years. Then, he held university appointments at the Western Australian Institute of Technology (now Curtin University), Mount Lawley College and Graylands College (now Edith Cowan University).

In the United States he had positions as tenured full professor at Florida State University (1987–1997) and the University of Pennsylvania (1997–2003). Tobin began a program of research in 1973 that continues to the present day. His current research interests include contemplative practices, wellness and wellbeing.

Tara Toye
has been an early childhood educator for 7 years. She holds a bachelor's degree and certification in childhood education, and a master's degree in early childhood education. Tara has taught kindergarten and has been teaching first grade for the last four years. She continues her love for teaching young children at a dance studio after school hours as well. She has a passion for educating and supporting children at the early stages of their life, where learning and growing is important academically, as well as emotionally and physically.

Yau Yan Wong
has a bachelor of science degree in psychology from Virginia Polytechnic Institute and State University in the USA and a master of science degree in research methods in psychology from University College London in UK. For the past ten years, Yau Yan Wong has been leading mindfulness research projects and providing mindfulness training to her fellow teachers, students and parents in a laboratory school in Thailand. In 2022, she completed a PhD in science education at Kasetsart University, Thailand. Her research interests include mindfulness, wellbeing, human adaptation, sustainable development, and science education as a lived experience.

Shequana Wright-Chung
is an Early Childhood Educational Administrator with the Division of Early Childhood for the New York City Department of Education. Within this role she supervises and partners with coaches that support school leaders and teaching teams on implementing best practices in prekindergarten and 3K programs. She also continues her research as an adjunct assistant professor at Brooklyn College (CUNY) by exploring with preservice teachers their emotional responses while teaching and learning early childhood mathematics to young children. She received her PhD from the Urban Education doctoral program at the Graduate Center of CUNY in the Spring 2018.

Grant Zouch
is a PhD candidate at Victoria University of Wellington | Te Herenga Waka. He was a primary teacher for fifteen years before a heart attack at school prompted a move into educational research. While Grant's wider research is centered on wellbeing, his doctoral thesis is a narrative inquiry into teacher attrition. It explores the personal narratives of former primary school teachers and how their experiences contributed to their decision to leave the classroom. Grant lives in rural Wairarapa with his wife and two furry friends.

CHAPTER 1

Attaining and Sustaining Wellness

Kenneth Tobin and Konstantinos Alexakos

Abstract

In this chapter we provide a context for *Contemplative Practices for Sustaining Wellness: Priorities for Research and Education* and review the constituent chapters. In so doing, key issues we address are physiological expression of emotion, balancing physiology and emotions, polysemia of the body, living with dis-ease, intervening as necessary to attain and sustain wellness, and contemplative practices to support healthy living. Among the lessons learned are the importance of knowing myself so as to facilitate self-care when it is desirable to do so and, as appropriate, to care for others. Several researchers also highlight the importance of learning to have productive lives within chronic illness, such as depression and kidney disease.

Keywords

wellness – self-care – contemplative practices – emotions – healing practices

1 Physiological Expression of Emotion

Wellness is a term we use when we refer to humans, although, as is obvious, wellness relates to all organisms considered to be alive. Possibly due to our research on teaching and learning, our initial focus on wellness concerned self-care and caring for others. We are not engaged to the same extent with wellness as it relates to Western doctors in the doctor's office, clinics, and hospitals. Nor have we studied the treatment of sickness and ill health through prescription drugs. Instead, our research transitioned into wellness in schools and classrooms, starting with expressed emotions and their relationships with student and teacher conduct and physiological changes (Roth & Tobin, 2010).

These foci led directly to self-help in that we wanted teachers and students to be more aware of their expressed emotions and ways in which they could ameliorate excesses if and when they considered it beneficial to do so. We learned from the work of Pierre Philippot, Gaëtane Chapelle and Sylvie Blairy

 | DOI:10.1163/9789004527348_001

(2002), that changing breathing patterns would change expressed emotions and vice versa. Accordingly, we began to use what we referred to as breathing meditation to release stuck emotions (Alexakos, 2015). We were surprised by the extremes we observed in pulse rate, blood oxygenation, and blood pressure. This awareness prompted us to assign higher priority to adopting an array of contemplative practices to ameliorate anxiety and stress, which we thought were most likely responsible for striking changes in oximetry data obtained from teachers and students as they prepared to teach and while teaching. Accordingly, we began to develop a toolkit of contemplative practices that could be used by teachers and students to harmonize their emotions and emotional responses. Importantly, our research on breathing and expressed emotions opened the door to the design and use of interventions such as breathing meditation, touch, and heuristics, so that all participants in our research could benefit from what we learned in our ongoing research. Our next steps were to undertake research on use of the breath to attain systems of equilibrium, hereafter harmony, in the mind and body (Powietrzynska, 2016).

This volume continues ongoing studies in which researchers have investigated relationships between expressed emotions, physiological changes in breathing patterns, blood circulation and wellness, living with dis-ease,[1] and use of interventions to live with chronic disease and, when possible, restore healthy functioning of the body (i.e., harmonize the body to be at ease). In their chapters, the authors afford unique pathways that address three broad questions: what is happening, why is it happening, and what more is there to complement what we have learned? The authors | researchers who contributed to the book consider their work as a learning resource for all participants (including readers), a chance to learn about perspectives that differ from their own, and a means to improve the quality of education for those who may need additional and/or different resources to reap the benefits of education. Unique aspects of the book's chapters include complementary approaches and practices for self-care, caring for others, living with chronic disease, and harmonizing universal energy. To ameliorate emotions and enhance wellness a variety of healing and contemplative practices are discussed, including breathing meditation and mindfulness in everyday activities. In doing so, authors also address a diverse set of critical issues, such as education, resilience, vulnerability, racism, misogyny, bigotry, and poverty.

However, in the workplace and everyday life, including schools, participants often do not have the power or even the knowhow, to stop what they're doing and initiate needed healing, and restorative practices. An implication of the research presented in the chapters of this book is that all participants should have the autonomy to enact appropriate contemplative practices if and when they are considered necessary. We conclude that extant structures may need to be replaced by alternatives that recognize the importance of self-help and place a priority in educating the population in healing and contemplative knowledge systems and practices.

2 Overview

In the remainder of this chapter we review the chapters of this book, highlighting key foci, contributions, and interconnections between chapters. We conclude the chapter with a look toward what we consider to be the highest priorities for research, policies, and practices in these turbulent times and in the years that follow.

3 Balancing Physiology and Emotions

3.1 *Anxiety, Stress and Pulse Rate*

Corinna Brathwaite (Chapter 2) examines anxiety in relation to the intervals of time prior to a person beginning to speak. Her research is consistent with earlier studies (e.g., Amat et al., 2016; Brathwaite, 2022) and was undertaken in a science teacher education class taught by Konstantinos. Corinna's research is an authentic inquiry in which she utilized video analysis, oximetry, cogenerative dialogue, and event-oriented inquiry. Corinna identified an event characterized by a student's heart rate rapidly increasing from about 90 bpm to a maximum of 164 bpm. This elevation of heart rate occurred prior to the class beginning. Then, as the student, Petra, approached the time in class when she was scheduled to make a presentation with two other students, her heart rate once again increased rapidly, as anxiety about presenting appears to have re-occurred and Petra's pulse rate entered the 150 bpm range.

A cogenerative dialogue, in which video segments from the class were reviewed, enabled Petra to discuss her rising anxiety and stress as the time approached for her to begin her presentation on what was regarded as a thorny issue – involving gender and sexuality. Petra explained that the topic itself was not the issue. She noted that her rising anxiety, evident in sweaty palms, built from a foundation of worry, nervousness, and strengths. Petra acknowledged that added stress may have been due to differences in expectations between she and her two co-presenters. Petra was afraid of failure, especially in regard to being unable to answer difficult questions asked by her peers and possible on-the-spot critique from Konstantinos.

In terms of next steps, it seems paramount for people to know themselves and what triggers anxiety, when triggering occurs, and contexts in which anxiety rises and falls. As well as developing knowledge, it is important to have the tools to harmonize blood oxygenation, heart rate, and blood pressure. It is assumed, but needs to be researched, that such activities are calming, while reducing anxiety and stress.

Corinna's research is reminiscent of a canary in the coal mine, a point addressed by Shequana Wright-Chung (Chapter 3). The results are eerily similar to those obtained by Tobin et al. (2016) when Donna King, an experienced science educator, had a high pulse rate prior to beginning her class, which required some knowledge of chemistry. Donna also expressed concern about being asked questions she was unable to answer because she considered herself out of field to teach chemistry. We make this point here because the physiological response to emotion is not necessarily related to length of experience as a teacher. We offer several points to consider. First, all teachers should have heightened awareness about the possibility of anxiety and stress occurring before and during teacher episodes. Second, teachers should know how to identify rising stress and take corrective actions in the moment. Accordingly, we regard it as a high priority to know myself, possess contemplative tools to correct adverse physiological responses to stress and anxiety, for example, and adopt flexible classroom structures so that changes can be made for the entire class, or for individuals, when it is appropriate to do so.

3.2 *Using Research and Contemplative Tools to Address Disillusionment*

In Chapter 3, as she addresses beginning teachers' emotional experiences associated with disillusionment and stress, Shequana Wright-Chung examines teaching and learning environments in terms of the presence of crypto positivism (Kincheloe & Tobin, 2009) and standardization. It is likely that disillusionment and stress relate to contradictions teachers experience when their lived experiences in schools are at odds with their expectations. This particularly applies to teachers' perceptions that they do not have control in their own classroom, including classroom practices and approaches to teaching and learning. In her study, Shequana utilizes free-writes and heuristics as contemplative tools to heighten awareness about characteristics of learning and teaching that are salient to participants' experiences of early childhood teaching and learning, and associated contradictions.

Shequana modeled how a free-write of her experiences as an elementary teacher can heighten awareness of crypto positivism. In her writing and subsequent discussions with the class, Shequana drew attention to her emotional responses as a beginning teacher to not having control of her classroom and associated teaching and learning practices. Work-related stressors associated with her lived experiences created emotions Shequana identified as stress, fear, anger, anxiety, and guilt. Importantly, she addressed the issue with not becoming stuck on emotions such as those she identified (Chödrön, 2013).

Shequana adopted the role of teacher | researcher, and in so doing, she modeled how prospective teachers can explore contradictions that arise in their own schools and classroom environments. Her approach drew attention to the salience of teachers conducting research in their own classrooms and adopting an authentic approach in which they identify crypto schemes (e.g., beliefs, rules, acceptance of standard practices for effectively teaching and learning) and enact changes that participants consider to be for the higher good. Once again, there is a clear need for tools to afford continuous change within a context of all participants in a class having roles as researchers while also being teachers and learners. Also, there is a case for agency, in which all participants can do what is necessary to ameliorate emotions when they decide it is desirable to do so. This includes getting unstuck. Accordingly, a set of contemplative tools, such as meditation, heuristics, and free-writes, might be available for participants to utilize in-the-moment. Having the agency to take a break for self-help is a novel idea in most classrooms, but it is a life skill we consider students should learn at an early age.

3.3 *Meditation and Mindfulness during a Pandemic*

Anna Malyukova and eight participants | researchers (Chapter 4) examine expressed emotions of an instructor and students from a graduate class during the COVID-19 pandemic. The authors of the paper employed narrative to glean insights into emotions and other experiences that arose in a context of troubled times. The multilevel study employed event-oriented inquiry to obtain an array of insights into changes that encompassed the lifeworlds of individuals, changes within the city of New York, and at a macrolevel, worldwide changes.

At macro-, meso-, and micro-levels there was evidence of trauma associated with required changes in a context of participants feeling overwhelmed, isolated, sad, and confined to their homes. Many of the graduate students in their professional roles as early childhood teachers of very young children, had the added challenge of learning to teach remotely in environments in which play, imagination, and storytelling all had to be modified and made extremely difficult. Despite narratives that depict stress, discouragement, lack of motivation, and depression, there were signs that Anna's graduate students made the most of what was available, adapting to new environments, including changed lifestyles and structural necessities. Evidence was provided of solidarity, joy, pride, and increasing respect for others.

The authors illustrate use of contemplative tools, such as soft breathing, to stay calm and work through challenges of poor health, limited financial resources, and being required to isolate spatially and socially. Meditation and mindfulness became potential tools while teaching during the COVID-19 pandemic.

4 Polysemia of the Objectified Body

4.1 *Lives Worth Grieving*

Carolyne Ali Khan (Chapter 5) begins her chapter with a discussion of vulnerability and raises the question of whose lives are worth grieving. Carolyne situates the conversation in a number of contexts that are critical to our lived experience in 2022, a time of uncertainty as we live in an era considered by some to be post pandemic and others as a calm before the storm. Whose lives have been and will be sacrificed is evident in the ways in which different communities address COVID-19, and decide what is necessary to sustain human lives. Carolyne connects vulnerability and whose lives matter to Black Lives Matter, #MeToo, and Trans Lives Matter.

Carolyne addresses a great deal in her autobiography, particularly reductivism – a tendency to oversimplify social life in terms of what are considered to be the most salient variables. For example, issues of objectification of the body are associated with metonymic distortions arising from understandings reduced to a small number of social categories, such as race, sexual desirability, socioeconomic status, religious affiliation, size, and age.

As Carolyne's writing of the chapter pivots to her autoethnography, she asserts that the body is central to hierarchies of privilege, and vulnerability she provides us with many pathways for research, education of self and others, and transformation. Finally, as constituents of wellness and wellbeing,[2] Carolyne addresses pain and pleasure.

We concur that there is pressing need for research focused on vulnerability and privilege within the domain of wellness, contemplative inquiry, and healing.

4.2 *Harmonizing Energy to Attain and Sustain Wellness*

Sister Tibebwa (Chapter 6) addresses energy in the body from multiple perspectives. In the tradition of contemplative practices, Sister Tibebwa examines energy as a life force, which she describes as composed of masculine and feminine energies. Though we may physically present ourselves in a particular gender, we all have both masculine and feminine energies within us. Feminine energy can manifest as dynamic, intuitive, surrender, receptiveness, creativity, and flexibility. In a complementary sense, masculine energy can emerge as logical, focused, direct, active, and willpower. Sister Tibebwa notes the importance to have a balance in the flow of these energies and provides examples of how ratios of masculine and feminine energies are fluid and change within different contexts.

While writing this work, Sister Tibebwa re-lived the experiences associated with imbalances of these energies. Imbalances between masculine and feminine energies contrast with engagement of being in the moment – when there is harmony between masculine and feminine energies. Harmonizing masculine and feminine energies within one body is possible, even though lived experiences might encourage and reward imbalances.

We regard it as important to view masculine and feminine energies as dialectically related in that they are co-present, contemporaneous, and interconnected. What may be constituted masculine or feminine is only labeled as such in relation to the other and is fluid. If there are ebbs and flows in masculine and feminine energies, the manifestation within a person will reflect a changing flux, which can be transformed agentically and passively (i.e., agency | passivity). As Sister Tibebwa notes, it takes considerable effort to be 100% one type or the other. In such cases, imbalances are created and these may lead to wellness projects associated with "doing" too much in one direction. At such times, contemplative tools are beneficial in restoring equilibrium.

5 Cultural Identity

5.1 *Using Sport to Build and Transform Cultural Identity*

Tabitha McKenzie, Joanna Higgins, Suskya Goodall, and Grant Zouch examine wellbeing in a context of Aotearoa, New Zealand (Chapter 7). The authors contextualize their research on wellbeing in terms of IronMāori, a sport created to attract Māori participants. The sporting event involves a swim of 2.4 miles, a 112-mile bicycle ride, and 26.2 miles of running. The event must be completed within a cutoff threshold of 17 hours. The authors discuss IronMāori in an historical context that emphasizes how European colonization and, in particular, disease, war and disconnection led to the decimation of the Māori and their culture. As the Māori developed immunity toward European diseases, the population decline reversed, but concerns for the wellbeing of Māori continue to the present.

The enactment of IronMāori was intended to be a sporting event that focused on a Māori worldview which considers wellbeing as existing within a web of interrelationships and associated obligations. The Māori perspectives embrace interconnection, interdependence, and balance. Of central importance is the

Māori relationship to land, which is considered foundational for interactions with others. A holistic frame for wellbeing involves physical, mental, emotional, social, and spiritual components. These components were built into the design of IronMāori. Approximately 6000 competitors, participated in the event. It is cross-age and inclusive – showing high value for the lifespan. Winning is not the goal. IronMāori is about getting ready for the event and being involved. The Māori holistic worldview emphasizes family and relationships with each other, with the community, and with the land.

Since IronMāori began in 2009, there have been ripple effects as IronMāori has served as a heuristic for the design of age and gender appropriate events for the population at large. Tabitha and her colleagues present positive insights concerning the impact of IronMāori in Aotearoa New Zealand, especially on the wellbeing of Māori people.

5.2 *Being Othered*

The autobiographical study undertaken by Theila Smith (Chapter 8) continues in the tradition of the important research we have done at Brooklyn College over the past decade. In particular, Theila's research picks up where Konstantinos Alexakos and Leah Pride (Alexakos et al., 2016) left us – dealing with emotions and thorny issues in science education – on this occasion issues associated with being an Afro-Caribbean, female, science teacher in a majority white school. Like so much of the autobiographical works in this book, Theila provides rich, and often gut-wrenching vignettes as a racialized "other" with engaging vignettes that provide deep insights into issues of race, identity and associated projects concerning intense emotions, and threats to wellness. As we are drawn into Theila's lived experiences, we too experience some of the emotional states she describes. We have a strong sense of admiration for this author, her courage, resilience, and humility.

What more is there? The question resonates with Harold Garfinkel's ethnomethodology (Garfinkel, 1967). We have an initial response that spurs us to action – there always will be more. The work of a researcher is never done. This is certainly the case in Theila's ongoing research. Among the contemplative practices we encountered were meditation and yoga. Although these practices make a positive difference, more are needed. Theila opted to receive therapy, but knowing herself, she also needed to receive acupuncture treatments so that she could ameliorate high intensity anger. In her ongoing research we are confident that already more contemplative activities have been added to the bricolage of possibilities.

In a chapter that offers so much, we note the power of the work on tokenism, imposter syndrome, and the pervasiveness of fear, shame, guilt, embarrassment, and inferiority. In a context of research on identity and ego, and wellness projects such as chronic depression, we highlight this cluster of constructs as priorities for research, not just in teaching and learning – but more generally, in society.

Theila's research on emotions connects with our early work that we address in the Foreword. It also aligns well with current studies in our research squads that involve contemplative practices in a context of thorny issues (Alexakos, 2022) and wellness, wellbeing, and sustainability.

Doing more research along the pathways in Theila's work is a high priority. As this volume is sent to production, there are ample signs that research in these areas is a high priority as humanity struggles with ways in which goals like freedom can be attained and sustained.

5.3 *Transforming Racial Identity through Dance*

In Chapter 9 Francie Johnson examines racism, anxiety, self-doubt and emotions and using dance as a wellness practice. In so doing there is an immediate connection with Theila Smith's research and its emphases on race and issues of identity (Chapter 8) and Hema Daswani's (Chapter 12) autobiographical work. It also complements Carolyne Ali Khan's chapter 5, as it addresses the body and kinesthetic memory. Francie describes how she employs dances from the African diaspora to reaffirm the value of her African American self-identity, ameliorate negative emotions, and replace internalized racism, doubt and anxiety with self-love.

An interesting event that Francie describes arose during a discussion around identity in her high school dance class. In response to her questions on identity, students bring up the connection between culture and country of origin. Her students politely ask Francie about where she is from. When she replies the USA, the students ask about the origins of her parents. As Francie points out, her ancestry is infused with a mixture of bloodlines that originate in Africa, Europe, and the USA, including Native American. Racism, as it is experienced by Francie, is associated with her skin color. Francie explains how dance allows her to build positive emotions and self-identity by connecting to Africa via dances from the African Diaspora. The strength of autobiographical research is evident throughout the chapter and enables Francie to communicate how and why she chose "to think, act and believe in what I do in learning to live as an African-American."

6 Living with Dis-ease

In this section we review four chapters that use narrative to address living with dis-ease, some of which was chronic and drastically affected the author's lifestyle. Each author presents possible pathways for others to consider, adapt and appropriate as they seek to attain and maintain wellness while proceeding with their lives.

6.1 *Finding the Right Path and Living on It*

Eleanor Miele (Chapter 10) presents a personal narrative that contains vignettes about her personal and environmental wellness. Ellie explores wellness, resilience, stress, and environmental health in a context of making a case for taking care of ourselves, and the environment. Ellie elaborates the theme of *know myself* in a story that explores aspects of her biography.

We are all too familiar with the notice given to passengers on an airplane prior to takeoff. "Should the oxygen masks come down, put your oxygen mask on first before you endeavor to help others." This advice is to avoid the peril of potential care-givers losing their ability to operate effectively, or at all, as oxygen-saturation levels drop to perilously low percentages. However, Ellie notes that most of us go through life giving priority to jobs, family, and then ourselves. Taking care of self before others, in everyday life, may be construed as selfish. And yet, there are many contexts in which knowing self and how to effectively self-care are priorities at a time in which we are also told to take care of our planet.

Ellie describes her constant coughing, production of phlegm, and eventual diagnosis of chronic obstructive pulmonary disease (COPD). In so doing, she addresses her interactions with Western doctors, diagnosis and prescription, and the importance of checking side effects of prescribed drugs. Importantly, Ellie noted: "Too much focus on caring for my family and doing my job left no room for me."

What we found interesting was that Ellie, who has a PhD in molecular biology, has the knowledge and associated tools to take care of her own wellness. But because of her professional commitments and obligations to provide care for others (friends and family) however, she found that there was insufficient time to appropriately care for her own health.

It was only when Ellie's condition was diagnosed as COPD that she changed her priorities and used her knowledge of self-care to change lifestyle and effectively address the COPD label. An interesting sidebar that Ellie addresses is the relative heft of Western and Eastern medicine. We regard this as an important issue that has implications for health and wellness throughout the world and across a spectrum that spans recently born through to those in hospice care.

6.2 *Living with Chronic Depression*

Piyanate Paeng Chuychai presents a narrative autobiography of living with chronic depression (Chapter 11). Throughout her educational life Paeng was talented in mathematics and physics but was not comfortable in social situations when she was called to present her work to her teachers and classmates. For example, it was apparent at high school, University undergraduate school, PhD studies, and postdoctoral experiences that Paeng's depressive symptoms were associated with her work and associated stressors of high-performance expectations. Lack of confidence in her own capabilities exacerbated health challenges that confronted Paeng as her life unfolded.

Features of Paeng's narrative about living with depression are thick descriptions of when depression appears, its manifestations, and ways in which Paeng and others treat the disease. Paeng addresses issues such as self-harm, suicidal thoughts, and lifestyle issues as well as details of psychiatric treatments, prescription drugs, and doubts about the efficacy of Western medicine. Among the lifestyle issues that emerge in the research are loneliness, diet, exercise, allergies, and side effects of prescription drugs.

Paeng's research on her journey provides researchers with ample issues that clearly are a priority for research, especially salient to science education and science educators. Clearly there is need for additional research on how people living with chronic depression balance the treatments adopted in Western medicine and lifestyle choices available to those having wellness projects.

6.3 *Intervening to Improve Wellness*

Hema Daswani (Chapter 12) explains how she used acupuncture and Jin Shin Jyutsu (JSJ) together with other complementary healing practices to address osteoporosis in ways that would not require prescribed medication. Expanding on her knowledge of complementary medicine in self-help situations, Hema opened a practice in which she used what she had learned to assist in healing clients' health projects. A feature of Hema's chapter is a plethora of suggestions for healthy lifestyles. In each case Hema advocates a course of action based on an ongoing autoethnography that views wellbeing as a series of commitments to changes in lifestyle – extending beyond acupuncture and JSJ to include activities such as dance, yoga, eating and drinking nutritiously, and adopting daily routines, such as cleaning the teeth, to maintain a healthy body and mind.

Hema describes a series of finger holds, as ways to ameliorate disharmonies in energy flows and expressed emotions. JSJ involves soft touch, does not cause pain, and does not require clothing to be removed. This is the exact feature that makes JSJ ideal for uses in classrooms, during commutes to school and work, while sitting at a concert, or acting in-the-moment when a person experiences dis-ease and needs to harmonize the body without drawing attention to what they are doing.

In an autobiographical narrative, Hema explains how she was diagnosed as having osteoporosis at a relatively young age, and experiencing a progressive step-by-step decline in her bones, connective tissue, and muscle. Projections of the doctors suggested that her physical decline would continue until she was confined to a wheelchair. Due to Hema's resolute search for potentially successful healing modalities, she gradually improved her health, by integrating promising possibilities from a number of complementary healing modalities. These included nutrition, acupuncture, JSJ, Eden's energy medicine, and yoga. Hema's integrative approach, embraces a perspective that her body will heal itself if she provides the resources it needs – that is, by living a lifestyle that sustains wellbeing.

6.4 *JSJ Complements Western Medicine*

Andre Poole (Chapter 13) presents what he learned from a study in which Ken administers JSJ to JP, Andre's daughter. Andre's study is a good example of ripple effects. Several of his colleagues had undertaken research on wellness and used JSJ as a complementary approach to healing (Proscia, 2017). Andre was encouraged about the potential efficacy of JSJ, derived from presentations, publications and conversations with fellow-researchers who had undertaken research in which JSJ was used. Accordingly, Andre decided he and his family might benefit from receiving JSJ treatments.

Andre asked Ken to use JSJ to treat JP, who was experiencing ongoing issues with her digestive system. Seemingly, Western medicine was not improving JP's wellness and hence, JSJ was used as a complementary practice. In the chapter, Andre utilizes oximeter data collected during JSJ treatments as well as narratives, video analysis, and authentic inquiry. The research adds to a growing number of studies our research squad undertook to explore the efficacy of JSJ in ameliorating excess emotions and seeking to heal dis-ease and/or have a role in alleviating discomfort – by complementing Western medicine, rather than providing an alternative.

Following the study, Andre engaged in workshops to learn how to use JSJ in self-care and also to administer treatments to family members. The workshops were presented by a JSJ practitioner, supported by text and an associated card set written by Waultraud Riegger-Krause (2014). Furthermore, in his teacher education courses at Brooklyn College, Andre taught students, all practicing and prospective teachers, about wellness and potential applications of JSJ.

In a second chapter in this volume (Chapter 14), Andre presents an analysis of personal wellness, in which he raises questions about his health as he integrates pranayama yoga and JSJ into a daily self-help regimen, that includes ongoing research. Andre endeavors to know himself in terms of his wellness, broadening and deepening his understandings of self. The text is noticeably reflexive, as Andre presents himself as a burnt-out teacher who had seemingly normalized the pain of stress. Throughout the chapter Andre alludes to a jam-packed lifestyle, which included a highly scheduled routine that began early in the morning and did not finish until late at night. Seemingly, little time was left for relaxation, including sleep.

Andre situates his inquiry in a context of his uses of pranayama yoga and JSJ as complementary healing practices and contemplative tools. Andre notes that he loves to find patterns in numbers and this is evident in his analyses of pulse rate, blood oxygenation and blood pressure. The numbers were obtained from a contemplative activity, referred to as dynamic meditation, a 20-minute pranayama yoga session in which Andre wore a finger pulse oximeter and could thereby relate pulse rate and blood oxygenation to specific moments in the activity, as well as documenting trends in blood pressure, measured before and after each daily session.

In a daily journal, Andre provides evidence of heightened awareness and growing curiosity about possibilities of complementary practices and contradictions that arose regularly. For example, while using the main central vertical flow, from JSJ, Andre noticed an elevation of body temperature. Also, he noticed he was eating less food, while at the same time not feeling hungry.

Andre's two chapters provide nice examples of a strong orientation towards self-help, that embraces the mantra of *Know Thyself.* When Konstantinos and Ken learned to practice JSJ, Mary Burmeister (1990), the person who internationalized JSJ, emphasized *Now Know Myself.* The *now* emphasizes the importance of knowing in the moment. To do so, a person needs to be present – to have heightened awareness of the body and mind, and from the perspective of JSJ, movement patterns of universal energy in, through and out of the body.

Andre explicitly questions his understandings about wellness, healing, and contradictions he does not presently understand. Andre's explicit questions of himself provide insights into an emergent and contingent design of his studies, which assign importance to seeking answers to questions that arise during the conduct of a study. Andre's style of writing his research with his emphases of knowing self and self-care provides links well to the other chapters in the book.

7 Intervening When and as Needed

7.1 *Agency to Act in the Moment*

Corie McCallum (Chapter 15), due to COVID-19 work from home requirements, was forced into a context that was not optimal. Although there were advantages associated with not having to commute to work, the blurred boundaries between work and home began to create dissonance in Corie's life. For example, Corie found that she checked her work email and responded right away irrespective of the time of day and day of the week. Because of quarantine at home rules that applied in New York, Corie made herself available for Zoom meetings even when they were scheduled at a time that usually was considered after work. These examples are consistent with others that Corie considered to reflect a lack of boundaries, and which became a source for stress and irritation.

Although Corie was proud of being flexible in regards to home and work, she was stressed by unprecedented access. Initially, she tried coping with the mounting stress by eating. Being at home however meant ample access to food. Caffeine, chocolate, and comfort food became the eating practice she used to manage emotions. Corie makes it clear that this was not a new management strategy. Prior to the pandemic she had managed emotions, especially stress, by eating and drinking with friends. However, in the changed contexts for work and home, the practice of eating and drinking to ameliorate excess negative emotions began to impact Corie's wellbeing.

Corie acknowledges that immediately prior to the arrival of the pandemic she was unwell. During the pandemic Corie began to gain weight, triggering further negative emotions such as guilt, shame, despondency, and anxiety. This is when Corie began to prioritize self-care. Accordingly, she began to go for outdoor walks when she felt it was beneficial to do so. When she needed to walk, to relieve stress or to free up her mind, she used her agency to do so. She did not regard it as necessary or desirable to wait until out-of-work time to do this. Walking not only tended to clear her mind, but it also enhanced physical fitness, and her health.

In knowing herself, Corie was aware of her poor dietary habits and she shifted to managing her emotions by walking rather than eating and drinking. She notes that, at least up until the time of writing, she had not changed what she eats, but had ceased a practice of eating to reduce stress and other negative emotions. Interestingly, Corie now walks as a daily holistic activity. That is, she walks for wellbeing rather than myriad reductive ways, which may be argued are primary reasons for walking – e.g., reduce stress, clear the mind, lose weight, maintain fitness, feel good, etc.

Considering the autobiographical approach Corie used in her chapter, it is a fine example of "knowing thyself." Corie uses writing as a reflexive tool that brings salient parts of her lived experience into the light. As her awareness of aspects of lived experience heighten, she opens up to learning from experience and changing as desirable. Importantly, Corie accepts ongoing contradictions as resources for further transformation and intentionally does not beat up on herself. Her writing serves as a good example of the relationship between knowing thyself and self-care.

7.2 *Living Well within an Illness*

Beatriz Panduro and Lizette Ramos (Chapter 16) undertake a study of chronic kidney disease among Mexican children and adolescents. The primary foci in their study are emotions, wellness, and health literacy. The research examines the incidence of kidney disease, relates the disease to poverty and other sociocultural factors, and explores education in relation to self-care, and education of caregivers, especially mothers. The use of narratives and polyphonia provide many examples of ways in which emotions are ever-present in cases of acute and chronic disease. No doubt, in this research, which is situated in hospitals, homes, and more generally in lived experiences, there are myriad avenues for follow-up work in an international context and in health projects beyond kidney disease. Importantly, the research investigates terminal disease and related lived experiences that include contexts of despair, abandonment and futility.

The stem of the title of their chapter, *Wellness during illness*, heightens our awareness of diseases that arise in childhood and are managed using Western technologies and prescriptions until death occurs. Even though an adolescent may have a terminal disease, such as chronic kidney disease, pain and suffering can be managed by maintaining lifestyles that reduce suffering from the disease and enhance wellness through diet, exercise, and other aspects of lifestyle.

Throughout the chapters of this volume, there are examples that parallel those laid out by Beatriz and Lizette. Interesting similarities are evident in: Chapter 10, in which Eleanor Miele describes her experiences with chronic obstructive pulmonary disease (COPD); Piyanate Paeng Chuychai's Chapter 11 of her struggles with depression; and Chapter 12, in which Hema Daswani illustrates an integrative approach to restoring good health while overcoming osteoporosis.

8 Contemplative Practices in Everyday Life

8.1 *Living Mindfully*

Yau Yan Wong (Chapter 17) provides a narrative of her upbringing at home and subsequent experiences as a teacher in Hong Kong. In so doing, she illustrates how teaching can be highly stressful, especially since it involves numerous hours of out-of-school work, associated with evaluating student work and planning lessons. Such work has serious implications for teachers' lives, impacting their wellness and the quality of life at home. Frayed nerves and anger can lead to deleterious forms of conduct and associated interactions with family and friends.

Later in Yau Yan's career, she become a resident of Thailand. It was there that she was introduced to mindfulness and, with other teachers in her school, participated in multi-day retreats and professional development activities. Together she and these other teachers developed a professional development community in their school so that they could share their experiences of using mindfulness in the classroom and thereby learn from one another.

Yau Yan provides detailed descriptions of her engagement in a variety of mindfulness activities and through her uses of narrative we are introduced to important dos and don'ts related to meditation and mindfulness. In so doing, readers have opportunities to learn about mindfully sitting, walking, eating, speaking, listening, and doing housework (e.g., cleaning dishes, toilets, and sweeping the floor). Having learned about mindfulness as an activity for everyday life, the teacher-participants in the research were able to adopt similar approaches in their classrooms. Among the salient issues addressed by Yau Yan are bullying at home and in school, and learning during the COVID-19 pandemic in which highly stressed students worked from home using computers and also were involved in hybrid models during which some of their learning was done at home and some was done at school. The emotional toll of learning via computers from home and also attending school during the COVID-19 pandemic, highlighted a need for research on the wellbeing of students, teachers, parents and others involved in hybrid teaching and learning activities, at school and at home.

The context in which research is embedded is always a mediator of what is happening, why it is happening, and what more is there to learn from this inquiry? This is especially the case during a pandemic like COVID-19, which has now been pervasively present for more than two years. In the case of the research included in this book, the researchers/workers were greatly impacted by COVID-19 as cities/countries throughout the world shut down as they isolated people from one another in attempts to save lives, control the creation and spread of variants of the virus, and then identify ways for citizens across the age spectrum to resume productive lives while working from home, utilizing the Internet and computer applications, such as Zoom, to afford face-to-face contact at a distance. Accordingly, there were new patterns of work and learning that catalyzed highly intense emotions and associated health projects. Yau Yan's research in Thailand connects, via its partial immersion in COVID-19, with the research presented in Chapters 4, 12, and 15, authored by Anna Malyukova, Hema Daswani, and Corie McCallum respectively. Perhaps in a less explicit way, all four chapters interconnect with the other chapters in the book in the sense that the pandemic was a critical component of shared contextually mitigating factors (Gallard Martínez, 2020).

8.2 *Learning from Everyday Life*

Wolff-Michael Roth (Chapter 18) was an active collaborator with Ken from the late 1990s until about 2009. Michael is a pioneer of sociocultural theories being applied in science education. While his research path has diverged from ours, his impact on our research squads has been highly significant. We view his chapter in this book as complementary to those that preceded it. Michael situates his research in everyday activities, including cycling, use of a computer, and weeding. Michael addresses a number of frameworks that underlie his extensive portfolio of research. These include coherence, consciousness, experienced time, and holistic experiences in which he describes and theorizes being-in-the-flow as it relates to weeding, and other forms of social involvement.

Michael's theoretical frameworks are considered as ways to experience a lifeworld – providing novel ways to notice and appropriate resources to support social transactions. Such a stance, oriented toward flow, would likely rekindle fresh curiosities that lead to new research pathways and possibilities. We believe that such aspects that can potentially expand others' visions to situate their work in mundane aspects of life to be a priority for research.

9 Next Steps

The contributing authors to this volume illustrate the importance of knowing self. This is a transcendent goal that can begin with the emergence of consciousness and, possibly end with the transition we associate with death – when the physical body ceases to function. Throughout the human lifespan, as a person lives and experiences life in myriad contexts, knowing myself now involves being aware of what is happening in the moment, in relation to mind body, and, for many, spirit. Although we are limited in what we know, what we know is a resource for navigating a lifeworld that is experienced as a dynamic flux of structures – resources we can appropriate to afford a purposeful life.

When we first opted to use oximeters to monitor pulse rate and blood oxygenation, it was difficult to procure oximeters, they were expensive, and considered to be medical equipment. In a relatively short time this situation changed dramatically. Nowadays, smart phones and Apple watches, for example, provide oximeter readings routinely, and hence it is relatively easy for people to know themselves in terms of these physiological variables. When there are sudden changes, a person can be informed by their mobile devices as the changes happen, allowing for more personalized care.

Given the accessibility of oximeter readings, it makes sense for teachers and students to know what is happening physiologically as they participate in school-related activities. Also, as part of education, it is reasonable to expect all citizens to know how their wellness can be affected by changes in pulse rate, blood oxygenation, and arterial blood flow. If blood oxygenation falls into the low 90% range, what might be expected for a teacher or student? What can an individual do, in the moment, to change their blood oxygenation back to a level that is normal for them? Other oximetry data also can, and should, be reviewed to ensure that individuals are informed and can act to attain and sustain wellness.

Since the 1970s at least, there have been efforts to enhance the quality of student engagement in classrooms (Capie & Tobin, 1981). Various labels have been used to highlight potential enhancements such as cooperative learning, student-centered learning, and peer teaching. Indeed, in our research on coteaching, we strongly advocated students as teachers, coteaching peers, and other variants that we considered to be highly effective (Tobin, Alexakos, & Powietrzynska, 2022). However, since 2012 it has been clear in our research that some participants get increasingly anxious when they are to teach or present to others (e.g., Brathwaite, Chapter 2, this volume; Tobin et al., 2016). The anxiety relates to teachers and peers. Immediately prior to getting involved in presenting to others, some people will experience increased pulse rate, lower blood oxygenation, and higher blood pressure. This may be accompanied by sweaty palms, panic attacks, dry throat, and other physical indicators of increasing stress, including dizziness and tears.

If participants experience anxiety, high stress levels, and physical signs of disharmony, these signs suggest they might benefit from changing how they engage – after dealing with the disharmony. As a basic life skill, all participants in education should know about wellness as it pertains to their own wellbeing – enabling each participant to know themselves to an extent that conscious monitoring affords self-care when it is desirable.

Considerable evidence supports uses of breathing meditation and soft touch approaches to healing, such as holding fingers and placing hands on the body so as to harmonize energy flows. In addition, mindfulness practices and their applications in everyday life show the potential of being mindful while eating, walking, jogging, dancing, cooking, sweeping the floor, taking a shower, and cleaning the toilet. Such practices can be considered, along with myriad others, as contemplative tools that potentially can enhance wellness.

9.1 *Now Knowing Myself*

The authors | researchers of the chapters in this book frequently employ autobiographical texts to present important insights into the salience of *Now Knowing Myself*. We feel it is a strength of the works published in the book that researchers often were puzzled by something that happened that did not fit with what was expected. That is, contradictions arose about expressed emotions, responses of their bodies, and emergence of dis-ease. As they sought to understand, they became more aware of the importance of contradictions in relation to wellness. In many of the chapters, contemplative tools and complementary healing practices were used proactively to address emerging health projects, and in other cases to re-harmonize flows of universal energy in the body, to attain a state of wellness that was sustained thereafter through healthy living.

As a collective, the chapters of the book illuminate what we know about emotions and ways in which they mediate not only what happens but also our understanding of what is happening. We are not medical doctors and what is presented in this book is for educational and research purposes only and should not be constituted as medical advice. We encourage readers to utilize the research presented in the book heuristically (i.e., as a guide rather than a template), to highlight wellness projects in their own lives and the extent to which they have the knowledge to live with chronic illness or to enact interventions for the purpose of attaining and sustaining wellness. We invite all readers to initiate research projects to contribute to ongoing research on wellness, not only in classrooms but in every part of their lives and the places they live, work, and be.

Notes

1 Frequently we use the term dis-ease to convey a lack of feeling at ease. We are not speaking of a diagnosis of a disease, which often accompanies a label and an associated prescription. In general, as practitioners of complementary healing practices, we are interested in identifying disharmonies in the functioning of an individual and using practices to restore harmony and a feeling of ease. We have a general concern that use of medical labels can catalyze a rise of emotions such as fear and sadness, which can serve as foundations from which further wellness projects can sprout and grow.

2 The way we conceptualize wellbeing is to consider individuals in a social collection in which resources for action are relationally and dialectically interconnected. It is not just the inner functioning of individuals that determine whether wellbeing occurs, but also harmony throughout an ecosystem. To maintain optimal harmony the quality of food, air, water, and soil all need to be considered as well as temperature changes, storm systems and other aspects of climate, such as air pressure. Also, societal structures, affordance, and social and economic disparities and inequities need to be addressed.

References

Alexakos, K. (2015). *Being a teacher | researcher: A primer on doing authentic inquiry, research on teaching and learning.* Sense Publishers.

Alexakos, K. (2022). Conscious spaces and self: Boundaries, core, me not me, and being in the heart. In K. Tobin & K. Alexakos (Eds.), *Transforming learning and teaching: Heuristics for educative and responsible practices* (pp. 362–381). Brill. https://doi.org/10.1163/9789004507609_018

Alexakos, K., Pride, L. D., Amat, A., Tsetsakos, P., Lee, K. J., Paylor-Smith, C., Zapata, C., Wright, S., & Smith, T. (2016). Mindfulness and discussing "thorny" issues in the classroom. *Cultural Studies of Science Education, 11*(3), 741–769. https://doi.org/10.1007/s11422-015-9718-0

Amat, A., Zapata, C., Alexakos, K., Pride, L. D., Paylor-Smith, C., & Hernandez, M. (2016). Incorporating oximeter analyses to investigate synchronies in heart rate while teaching and learning about race. *Cultural Studies of Science Education, 11*(3), 785–801. https://doi.org/10.1007/s11422-016-9767-z

Brathwaite, C. (2022). Exploring hidden anxiety-provoking experiences through the use of oximeter analysis and cogenerative dialogue. In K. Tobin & K. Alexakos (Eds.), *Transforming learning and teaching: Heuristics for educative and responsible practices* (pp. 256–278). Brill. https://doi.org/10.1163/9789004507609_013

Burmeister, M. (1990). *A and Q text: Know myself.* Jin Shin Jyutsu, Inc.

Capie, W., & Tobin, K. (1981). Pupil engagement in learning tasks: A fertile area for research in science teaching. *Journal of Research in Science Teaching, 18*, 409–417. https://doi.org/10.1002/tea.3660180505

Chödrön, P. (2013). *How to meditate: A practical guide to making friends with your mind.* Sounds True.

Gallard Martínez, A. J., Pitts, W. Brkich, K., & Ramos de Robles, S. L. (2020). How does one recognize contextual mitigating factors (CMFs) as a basis to understand and arrive at better approaches to research designs? *Cultural Studies of Science Education, 15*(2), 545–567. https://doi.org/10.1007/s11422-018-9872-2

Garfinkel, H. (1967). *Studies in ethnomethodology.* Prentice Hall.

Kincheloe, J. L., & Tobin, K. (2009). The much exaggerated death of positivism. *Cultural Studies of Science Education, 4*, 513–528. https://doi.org/10.1007/s11422-009-9178-5

Philippot, P., Chapelle, G., & Blairy, S. (2002). Respiratory feedback in the generation of emotion. *Cognition & Emotion, 16*, 605–627. https://doi.org/10.1080/02699930143000392

Powietrzynska, M. (2016). From the grip of depression to a newfound euphoria for living: Gliding across the spectra of resilience and outlook. In M. Powietrzynska & K. Tobin (Eds.), *Mindfulness and educating citizens for everyday life* (pp. 213–234). Sense.

Powietrzynska, M., Noble, L., O'Loughlin-Boncamper, S., & Azeez, A. (2021). Holding space for uncertainty and vulnerability: Reclaiming humanity in teacher education through contemplative | equity pedagogy. *Cultural Studies of Science Education, 16*(3), 951–964. https://doi.org/10.1007/s11422-021-10035-x

Proscia, P. A. (2017). Coming face to face with fear: journeying to wellness. In M. Powietrzynska & K. Tobin (Eds.), *Weaving complementary knowledge systems and mindfulness to educate a literate citizenry for sustainable and healthy lives* (pp. 291–303). Brill.

Rieger-Krause, W. (2014). *Health is in your hands: Jin Shin Jyutsu – practicing the art of self-healing (with 51 flash cards for the hands-on practice of Jin Shin Jyutsu)*. Upper West Side Philosophers Inc.

Roth, W.-M., & Tobin, K. (2010). Solidarity and conflict: Prosody as a transactional resource in intra- and intercultural communication involving power differences. *Cultural Studies of Science Education, 5*(4), 807–847. https://doi.org/10.1007/s11422-010-9272-8

Tobin, K. (2016). Mindfulness as a way of life: Maintaining wellness through healthy living. In M. Powietrzynska & K. Tobin (Eds.), *Mindfulness and educating citizens for everyday life* (pp. 1–24). Sense.

Tobin, K. (2018). The role of mindfulness in harmonizing sustainable lifestyles. *Learning: Research and Practice, 4*, 112–125. https://doi.org/10.1080/23735082.2018.1435039

Tobin, K., & Alexakos, K. (2021). Global challenges need attention now: educating humanity for wellness and sustainability. *Cultural Studies of Science Education, 16*(3), 651–673. https://doi.org/10.1007/s11422-021-10080-6

Tobin, K., Alexakos, K., & Powietrzynska, M. (2022). Coteaching: then, now, and in future. In K. Tobin & K. Alexakos (Eds.), *Transforming learning and teaching: heuristics for educative and responsible practices* (pp. 18–38). Brill.

Tobin, K., King, D., Henderson, S., Bellocchi, A., & Ritchie, S. M. (2016). Expression of emotions and physiological changes during teaching. *Cultural Studies of Science Education, 11*, 669–692. https://doi.org/10.1007/s11422-016-9778-9

CHAPTER 2

Exploring Hidden Anxiety-Provoking Experiences through the Use of Oximeter Analysis and Cogenerative Dialogue

Corinna Brathwaite

Abstract

In this chapter I discuss my investigation of a student's (Petra's) anxiety during her group presentation using event-oriented inquiry. This event was selected because of the increase in her heart rate 60 seconds prior to the moment she began speaking. A combination of video recordings, oximeter readings and cogenerative dialogues are used to explore anxiety-provoking experiences even when such emotions may not be outwardly visible through other means, like facial expression, gestures, and tone.

Keywords

emotions – heart rate – teaching – learning – oximeter – anxiety

•••

> *Corinna: Many times in a classroom, having to present makes me feel sick to my stomach. The experience of even knowing that I will have to present in public is dreadful regardless of the size of the audience. Not really understanding the need for it outside of business meetings, I felt that it could be a practice that educators would stop using. While there are great reasons to have presentations assigned – even group assigned presentations – my anxiety built a wall of intolerance.* [Author's thoughts and way of interacting with reader (Van Maanen, 2011)]

Petra, a young woman studying to become a science teacher, was taking a course with Konstantinos Alexakos, the professor of the science education course, at CUNY Brooklyn College in the spring semester of 2012. The class participated in a study that incorporated video recordings and finger pulse oximeters, to collect data on physiological responses to emotional stimuli

 | DOI:10.1163/9789004527348_002

heuristics, cogenerative dialogues (hereafter cogens) and clickers to gather participant feedback of experienced emotions and climate in the classroom. Kenneth Tobin and Alexakos were the lead researchers exploring emotions and emotional climate in teaching and learning. In this chapter, I identified a salient contradiction as an event to explore the anxiety Petra experienced at the beginning of her co-presentation in front of her class.

Sometimes we have nothing to be scared about, but the mere anticipation of what could possibly go wrong worries us to the point of fear, otherwise known as anxiety (Frazzetto, 2014). Adapting Van Maanen's (2011) narratology, I weave in my own experience and thoughts on anxiety over presenting and public speaking, as I investigate and learn from Petra's experience. Introducing my own voice allows me to become more aware of how I feel about presenting, although I also was told that I did not look nervous.

To investigate Petra's anxiety experiences, this study was grounded in Interaction Ritual Chains (IRC), Event-Oriented Inquiry, and Hermeneutic Phenomenology.

IRC require four elements: there has to be one *other*; there must be a connection or solidarity associated with the *other*; a distinct barrier that connects the associated group; and there must be an emerging emotional output shared by all members of the associated group (Collins, 2004). IRC grounds this study, because interaction does not restrict itself to a physical *other*. Collins (2004) does acknowledge the internal self, or inner voice, as part of the *other* as well. Hermeneutic Phenomenology is the exploration of what happened from the perspective of the person who experienced it and why it happened (Roth, Tobin, & Zimmermann, 2002). Hence, hermeneutic phenomenology is a major part of this study.

This study is grounded in Event-Oriented Inquiry (Tobin, 2013). Tobin's development of Event-Oriented Inquiry is grounded in Sewell's understanding of culture and event – an event being interpreted as a spike in the curve, which highlighted change or conflict in what was happening in the moment. Tobin's study with oximeters incorporated analyzing Donna's heart rate (HR), blood pressure (PLETHY), and blood oxygenation (SpO_2) before and while teaching. Donna King, a professor for pre-service science teachers, wore an oximeter, permitting Tobin and colleagues to research her HR, PLETHY, SpO_2, and the emotional climate (EC) of the class. Tobin used event-oriented inquiry, identifying events by searching for salient contradictions, and hermeneutic phenomenological methods to investigate Donna's emotional experiences on multiple levels, but grounded his study with polyvagal theory, whereas this study focused on Collins' interaction ritual theory and interaction ritual chains. Tobin, as in the event discussed here, used descriptive statistics in addition to looking at both HR and PLETHY to identify events (Tobin, 2016).

The event discussed here took place during the fifth week of the course. Petra was having an internal conversation with herself as she was about to take her turn at presenting. The internal conversation, between herself and her inner voice, was an inner interaction ritual chain within another interaction ritual. In the minute before she began presenting, the emotional experience was surreal for her, because this emotion surfaced as she was waiting for her moment to speak in her presentation. It was through the cogen following the presentation that Petra communicated her emotional experience at that moment. In the video, she displays visible coping strategies like fidgeting fingers, or rotating a ring on a finger. Nervousness and stress are symptoms of anxiety (Frazzetto, 2014). Two of the questions arising in this research were: Why was Petra anxious about presenting? What about this presentation made Petra anxious?

1 Oximeter Analyses in Teaching | Learning

> *Corinna: I had hoped to find something interesting about it as well, and I did. Petra's experience became not just a point of interest for me, but also a reflective experience about my own public speaking.*

The class incorporated oximeters for presenters to wear each week. Oximeters are devices that collect three readings: heart rate [HR], blood oxygenation [SpO_2], and strength of the heartbeat [PLETHY] (Calderón, 2014). The data would be saved automatically as an Excel file if the device was connected properly to a computer with Bluetooth access. After observing the HR column, Petra's heart started to race. It contradicted the HR pattern Petra had at the beginning of the oximeter file, collected during the class session. After identifying the event, the data, along with transcripts from the video recordings, helped in further investigating what happened during the event. Thus identified, this event was further analyzed on a macro-level, meso-level, and micro-level.

When I next looked at the video, what I saw was amazing. Petra was about to present with two other students, when her HR went up before she began speaking.

> Corinna: *You see, when I present I am completely nervous. My palms start to sweat and/or feel cold. My heartbeat seems to drown out the sounds of the room to the point where I am no longer involved in what the class is discussing. I have always struggled in some way with presentations. I felt like I understood what could have been potentially what Petra was experiencing; however, I am not her. She had her own feelings and I was very curious to find out what she felt she was going through.*

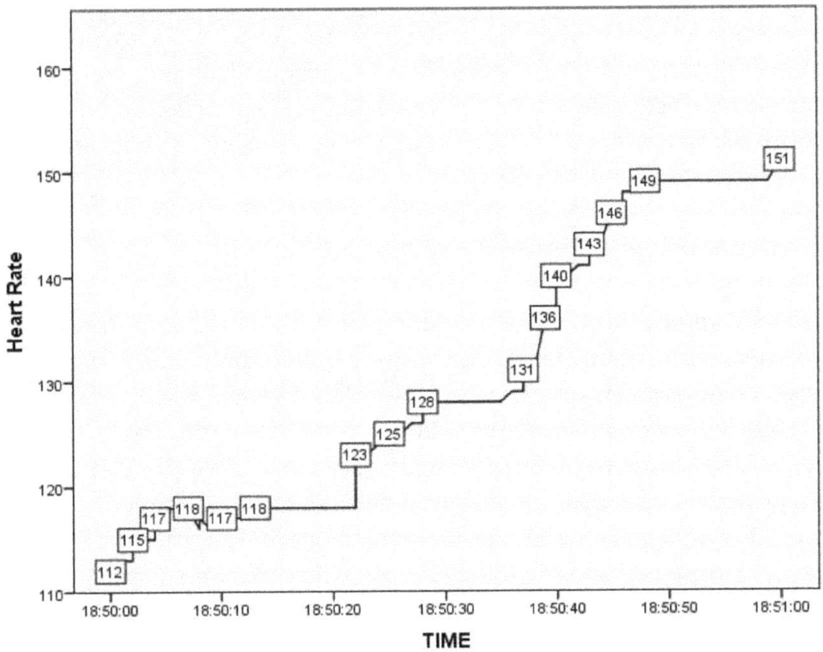

FIGURE 2.1 Petra's HR sixty seconds before leading presentation

This particular chapter investigates Petra's physiological responses to her anxiety in the classroom and focuses on the data collected from the videos, oximeters, and cogens during the fifth week of the course. Finger-pulse oximeters offer three readings per second.

I found it interesting that what seemed steady and normal HR started to increase rapidly a minute before Petra began to speak (Figure 2.1). It has been found from the work of others that free speaking causes the HR to increase (Bernardi, 2000). Petra had not yet started to outwardly verbalize her thoughts, when her HR began to increase steadily. With Petra's HR accelerating rapidly during the sixty seconds, this rapid change of beats per minute (bpm) revealed a salient contradiction to the consistent HR that was below 100 bpm in class.

After identifying the event and watching the video of Petra's presentation, I used a cogen Petra had done with Alexakos to gain further information about what Petra felt, from the participant herself. Cogens are low-risk communal sessions that occur as either a reflection on evidence of what occurred or collective reflection upon what occurred throughout the experience of the research. Events need further understanding and unpacking from those that experience it and cogens offer a low-risk, safe space (Tobin, 2012). Wolff-Michael Roth and Tobin (2001) investigated a teacher's approach to teaching and learning in a science classroom through the use of cogens, as it was a shared experience between the members who partook in the class.

In this study, the video recording allowed insight to what occurred in the classroom during the event and the cogens. In this chapter I discuss Petra's anxiety from a minute before her turn to talk came during the presentation with two co-presenters, Paula and Ian, on the topic of gender, sexuality, and education.

2 What Happened to Bring about This Salient Event?

The video recordings along with oximeter readings were used to capture data. Petra and her co-presenters prepared to speak to their peers about gender roles and how stereotypes may affect the success of each gender within the classroom. While Petra stood in the front left corner and faced the class, another student, Laura, a classmate being presented to, started to talk to the class about her own personal experience as a female and her knowledge of tools.

Petra's HR throughout the minute is indicated in the brackets. Petra, who was the only presenter wearing a finger pulse oximeter, was standing at the front left of the classroom next to her co-presenter while Laura, their classmate who was not presenting, spoke for about 60 seconds (detailed in Table 2.1). Petra's HR increased steadily to 151 beats per minute (bpm) where she exhibited a high level of oxygenation at 98%.

The first moment that Petra's PLETHY peaked was between 18:50:08 and 18:50:09. Petra had clicked her data on her clicker and positioned herself next to her female co-presenter, Paula, right before her PLETHY rose. Laura was talking about her experience with gender roles in her example about tools. The timer sounded, alerting the students to make a note of their emotional state in the classroom.

The second moment her PLETHY peaked happened 3 to 4 seconds later as Laura was saying "my aunt." Her HR maintained a bpm of 128 throughout the 4 to 5 seconds along with her SpO_2 remaining at 98%. Petra was rotating the clicker in her hands as described about the prior second. Petra started touching her nose, then her right cheek. Following that, her hands were in front of her stomach, and she started rotating the clicker with both hands for approximately 23 seconds. While rotating the clicker, 4 to 5 seconds were spent scanning the classroom. Five seconds later, Petra was seen looking down at the rotating clicker for another 3 to 4 seconds. After that, Petra looked at the class, shifted on her right foot, and was just holding the clicker for 17 seconds. In order to understand what Petra was feeling during the event, a cogen was necessary, because it was the only way Petra would be able to not only reveal her anxiety, but also explain it in greater detail. Observing the change in Petra's HR caught my attention and was the catalyst that led to me watch the video and

TABLE 2.1 Transcript during 60-second event

Time	What was said?	What was heard?	What action was done?
18:50:00	*Laura: [118] … Well*	Phlegmy coughing	Everyone was looking forward. A coughing student was seen covering mouth. Female co-presenters were looking at projected slide on screen and male presenter was looking at his female co-presenters.
18:50:01	*Laura: I'm the oldest.*	Student was still coughing	Petra was touching something on the table in front of the board where the projection screen was.
18:50:02	*So he used to kinda like*		Petra was going back to where she was standing with her co-presenters
18:50:03	*[123] call me*		Petra was completing her placement by her female co-presenter and both were looking at the projected PowerPoint (PPT) slide
18:50:04	*to … – if he had – he had*		Female co-presenter, Paula, was looking at the class and towards the end of this moment Petra started to also look at the class
18:50:05	*this *inaudible* [125]*	Sound (timer?) sounded off	Students reached for their clickers to indicate their emotional level in the class at that moment. Petra used the clicker that was already in her hand then took a step forward. She looked like she was about to place it on the front table, but then was seen stepping back while keeping the clicker in hand. After they clicked, the class seemed to either look at Laura (including presenters) or to the front of the classroom.
18:50:06	*so he would call me to like*		
18:50:07	*identify [126]#*		
18:50:08	*like specific tools [128]*		Between the period when Laura was heard saying "tools" and "and stuff," Petra's PLETHY was really high. As "tools" was heard, the last chime of the timer sounded also.
18:50:09	*and stuff like*		Students finished clicking.
18:50:10	*that.*		
18:50:11	*So, but in some*		
18:50:12	*cultures like my*		Petra was shifting clicker from hand to hand, like very slight juggle
18:50:13	*Aunt in their*		When "my aunt" was heard, Petra's PLETHY was very high again.

(*cont.*)

TABLE 2.1 Transcript during 60-second event (*cont.*)

Time	What was said?	What was heard?	What action was done?
18:50:14	*home the girls*		When "home" was heard, Petra touched her nose, and remained touching her face. Her hand moved from her nose to her right cheek by the time "tools" was heard, while Paula began to scratch/touch nose.
18:50:15	*are not allowed to be*		
18:50:16	*anywhere around tools* [*129*]		
18:50:17	*that was*		Petra and Paula brought their hands down at the start of this moment completing the action by the time "masculine" was heard. Petra kept both hands in front of her stomach holding clicker and Paula had her hands behind her back.
18:50:18	*really* [*131*] *a –a*		
18:50:19	*masculine*		
18:50:20	*thing* [*136*]. *Right?*		Petra was steadily rotating clicker with her hands holding both ends of the clicker. (between second 20 and 29)
18:50:21	*So,* [*140*] *now that I've become*		
18:50:22	*my own …*		
18:50:23	*an adult* [*141*]		
18:50:24	*if I need* [*143*] *to find something*		
18:50:25	*in my home* [*146*]		
18:50:26	*tighten a screw* [*148*] *or something*		
18:50:27	*I don't have to call my*		Ian adjusted his shirt.
18:50:28	*husband* [*149*]		
18:50:29	*I know how to do it.*		
18:50:30	*But in some cultures, if*		When "cultures" was heard, male co-presenter looked down to the floor or at his feet quickly then looked back up, adjusted his shirt and massaged his left wrist. Petra was still rotating clicker. While Laura was saying "male in the home … idea" Petra started to scan the class from her right to her left (4 to 5 seconds).
18:50:31	*There isn't a male in the*		
18:50:32	*home,*		
18:50:33	*they can't do it. But if*		
18:50:34	*the um – the um*		

(*cont.*)

TABLE 2.1 Transcript during 60-second event (*cont.*)

Time	What was said?	What was heard?	What action was done?
18:50:35	*idea is that both men and women*		Petra was still rotating clicker. When "idea" was heard, male co-presenter, Ian, brought left hand to right ear (the top part) while right hand remained on left wrist. Then, he shifted his left hand to right wrist and massaged it really quickly. He next rested his left wrist over his right wrist on top of what looked like a container on the front table.
18:50:36	*can learn to do the*		
18:50:37	*same things. Right?*		
18:50:38	*Anthony: Right.*	*Some students nod in agreement.*	
18:50:39	*Laura: Because if you*		Petra looked down at the clicker while she continued rotating it.
18:50:40	*ask one [151] of my*		When a student researcher saw HR go to 151 he drew the attention of another researcher sitting next to him. Petra was still looking down at clicker she was rotating.
18:50:41	*small sisters who*		
18:50:42	*never used to be around*		Petra looked at the class.
18:50:43	*'Okay, come fix this screw.'*		Petra shifted to her right foot and was just holding clicker in place – not rotating (17 seconds).
18:50:44	*It will keep falling all the*		
18:50:45	*time on the*	*Some students laughed*	
18:50:46	*ground.*		
18:50:47	*Right? [152] So I'm like*		
18:50:48	*'Okay -*		
18:50:49	*We both can do [151] the*		
18:50:50	*same thing male or*		
18:50:51	*female. You don't*		
18:50:52	*need to have a maleness.*		
18:50:53	*We learn,*		
18:50:54	*But just different*		

(*cont.*)

TABLE 2.1 Transcript during 60-second event (*cont.*)

Time	What was said?	What was heard?	What action was done?
18:50:55	*Ways. Right? I might*		
18:50:56	*have taken a longer*		
18:50:57	*time to know what is*		
18:50:58	*a hammer*		
18:50:59	*whereas a-a*		
18:51:00	*a male*		

listen to the cogen. The cogen for presenters was set up for the students to discuss anything they recalled going through or happening during their time presenting. I focused on the cogen that explained what Petra was feeling during this minute from her own perspective.

2.1 *What Happened during the Cogen?*

This cogen between Petra and Alexakos was recorded two weeks after her group presentation in the class. The group's presentation was about gender and sexuality, both of which can be *Thorny Issues* (Alexakos et al., 2016). For the cogen, Petra met with Alexakos, aware that the topic was observing and discussing her experience of her own presentation.

At the start of the cogen, Alexakos began by asking Petra how the overall classroom experience had been, in her opinion. The conversation then transitioned specifically to the recordings with her wearing the oximeter in the classroom, where Petra recalled her emotional experience of her own presentation. Upon being asked if what Laura said made any impact, Petra responded that there was a mental block because of the preparation needed for her to begin speaking soon. Petra was not aware of what Laura said. Petra focused on her own emotions and her racing thoughts while Laura was speaking. Bakhtin interpreted inner feelings and inner speech as being dialogic, since all utterances are a form of language and contribute to continuous dialogue (Bakhtin, 1994).

When Alexakos began the video clip in Table 2.2, Petra admitted that her nervousness intensified as her turn approached. Paul Ekman classified the following as basic emotions: anger, disgust, contempt, fear, joy, sadness, and surprise (Ekman, 2003). Although anxiety is not one of the primary emotions,

TABLE 2.2 Transcript of Petra admitting to nervousness

[0:54] Alexakos: This is actually ... we spent a lot of time talking, and probably I shouldn't have done that cause I learned from Angie the other day ... cause people get anxious, and then ... Like *you* stay stressed the whole time. It's not like *you* just get stressed when you're about to speak ... *You* stay stressed when you're about to speak.
Petra: Oh me? Yeah.
Alexakos: That happens with a lot of bodies, like Angie [1:44]

it is a subcategory of fear, as fear comprises of both terror and nervousness (Frazzetto, 2014).

Ekman defined fear as a learned emotion mostly used to identify the feeling or emotion experienced, and defined by the collective or social structures when most or all have experienced the same feeling caused by the interaction (Ekman, 2003). Giovanni Frazzetto (2014) defined fear as a fight for survival where we have to fend off enemies, whereas anxiety is anticipation of fear built on worry, nervousness, and stress. Similarly, Petra was nervous before her turn to talk.

> *Petra: I feel the same way every time I am about to speak in front of a group of people. I have had classmates and colleagues who shared their feelings of nervousness when it came to presentations or even just speaking in front of any size group in and out of the classroom. However, I have met one person as an undergraduate who expressed that he enjoyed presenting as it gave him an adrenaline rush. I did look at him completely surprised because he was the first person I heard that from. Even celebrities, well singers, spoke candidly about having stage fright before their performing for a crowd even if the crowd bought tickets because of their artistry.*

Inner thoughts and inner voice can be described as symbolic interaction (Collins, 2004). Collins made clear that IRs are everywhere and can expand or apply to every type of interaction, which is why this internal conversation is an inner IR chain (Collins, 2004). Collins defined an IR as being positive if the emotional energy (EE) transformed into a positive emotion, and negative if the emotional energy transformed into a negative emotion. EE is what an individual looks for as an outcome of their IR, which is also an outcome of this event. This emotional experience that Petra is experiencing is the influx of emotion during the IR. Based on a positive experience of an IR, individuals will have a successful ritual outcome of feeling as a part of the group. Through feeling a part of the group, there would be this group identity that forms, with its own set of morals and symbols (words, visual icons, or gestures) that are assigned to the group, and EE shared by the group that molds into strong group solidarity (Collins, 2004).

Alexakos goes on to ask Petra about the presentation, in Table 2.3. According to Petra, content was not a factor in what made her nervous. Additionally, her group spoke about the provocative nature of the content and wondered how the class would receive the information and react. The collective thought process of the three co-presenters doing either really well or really poorly was on her mind. There was no middle ground on her evaluation scale; her

TABLE 2.3 Transcript of Petra anticipating the reaction of the classmates

[13:08] Alexakos: So, this is you, you're about to start talking and look and see what happens here. So, tell me what it was like going into the presentation?
Petra: Ummmmm It was ner – Like, I felt we were prepared, and I felt we were like synced. And that made me feel more comfortable with my group, but I was still nervous – just by the fact that I had to talk.
Alexakos: How about the topic itself?
Petra: The topic – it was just – like I don't, didn't feel bad talking about it because we like (um. Can you see me? Alexakos: Yeah. It's just that you stopped so I was wondering if that was you.) Oh um so like we were prepared. I was prepared with the topic. I was comfortable with it – I just – we had this thing in our minds, "Like how will the class take it?" Like we knew it was either going to go really bad or it's either going to go really well. Like we were actually expecting some good debates the whole sexuality part, whether we should teach it in school or not, bullying. Like we weren't sure how people were going to react to that.
Alexakos: What did you think was going to happen?
Petra: I … I really didn't know. Like – I didn't know. Like I know it was going to be a good debate so that's why we had all those questions, but I didn't about the people's opinions cause we just hadn't talked about it. Like we have a couple of people in the class that like to really express their opinions; we knew they were going to, but we weren't sure. Just because I didn't know about religious backgrounds, you know everybody is from a different country, and bringing in the gay topic
Alexakos: It's one of those topics that could've …
Petra: Yea, it could've easily went the way the video was going. The parents were like: "Do not talk about sexuality in the classroom" "Do not do this" Y'know? "This is wrong" [15:30]

expectations, and that of her group, were two extremes. Alexakos then asked her to elaborate by detailing what was anticipated. Her response was not knowing if they would actually interact, not knowing their beliefs, and knowing that it could be possible that the response could be similar to a video the group had shown earlier in the presentation. Even knowing that a couple of her classmates interacted and participated in the class discussions consistently, there was always the chance that even they might choose not to.

Table 2.4 details what the event higlighted in this study considered significant. Petra's HR is increasing before she opens her mouth to speak to her classmates. Petra forgot for a brief moment what her co-presenter, Paula, said to her as Petra was getting the clicker for the screen projector. Paula was letting her know that it was about to be Petra's turn to speak. As soon as that happened, Petra's HR started to increase. In describing what that felt like for her, Petra recalled feeling like, "I'm getting ready to *brief pause* fly" followed by a bit of laughter. Alexakos said, "You're getting ready to," before Petra interjected saying, "Escape." Paula spoke to Petra right before the event occurred. What we looked at in the graph in Figure 2.1 and the transcript in Table 2.1 is a result of the exchange. We saw and read what was occurring in the class as Petra was *flying*. As Petra was *flying*, so was her HR.

TABLE 2.4 Transcript of Petra's emotional experience as her HR increased

Alexakos: What's happening here? Paula turns and talks to you? What is she saying to you? That it's time to get ready? Is that what she's saying?
Petra: Um, no. It's just "Was that good enough?" I don't know. I don't know what she said.
Alexakos: Because after she talks she turns to you.
Petra: Ohhhh because I wasn't sure if she was going to
Alexakos: Yea see. As soon as you picked that up. Now see you picked up the remote, right?
Petra: Because I wasn't sure if she's actually going to present a couple of slides that related to that topic that we actually forgot to discuss. I was ready to present all of the history. That. That was no issue for me. I just thought she might talk about that a little bit like just the schooling part. So that moment I picked it up, that's when she told me like okay it's going to be my turn.
Alexakos: As soon as that happens now you're 128.
Petra: I'm getting ready to .... Fly? (she laughs a little bit) (Alexakos: You're getting ready to ...) Escape. [29:23]
Alexakos: See look at that ... Laura is still talking and now you're ...
Petra: Because now I'm preparing in my mind ... to talk. [29:32]

TABLE 2.5 Transcript of Petra's focus on Laura

Alexakos: Look at that it's at 152 in the video
Petra: Yeah ... I was listening to what she was saying but I wasn't focusing on her.

When during the cogen Alexakos pointed out to Petra that her HR reached 152 while Laura was speaking (Table 2.5), Petra began to reflect on her emotional experience. Petra mentioned the difference between how the presentation went in her thoughts versus how the presentation would be understood in actuality. The level of uncertainty Petra had about the class understanding her caused anxiety, and the cogen experience of replaying the presentation was the first time Petra heard herself. Alexakos asked if the HR activity had to do with feelings of stress or anxiety. Petra agreed to both feelings. When asked why there was anxiety, Petra said the following: "I'm still [anxious] because I'm constantly focusing on what I have to say next and how I should recover from a slide, and am I missing something, and what's on the slide, what do I have to say, and how is it going to come out of my mouth?" Petra listed seven points of concern about how the class would better understand her content knowledge. Alexakos then asked for confirmation of his understanding that her anxiety was more about the act of presenting and not about the content itself, to which Petra responded, "No." While the earlier part of the concerns were class participation and interaction with the content delivered in the presentation, in Table 2.6 Petra added that the concerns were as follows: her peers asking questions that could not be answered by the co-presenters; and correction by the professor on the spot.

It is evident in this cogen that Alexakos' teaching had transformed in him becoming more aware of how students felt about being corrected in the classroom. Alexakos did admit that in his teaching he found that students at times took issue with correction from him. Petra added that being corrected by Alexakos was no longer much of a concern. There was clarification that content knowledge was a small part of the concern, and that being understood was a much greater concern. Going into this class session, the class was expecting a group presentation. The three presenters were the collective group presenting to the rest of their class of peers, and those peers and the professor were the outsiders. The mutual focus from the collective was to have a successful presentation by making it as interactive as possible which would contribute to its being clear and understood. The shared mood came across as driven and of excitement to lead an engaged, interactive, and clearly understood presentation. Since this was during the IR, the IR outcomes were unknown. Solidarity

TABLE 2.6 Transcript of Petra detailing why she felt nervous before even speaking

[32:19] Alexakos: So, while you're watching something that went up from 158 to 164, here ... now that I stopped it actually it went up, but before as you were watching this it went from 88 to 91. And as I paused it, it went up to 94 ... 95. So how does it feel? Here, you don't have to wear this anymore (removes oximeter). So how does it feel watching this?
Petra: I'm curious now.
Alexakos: About what?
Petra: How I talk ... It feels weird. I don't watch myself ever. Ever.
Alexakos: Yea it took me a while to get used to myself. Now I just ... Before, when I used to record my class. I used to watch me first ... You have a very good voice.
Petra: I'm glad. It sounds clear in my head. [34:30]
Alexakos: It still stays up though. You're at 148. So even when you're not talking, I guess you're still stressed? (Petra nods yes) You're very anxious?
Petra: Yes I'm still because I'm constantly focusing on what I have to say next and how I should recover from a slide, and am I missing something, and what's on the slide, what do I have to say, and how is it going to come out of my mouth?
Alexakos: And you can see it here. You're between 148 and 150.
Petra: So even when someone else talks, because I know how many slides I have I know I'm still going to be talking. So, it's like ...
Alexakos: So, this is mostly about the presentation not necessarily about the content at this point?
Petra: At this point no. The content comes in ... because this is mostly history. So, I was comfortable presenting the history. The content comes in with African-American and Black. Um. I mean. If it's content, it's just a hint of it because I'm always nervous about if the class would ask me something. If you're going to ask me something and I may not know. (She laughs) Or you tell me, "That's wrong." (She laughs) [36:08]
Alexakos: I used to do that more often. I don't do it as much anymore ... you know? It's always a hard question to balance. I've been scaring people, and ... (Both laugh) ... and correcting people
Petra: (she laughs) Yea.
Alexakos: You know so some of my students may take issue with that. I don't mean ... and it's like okay ... If you do, then what happens?
Petra: I don't mind your comments anymore ...
Alexakos: Yea ... I try not to make them.
Petra: But here, I know I'm focusing on really the PowerPoint and what's on it and try to remember everything I have and just putting it together to ... to speak clearly
Alexakos: To speak?
Petra: Clearly? With ... Less of an accent. [37:03]

was identifiable because Petra spoke on the co-presenters' collective presentation goals. Petra's inner voice, led by anxiety, focused on clarity via preparation and communication and her accent. The weight of communication was heavier for her than the content itself.

3 Seven Anxiety-Ridden Concerns for Petra

The interaction between student presenter and the audience emphasized that the act of presenting is not solely about the student presenter while speaking aloud, but also about the inner voice. During the above cogen, Alexakos invited Petra to recall what was happening during her presentation and why this was happening. Upon seeing her HR increasing, Petra was alarmed. When asked about her experience of seeing her HR increasing, Petra responded that seeing high numbers was unexpected. When asked if there was any nervousness during the presentation, Petra agreed. Petra recalled what was happening while Laura was talking about tools. While Petra mentioned that there was a bit of self-consciousness about her English-speaking abilities, there was also concern about what would be said next, recovery methods should a mistake be made, doubtfulness of being fully prepared, what was on each slide, what to say, and how to actually form the words necessary to be understood.

> *Corinna: Being anxious neither takes away from nor adds to how passionate you are about the content you are discussing or trying to discuss. Passion, after all, can underpin feelings of either excitement or anger.*

The questions Petra asked herself are listed as categories in Table 2.7. The weight of each can vary as Petra did clarify that the concern was more about how to better communicate her points than her content knowledge. Each concern was categorized as an interaction skill. Interaction skills attempt to deal with academic tasks that take place in a learning environment, like presentations. Alexakos asked Petra if the anxiety was related to preparedness or about talking to the class. Preparedness represents content knowledge based on research and preparation of slides, and communication represents how the content knowledge will be shared with the people in the learning environment.

In Table 2.7, I highlight which points focused on preparedness on the content of the presentation and which focused on clearly communicating the knowledge to her peers.

> *Corinna: Looking at Petra's questions, I see it as possible fear of failure, more specifically of being misunderstood. I think when I presented I was*

TABLE 2.7 Seven points Petra was anxious about during 60 seconds

Points of concern during presentation	Interaction skill	Tense
How will my English-speaking skills be interpreted? (accent)	Communication	Future (frontstage)
What do I say next?	Communication	Future (frontstage)
How do I recover if I make a mistake?	Communication	Future (frontstage)
Am I prepared?	Preparedness	Past (backstage)
What is on each slide?	Preparedness	Past (backstage)
What should I say?	Communication	Current
What are the necessary words to say for me to be understood?	Communication	Current

> *afraid of failure, period. Since I knew I was being graded after all. I understand Petra's point in being sure of the content. I never stopped to disseminate what it was about the presentation that bothered me so much. I much prefer just exchanging my thoughts with one person at a time rather than a group of people at a time, especially if I am still at a point where I am still learning it.*

Petra worked with her group to not only share information, but to have the class interact and openly share their thoughts on the content in a scholarly capacity. Any point that addressed her having to speak to the class was classified as communication, while anything that was based on recall was classified as preparedness. Petra was, as stated in Table 2.6, more concerned with her delivery. In her case, there was a lack of confidence about how good her English was. Petra thought her accent would be too strong.

Expanding on Collins' IR theory I have added Tenses in Table 2.7; IR theory entails bringing in prior experiences of EE with interactions into the next experience. Since Petra's worry was about her accent, her awareness that English is not her first language impacted the delivery of her content knowledge. This is highlighted as *Future tense,* as Petra had yet to speak. Past speaking experiences caused her to anticipate being unclear and misunderstood. There was also mention of uncertainty about which terminology to use, as parts of the conversation included race: "Black" or "African-American."

Petra anticipated the potential reaction of her class to her content, as she planned how to transition from one point to the next, rendering this point also in the *Future tense*. Recovery from making a mistake is also *future tense,* as being unclear was an anticipation. Preparation here was about being ready to correct any misunderstandings. This is over-preparation, because being misunderstood is not something that can be calculated. Anxiety is great worry as to the possibility of failure (Frazzetto, 2014). It is important to highlight here that while there was no likelihood of her making a mistake, given that Petra was confident of her content knowledge, there was still preparation for recovering from mistakes before even speaking, and the possibility of being corrected by the professor. In the cogen with the professor, Petra mentioned being corrected by the professor and being no longer anxious about that possibility, which reinforces the IR characteristics of bringing in prior experiences and the emotions that came from these into the next.

The next two points are about preparedness, addressing readiness and recall. Readiness to present with technology (i.e., PowerPoint slides, Prezi, Posters, note cards, etc.) that helps us, necessitates that work be done beforehand. Recall, on the day of the presentation, has to do with remembering the points needed to be made that are connected with what has been gathered together for the presentation. Since both readiness and recall require prep work and research before the day of the presentation, both are categorized under *past tense* as Petra and the co-presenters had to have both done by presentation time. When preparing to say or do something, a quick mental check for readiness may occur. Petra went even further, asking herself how well each slide was stored in her memory.

Petra was concerned about what to say, which is labeled as *current tense*. Petra wanted to start putting her words together now before speaking, which leads to her final point of what words to use. The final point is also identified as *current tense*, as the majority of the concerns were about being understood, and being able to express her main points to the class clearly and correctly.

Tenses and *Interaction Skills* are used to categorize Petra's concerns on how to complete a task assigned to her in a learning environment. Navigating how to co-present on a difficult topic such as gender and including talking about race in a way that would bring about dialogue in the classroom is stressful. Petra mentioned during the cogen that Paula wanted to revisit, or clarify, a point that was misunderstood before Petra's turn. There is a possibility that Paula's need to clarify a point may have added to Petra's anxiety, justified her being anxious, or caused the anxiety Petra experienced. In either case, the co-presenters collectively attempted to present in a way that would goad their peers into joining the conversation. Petra wanted to maintain the goal of her co-presenting group. The moment right before starting the presentation is a moment where there is potentially an influx of emotions or, as some people may express it, "the moment of truth." This significant event revealed a pivotal moment in an interaction, which is lacking in research on teaching | learning.

Presentations are common in the classroom, both individual and group assigned, and definitely understood by many who have been in classrooms before as either teacher or student. The emotional outcome that Petra would be looking for in this IR would be that the presentation went really well, as stated in the cogen. Success would equate with being understood by her own standards. There were two extremes also as defined by her group, that the IR would either be a positive or a negative experience. Petra wanted to give herself the opportunity to ensure a positive emotional experience, so the thoughts caused doubt and uneasiness, which is why at the start of her portion of the presentation there was stress and anxiety. To suppress her stress and anxiety, the seven points of concern offered a mental check that would ensure a successful presentation experience for her. Two of her points could not be changed on the day of the presentation and they were labeled in the *Past tense.* The remaining were aspects that would be dealt with during the presentation that would positively impact the IR, as it depended on her communication with the class and clarity. Her concern in the latter was her language accent as a non-native English speaker and about using the right words. Language was a concern and there was a distinction made between the concerns about sounding clear in your own thoughts versus being uncertain of how you sound to others.

> *Corinna: I concur, I sound amazing in my own thoughts as well. Plus, I know what I mean to get across and the intentionality behind how I structure my sentences.*

With the *current tense*, Petra was focused on how to begin her presentation. Just like first impressions are important, what's said at the start and end of a presentation are important. The *future tense,* would be how to progress and transition through her points. Anxiety is focused on both the *current tense* and the *future tense* as the apprehension is built by anticipation and worry of her communicating the content. Also, she would have deepened her sense of anxiety had she felt unprepared.

3.1 *Preparedness versus Being Understood*

The mere awareness that the moment to present was just a few seconds away triggered Petra to become anxious and immediately concern herself with how to express herself clearly and finish her presentation feeling understood by her peers and teacher. Her seven questions are broken into three main concerns

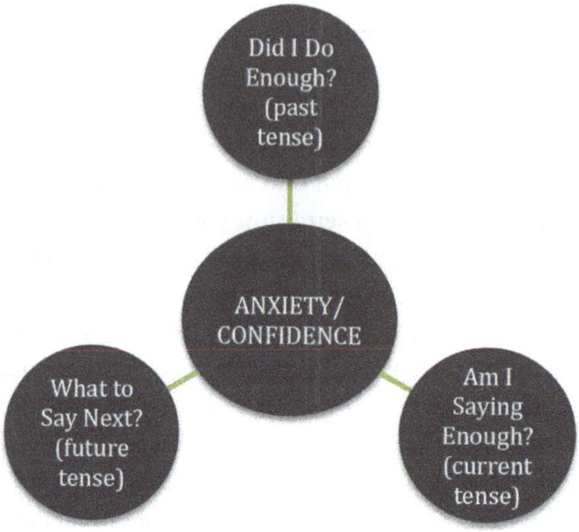

FIGURE 2.2
Emotion in IR

that can either lead any student presenter to feeling anxious or confident (Figure 2.2).

The main ideas from the tenses are placed in three categories, in Figure 2.2, with regard to the following three questions: Did I do enough; Am I saying enough now; and What to say next? *Past tense* is what cannot change, *current tense* is what can be said now to prevent any misunderstandings, and *future tense* is recovering and clarifying based on the anticipation of failure or messing up our point. In the moment, there was concern on whether enough would be said and what to say next, even though the co-presenters felt prepared. Speaking to her peers and to the professor clearly was more of a concern for Petra, to the point of anxiousness, or nervousness. Worries about what to say next, how to recover from a slide, what to do if we miss something, remembering what's on the slide, what to say, and what actually comes out was all Petra was thinking about in the minute leading up to her own presentation, as detailed during the cogen. Due to changes in her HR being statistically significant ($p < 0.01$) during this event, this emotional experience that Petra had is evidence that emotions and HR do have a dialectical relationship to one another. There are many who have gone through what Petra has gone through before presenting in the class, myself included. If I had looked at the oximeter readings alone, I would not have known that the experience had no audible verbal interaction on her part. The fact that Petra was just standing there in front of the room with two other presenters just waiting for her turn to present was remarkable and unexpected for me. The interaction Petra had during this event was with herself before starting her part in the presentation to the rest of the class. While Laura was speaking, her HR was already increasing as her emotions and inner voice were engaged in an anxious exchange, or dialogue. That engagement between herself and her inner thoughts may have been a way of coping to reassure herself that Petra did and can in fact address those seven points of concern. The influx of emotion that occurred before doing an assigned task such as presentation points out that there is something that occurs between the backstage and frontstage within an interaction.

Reflecting on the evidence found in Petra's case and relating to her experience as a shy person myself, at first, I tended to think of her experience while waiting to present as solely what a few unlucky students feel. I did not think of the act of being nervous while presenting as a phenomenon to look more closely at, because I personally know of others who enjoy presenting and feel they never get nervous. However, Petra learned about her clarity in speaking to others because of the cogen. Wearing an oximeter helped, because seeing her HR rising during the playback of the presentation brought awareness. The three points, "Did I Say Enough," "Am I Saying Enough," and "What to Say Next" can be talking points in the classroom for grades of any level before presenting, to build a stronger collective effervescence to transform anxiety into confidence when it comes to sharing knowledge and learning in the classroom, impacting both teaching and learning. Also, attaching weights to it would individualize the experience for each student. "Am I Saying Enough" and "What to Say Next" can be emotional, and these are in the moment circumstances in communication and interaction. While as teachers we may discuss presentations with regard to presenting skills and stress preparation, it may not be at the forefront as an issue to allow discussions in perhaps all classrooms. Through this investigation I hope to bring about more discussions on anxiety experiences in the classroom, even if it needs to begin with oximeters in the classroom, video recordings, and cogens.

References

Alexakos, K. (2015). *Being a teacher|researcher: A primer on doing authentic inquiry research on teaching and learning*. Springer.

Alexakos, K., Pride, L. D., Amat, A., Tsetsakos, P., Lee, K. J., Paylor-Smith, C., Zapata, C., Wright, S., & Smith, T. (2016). Mindfulness and discussing "thorny" issues in the classroom. *Cultural Studies of Science Education, 11*, 741–769. https://doi.org/10.1007/s11422-015-9718-0

Bakhtin, M. M., Voloshinov, V. N., Medvedev, P. N., & Morris, P. (1994). *The Bakhtin reader: Selected writings of Bakhtin, Medvedev, and Voloshinov*. E. Arnold.

Bayne, G. U. (2007). *Identity, culture and shared experiences: The power of cogenerative dialogues in urban science classrooms.* CUNY Graduate Center Retrospective Dissertations and Capstones. https://library-gc-cuny-edu.central.ezproxy.cuny.edu/legacy/items/show/3859

Bayne, G. U. (2012). Capturing essential understandings of the urban science learning environment. *Learning Environments Research, 15*(2), 231–250.

Bernardi, L., Wdowczyk-Szulc, J., Valenti, C., Castoldi, S., Passino, C., Spadacini, G., & Sleight, P. (2000). Effects of controlled breathing, mental activity and mental stress with or without verbalization on heart rate variability. *Journal of the American College of Cardiology, 35*(6), 1462–1469.

Calderón, O. (2014). *Transformative science education through action research and self-study practices* [PhD dissertation]. CUNY. http://works.gc.cuny.edu/etd/22

Calderón, O. (2016). Oximetry: A reflective tool for the detection of physiological expression of emotions in a science education classroom. *Cultural Studies of Science Education, 11*(3), 653–667.

Collins, R. (2004). *Interaction ritual chains.* Princeton University Press.

Ekman, P. (2007). *Emotions revealed: Recognizing faces and feelings to improve communication and emotional life.* Macmillan.

Ekman, P., & Friesen, W. V. (2003). *Unmasking the face: A guide to recognizing emotions from facial clues.* ISHK.

Frazzetto, G. (2014). *Joy, guilt, anger, love: What neuroscience can—and can't—tell us about how we feel.* Penguin.

Hermans, H. J., & Kempen, H. J. (1993). *The dialogical self: Meaning as movement.* Academic Press.

Roth, W. M., & Tobin, K. (2001). Learning to teach science as practice. *Teaching and Teacher Education, 17*, 741–762.

Roth, W. M., Tobin, K., Zimmermann, A., Bryant, N., & Davis, C. (2002). Lessons on and from the dihybrid cross: An activity–theoretical study of learning in coteaching. *Journal of Research in Science Teaching, 39*(3), 253–282.

Sewell, W. H., Jr. (2005). *Logics of history: Social theory and social transformation.* University of Chicago Press.

Tobin, K. (2006). Learning to teach through coteaching and cogenerative dialogue. *Teaching Education, 17*(2), 133–142.

Tobin, K. (2014). Using collaborative inquiry to better understand teaching and learning. In J. L. Bencze & S. Alsop (Eds.), *Activist science & technology education* (pp. 127–147). Springer. https://doi.org/10.1007/978-94-007-4360-1_8

Tobin, K. (2015). The sociocultural turn in science education and its transformative potential. In C. Milne, K. Tobin, & D. deGennaro (Eds.), *Sociocultural studies and implications for science education* (pp. 3–31). Springer. https://doi.org/10.1007/978-94-007-4240-6

Tobin, K., King, D., Henderson, S., Bellocchi, A., & Ritchie, S. M. (2016). Expression of emotions and physiological changes during teaching. *Cultural Studies of Science Education, 11*(3), 669–692.

Tobin, K., & Ritchie, S. M. (2012). Multi-method, multi-theoretical, research in the learning sciences multi-level. *Asia-Pacific Education Researcher, 21*(1), 117–129.

Tobin, K., Roth, W. M., & Zimmermann, A. (2001). Learning to teach science in urban schools. *Journal of Research in Science Teaching, 38*(8), 941–964.

Turner, J. H. (2009). The sociology of emotions: Basic theoretical arguments. *Emotion Review, 1*(4), 340–354. https://doi.org/10.1177/1754073909338305

Van Maanen, J. (2011). *Tales of the field: On writing ethnography*. University of Chicago Press.

CHAPTER 3

Ameliorating Disillusions

Navigating Stress Emotions in Teacher Education

Shequana Wright-Chung

Abstract

A beginning teacher's emotional experiences in the classroom can be negatively influenced by a sense of disillusionment and stress. Therefore, it is pivotal for individuals to become more aware of and explore how experiences and beliefs influence the emotions and emotional responses in teaching and learning environments. I employ authentic inquiry to frame the experience, interactions, interpretations, emotions, interests and curiosity of a teacher-educator | researcher and groups of preservice teachers. More specifically, I apply responses from heuristics, free-writes and class discussions to make meaning of emotions and emotional responses while teaching and learning with preservice teachers in my courses. In using authentic inquiry, I explore how the historical origins of positivism and standardization in schools have impacted emotional experiences in teaching and learning environments. Through this research, I have learned of strategies for uncovering the hidden positivistic structures that are often times embedded in the school system.

Keywords

authentic inquiry – disillusionment – stress emotions – free-writes– heuristics – positivism

1 Stress and Emotions

Every emotion exists in response to a complex combination of factors in the social and physical environments. The experiencing of fear, anger, guilt and anxiety can promote actionable changes in practices when they are identified and navigated (Frazzetto, 2014). Consequently, beginning teachers may experience emotions such as fear, anxiety, guilt and anger without receiving

 | DOI:10.1163/9789004527348_003

any preparation or support with exploring and managing these emotions. Emotions such as fear, anxiety, guilt and anger may lead to stress as teachers become stuck on these emotions and struggle with ways to navigate them. Stress impacts a teacher's mental, physical and emotional responses to the demands of teaching and learning (Kyriacou, 2001).

Tobin and research colleagues' adaptation of Stephen Porges (2011) ideas on polyvagal theory (PVT) suggest that the nervous system evaluates risk of social interactions by processing information in the environment using the senses (Tobin et al., 2016). When an environment is perceived as physically or mentally not safe, a fight-flight mode can occur. Within this flight or fight mode a teacher might respond to stress emotions by either attacking or retreating. Both responses may not be conducive to a productive teaching and learning environment due to the impact they have on a teacher's tone of voice, breathing patterns and facial expressions (Tobin et al., 2016). Therefore, a heightened awareness of how the experiencing of emotions can affect the physiological and mental states of all individuals in a teaching and learning environment and investigating strategies for not becoming stuck on emotions are pivotal.

2 Teachers' Stress Factors

There are many factors attributed to teachers' stress levels. According to the American Federation of Teachers (AFT) Quality of Work Life Survey (2015), 73% of teachers reported that they often find their work stressful. Significant factors of workplace stress were connected to the overall school climate and included excessive workloads, lack of support, constant changes at work, role uncertainty and lack of control, respectively. Additionally, teacher attrition rates have been linked to the measuring of teacher quality based on how well students perform on high stakes standardized tests (Ryan et al., 2017). Working in such high-stakes environments with little to no preparation or support can lead teachers to experience stress that stems from emotions such as fear, anxiety, guilt and anger (Roeser, 2013). More specifically, teachers may develop stress when they struggle with ameliorating and navigating emotions, they are experiencing due to workplace pressures and lack of control over their practices.

Experiencing stress emotions, as well as all other emotions, influence how teachers interact in teaching and learning experiences. However, there is little emphasis on the exploration of preservice teachers' emotional responses in teacher education courses. Leigh McLean, Tashia Abry, Michelle Taylor, Manuella Jimenez and Kristen Granger (2017) assert that the mental health of preservice teachers should be explored in efforts of helping them navigate and ameliorate some of the emotional struggles they may face as they enter the classroom. They associate a teacher's mental health to how they coped with experiencing stress emotions (McLean et al., 2017).

3 Disillusionment

A sense of disillusionment may emerge as teachers realize that the reward of personal satisfaction and sense of accomplishment promised by the media and many teacher-education courses, are in conflict with the increasing workload pressures and stress they are actually experiencing (Alexakos, 2015). The extensive time commitment, developmentally inappropriate expectations and realizations that a teacher is not in control of her own classroom and classroom practices, also contributes to the stress and disillusionment many new teachers experience.

During my experience as a preservice teacher, there was minimal focus on how emotions and emotional responses impacted the teaching and learning environment. Even when emotions were discussed, it was focused on how preservice teachers can express empathy and compassion to students without contextualizing and exploring the emotions that teachers may face in response to work related pressures. However, as preservice teachers become teachers in their own classrooms, preconceived beliefs and expectations may come into conflict with what they actually experience (Zembylas, 2013). These conflicts can lead to experiencing and expressing stress emotions that negatively impact the teaching and learning environment. Therefore, my research focus is on strategies for ameliorating some of the conflicts between what preservice teachers learn in their teacher education programs and the emotions they may experience as they enter the classroom.

4 Exploring Various Emotions through the Use of Heuristics and Free-Writes

As a teacher-educator and beginning researcher, I believe that it is important to encourage the critical exploration of emotions preservice teachers may experience as they enter the classroom. Moreover, in the teacher education courses that I teach, I collaborate with teachers to actively develop possible strategies they can use to make meaning of, navigate and ameliorate emotions that may negatively impact them and their students' physical and mental wellness.

Additionally, I used free-writes and heuristics as tools to make sense of my past and present emotional experiences and promote change in practice.

One tool that I introduce preservice teachers to are heuristics. Heuristics are tools that encourage teachers to explore, focus and raise awareness of characteristics teacher | researchers are interested in investigating or would like students to reflect on. Heuristics also provide ideas on how to change when and if change is desirable (Alexakos, 2015). The characteristics of a heuristic encourage teachers to become aware of emotions they experience as they interact in teaching and learning spaces. Through this awareness, teachers are transformed even if they do not actively explore this awareness in the moment (Alexakos, 2015). Additionally, heuristics are also used as a 'group symbol of solidarity' that is iterated over time (Turner & Stets, 2006). Each time the heuristic is introduced, preservice teachers are encouraged to make meaning of the characteristics and challenge ideas based on their own emotional experiences within society.

Free-writes and class discussions about characteristics on the heuristics were also used as tools to support teachers with expressing and making meaning of the many emotions they experienced as they interacted in teaching and learning environments. In this research, individuals spent ten to fifteen minutes at the beginning of class, freely writing down their ideas about characteristics on the heuristic. More specifically, in both the Spring 2015 and Spring 2016 semesters, teachers were encouraged to free-write about characteristics that were salient to their practices and why. After analyzing preservice teachers' responses, identified patterns and/or contradictions were highlighted as prompts for further class discussions and follow-up free-writes during subsequent weeks in the courses.

5 Flow of This Research

In this section, I describe the shifts I have made in my teaching and learning practices in regard to the exploration of emotional experiences. First, a free-write was shared and analyzed to illuminate how my experiences as an elementary school teacher influenced my interest in exploring teacher emotions. The free-write also illuminated my growth in exploring and making meaning of my emotions as I taught and learned with preservice teachers in my courses. Second, a description of my approach to critically exploring emotions is described to provide a context to my research. Third, an investigation into the historical aspects of positivism and the affects it has on the exploration of emotions in teaching and learning is highlighted. I also discuss how positivism is embedded in many of the standardized approaches that are present in teacher education programs.

Below is a free-write that I wrote on July 17, 2017. This free-write was based on my remembering the emotions I experienced as a teacher in the elementary school system. I share this free-write to preface the importance of engaging in a type of research that acknowledges the emotional experiences teachers may face as they teach and learn with their students and work within a school system. The emotional understandings I developed through my interactions with preservice teachers, advisors, research squad members and theoretical frameworks I have studied during my research are embedded in how I remember and make meaning of my previous experiences as an elementary school teacher. I highlighted the emotional responses, fear, anxiety, anger and guilt to emphasize how contextualizing these seemingly negative emotions led me to actively explore emotions with preservice teachers in my research. Concomitantly, I acknowledged the importance of not becoming stuck on these emotions. Becoming stuck on these emotions can negatively impact the physical and mental wellbeing of teachers, students and the teaching and learning environment (Tobin & Llena, 2014).

5.1 *Free-Write (July 17, 2017)*

The last five years of my profession as a teacher, teacher-educator, doctoral candidate and beginning researcher has been a journey into becoming more aware of the emotions I experienced as I interacted with others in teaching and learning spaces. The term 'journey' is used to emphasize the progression of my emotional understanding as I began to acknowledge and make meaning of many emotions that I had often learned to suppress.

As a teacher in the elementary school classroom, I realize that teaching and learning during initiatives, like the *No Child Left Behind Act* and the introduction of the *Common Core Standards* made me feel like I was part of a mass production. Within this mass production, emotions such as fear, anxiety, guilt and anger were present because I felt like I was not in control of my classroom practices. Instead, I was continuously reproducing large amounts of standardized products that were based on the interests and goals of those with power over the educational system. In order to deal with the emotions being experienced, I often times internalized the standardized ways of knowing, leading me to place value on cognition and disregard my own emotions and the emotions of my students.

The emotional struggles that I experienced as a beginning teacher in the elementary school classroom were not discussed in my teacher preparation courses. During my undergraduate and graduate studies in childhood education, most courses were focused on helping teachers develop an understanding of the content and providing strategies for how to teach the content to young students. I had one course that acknowledged some of the political structures that were embedded in the New York City school system, but I do not remember discussing how teachers would emotionally respond to or navigate these structures.

Student teaching was focused on planning and implementing lessons and managing paperwork and behaviors in the classroom. My supervising teacher's responsibilities were to model and provide strategies for effective teaching and classroom management. Teaching strategies included preparation of instructional materials and development of bulletin boards, supervising students as they work independently or in small groups, evaluating student work and writing feedback to students on next steps, and reflections on how successful the teaching strategies were and what I could do to improve them. My field work supervisor observed lessons I planned four times for the semester. Components of the observation were similar to the teaching strategies that the teacher modeled. During my student teaching I appreciated all of the teaching and classroom management strategies, I developed from my student teacher. However, there were many internal aspects, such as stress emotions in response to implementing the learned strategies that were not discussed. As I entered my own classroom in a different community from my student teacher placement, I began to struggle with stress emotions. Since navigating emotions in teaching and learning were not discussed as part of my teacher education preparation or student teacher experiences, I decided to explore my own strategies for navigating these emotions based on my emotional responses in my everyday life.

As a new untenured elementary school teacher, I experienced fear because I felt like I had no power or agency to focus on what I valued in my classroom practice. More specifically, even though my values were focused on acknowledging the different types of knowledge students brought to the classroom, I was fearful that if they did not do well on city- and statewide reading and math assessments my teacher evaluations would be negatively impacted.

My fear led to anxiety based on the experiences I observed from colleagues. I observed many teachers with years of experience, struggling to keep up with all of the political changes and mandates in education. Teachers who were once my mentors were now being rated as ineffective and their ideas devalued due to changes in citywide expectations. I also knew that an underlying reason for rating these experienced teachers ineffective was that their individual salaries would pay the salaries of two or more new teachers. Observing their experiences made me anxious about my future in teaching within a system where one year I would be meeting all expectations and my ideas were valued and the next year I would be seen as ineffective. Therefore, for the first few years of my teaching career, I attempted to remove my values from teaching in efforts to ameliorate my fear or anxieties. I believed that if I followed what was expected without challenging any of the ideas suggested by administrators or policy makers, I would survive teaching.

From my experiences as a student, a focus on emotions and emotional responses were viewed as a disturbance in the teaching and learning environment. Students or teachers who struggled with managing their emotions were either removed from the classroom or had to seek some sort of therapy or counseling. As a beginning teacher, I did not want to be ostracized for not being able to manage my emotions. Therefore, I attempted to not acknowledge or make meaning of the emotions I was experiencing and became a conformist with a focus on raising assessment scores. I believed that if I could detach myself from making emotional connections to what was happening in my classroom and the school, I could avoid addressing the emotions toward inequities that were present. However, trying to become emotionally detached did not work. My emotions were bottled up inside, and many times I would experience moments of anger or guilt toward myself and others.

There were times when I experienced guilt because I knew a focus on test scores was not benefiting my students. Students demonstrated a variety of ways of knowing and making sense of the world in the classroom and focusing on only a specific type of test did not privilege students' understandings and interests. Sometimes my kindergarten students would state: "We have to take another test again. I did not even get to play." I would respond to students by saying "after we take this test you can play," even though often times that was not true. My second and third grade students would ask me how they could use what they were learning in real life and I would struggle with giving them an answer.

Sometimes my guilt subsided when I was busy with the everyday routines of teaching. But during my quiet reflections, the feeling of guilt would rush through my body. Experiencing guilt caused me to become angry with myself for not privileging the many ways that students made sense of their world and disregarding the social and emotional needs that were present.

I experienced anger toward myself, administrators and the educational system as a whole. I experienced anger toward administrators because I believed that they were aware of struggles teachers were facing in and out of the classroom, but still demanded more from us. Anger was experienced toward the educational system because I believed that just as teachers were pressured by administrators to produce more, the educational system also pressured administrators to get more from their teachers and students without addressing the challenges that were present. I experienced anger toward myself for not having the power and courage to explore the variety of experiences students were facing in and out of the classroom, such as gang violence in their neighborhoods, abusive homes, malnutrition and going along with ideas that I did not value.

In 2012, my anger and guilt influenced thoughts of leaving the teaching profession. Even though I loved working with my students I felt like I was unable to make a change. After opening up to colleagues about the emotions I was experiencing, in 2013 I was encouraged to transfer to another elementary school. This school was a new school with untenured administrators. At first, the administrators encouraged me to incorporate my ideas and the ideas of my kindergarten students into teaching and learning practices. I had time to explore the emotional responses. However, when the third through fifth grade test scores came back below average at the end of the 2013–2014 school year, the administrators became more involved with raising test scores than encouraging creativity. During the 2014 school year, increasing test scores became a focus for the entire school, grades prekindergarten through five.

My emotional response of anger and guilt was more intense during the 2014 school year because I had experienced having my ideas valued during the previous year. I experienced students entering the classroom, sharing their ideas, smiling and laughing. Now my values and control over my classroom practices were once again being silenced due to test scores that were influenced by so many external factors. As the administrators began to focus on test scores, each teacher was micromanaged. Each morning, all teachers had to display and follow a predetermined schedule with the objectives for each component of the day. At different times of the day, one of the administrators would check to see if teachers were on the task that was displayed on the schedule. This left little to no time for students and me to explore any emotions that emerged in the classroom. Having little to no time to explore emotions led to more fights between students in the classroom and more frustration for me as the teacher because I knew that if students and I explored the emotions they were experiencing beforehand, it would not escalate to fights inside or outside of the classroom. I once again struggled with what I should do in response to the anger and frustration that I was experiencing in the classroom.

It was through my experiences as a second-year doctoral candidate in 2014 that I began to reevaluate how I made meaning of the emotions experienced in teaching and learning spaces. More specifically, I began to realize that I could not detach myself from my emotional experiences, but I should not become stuck on them either. When I was first introduced to a mindfulness heuristic, I started to reflect on what was happening in my classroom and why in a whole new way. The use of heuristics provided a framework for me to investigate the underlying causes of the emotions I was experiencing, and

I developed strategies for making changes in my practices based on the emotions I was experiencing. In 2012, when I reflected on my emotions, I viewed emotional responses such as anger, guilt, and fear as negative emotions that should be avoided and struggled with, while navigating these emotions when they emerged. However, as I began my work with heuristics in 2014, I started to develop a different understanding of the underlying causes of my emotional experiences and realized that experiencing these emotions can lead to active changes that promote the mental and physical wellness of myself and others.

Based on my experiences with using heuristics, I was better prepared to navigate the anger, guilt and frustration I experienced in the kindergarten classroom during the 2014 school year. I focused on exploring how my emotions influenced the emotions of my students and vice versa. I decided to take time throughout each day to actively explore emotions and emotional responses of my students and me. As children entered the classroom, I incorporated discussing our emotions as a part of the morning routine. To promote my own emotional wellness, I investigated the underlying causes of the stress emotions I was experiencing. I realized that not being encouraged to incorporate my ideas and the excessive testing of kindergarten students really impacted my emotional experiences as I interact with others in the classroom and school. I then thought of strategies that would help me ameliorate some of the stress emotions I experienced during the morning session of the day. One strategy included meeting with colleagues/ friends during lunch, rather than remaining in the classroom to grade papers or display bulletin boards. Another strategy I used was walking at least two laps around the nearby park while listening to my favorite type of music. Sharing stories, laughing with friends, and walking helped to ameliorate some of the emotions I experienced and rejuvenated me as I entered the classroom for the afternoon session of the day.

Since I noticed the emotions of my students changed from before to after lunch, during the afternoon session of the day I decided to take ten to fifteen minutes each day to turn off the classroom lights and invite students to sit with me or a friend and discuss the emotions they were experiencing and why, read a book, draw a picture or relax their bodies and listen to music. Engaging in the exploration of emotion during these components of the day, influenced how students and I responded to each other and ourselves. We began to become aware of the emotions of the other and often time changed our actions to benefit the overall mood of the class. Teaching the content also became less frustrating because students and I had an emotional understanding and shared our ideas throughout the learning process.

In 2014, I shifted careers from a classroom teacher to instructional coach. I chose to shift careers because I wanted the opportunity to share my experiences with other teachers who may be struggling with navigating their experiences as they interacted in the classroom. Teaching, learning, emotions and cognition are four interrelated constructs that cannot be separated. My emotional journey had become an intentional lifestyle of acknowledging and exploring different aspects of emotions as I formulated relationships within myself, with others and within the world.

6 Critically Examining Stress Emotions Illuminated in My Free-Write

Guiding my research is the belief in the importance of contextualizing emotions in preservice teacher education courses. Contextualizing emotions support how teachers navigate the many emotions they may experience as they enter the classroom. Making meaning of the emotions I experienced as an elementary school teacher, helped me to realize that when stress emotions such as fear, anger, guilt and anxiety are explored and contextualized, they can promote actionable changes in practice. Experiencing fear, anxiety, guilt and anger can be helpful because it sharpens a teacher's senses and prepares the body and mind for navigating potential life-threatening situations (Frazzetto, 2014). Heightened senses can lead teachers to become more aware of structures that might be negatively impacting the teaching and learning environment. However, without support and encouragement in exploring these emotions, teachers may become stuck and not understand how they can use these experiences to promote changes in practice (Powietrzyńska & Gangji, 2016).

Although stress emotions can promote actionable changes, remaining stuck on these emotions can be damaging to a teacher's mental and physical wellbeing. Experiencing stress emotions increases the heart rate and decreases oxygen levels, leading to physiological responses that may negatively impact the teaching and learning environment (Tobin et al., 2017).

From a neurological lens, Richard Davidson (2012) suggest that it is more difficult to access parts of the brain that promote clear communication when stress is overwhelming the mind and the body. Tobin and his collaborators in NYC and Australia, have also engaged in many studies that emphasize how a teacher's emotions can affect their tone of voice, body language, heart rate, facial expressions and overall emotional climate of a teaching and learning space. For example, as Tobin et al. (2013) collaboratively reported what they learned from studies with a high school teacher named Vicki, it was shown that a teacher's pulse rate is an indicator of changes in the power of the voice. When teachers resort to using a high pitch tone of voice as a means of communicating with students in the classroom, productive teaching and learning experiences cannot continue. The tone of voice also connects to the orientation of the head and the body. In the study with Vicki the orientation of her head and body were resonant structures for creating stress emotions, such as frustration.

In another study with Reynaldo Llena, Tobin (2014) reported emotional stress can weaken the immune system and lead to long term health effects. In each study teachers navigated their stress emotions by resisting to collaboratively work with their students. Instead they resorted to controlling the lesson and feeding their students information. Increased disparities between teacher and students may lead to intense emotions lasting for long periods of times. Kenneth Tobin, Stephen Ritchie, Jennifer Oakley, Victoria Mergard and Peter Hudson (2013) quote Jay Lemke (1990) in highlighting Reynaldo and Vicki's interactions as initiate-respond-evaluate patterns of teaching that are similar to what is seen in teacher education programs today. In these instances, a teacher asks a question, a student answers the question and the teacher evaluates the answer to the question. Consequently, when teachers enter their own classrooms the emphasis on maintaining control over students is enacted as they work in a system of accountability models and assessment (Tobin et al., 2013). In many teacher-education programs, the importance of teachers establishing and maintaining control over their students' cognitive and emotional abilities is constantly emphasized, without discussing the health effects that follow. As a teacher-educator and mentor, I push for contextualizing and critically exploring the underlying causes of why a teacher might be experiencing stress emotions and develop possible strategies for supporting teachers as they actively enact changes in practices if necessary.

7 Emotion Rules: Decontextualizing Emotions in Preservice Teacher-Education

When isolated from a context, stress emotions are often viewed and standardized from a negative perspective based on emotion rules. Teachers can experience stress emotions on a daily basis and manage these emotions based on the emotion rules aligned with the teaching profession (Hoschild, 1979). Emotions rules are based on how teachers should react to the other, without acknowledging the interrelationship between the self and the other in an interaction (Zembylas, 2002). In many helping professions such as teaching, employees may present themselves in strategic ways to express the emotions that are dictated by emotion rules (Turner & Stets, 2006a). In Arlie Hoschild's (2003) book, *The Managed Heart*, she describes how flight attendants were trained on how to emotionally respond to passengers. Yet there was a disconnect when flight attendants worked in the field. They were exposed to strategies for expressing emotions such as empathy to others, without a focus on how the others' emotions affect their own emotion. This is similar to the disillusionment between the emotions and emotion rules that many preservice teachers experience. Teachers discuss strategies for showing compassion and are responsive to the needs of their students without contextualizing their own emotional experiences in the classroom based on the workload pressures that are existent. Jonathon Turner and Jan Stets (2006a) include Susan Shott's (1979) theory to further discuss the emotions experienced when a teacher's identity does not align with emotion rules. Shott's theory closely aligns to the emotional experiences I highlighted in my free-write. According to Shott's theory, the arousal of guilt, shame and embarrassment signals to a teacher that she has deviated from the norm and that she must correct her behavior. The arousal of guilt, shame, etc. is due to social norms that create pressures to establish the appropriateness of an emotion in a particular situation. Shott defines culture as a stagnant force that controls the expression of emotions. However, I believe that cultural practices do not have a uniform meaning across time or people (Sewell, 2005). Tobin (2009) explains that even though there may be shared understandings of symbols within a culture, meanings themselves are ever changing across and within participants. Therefore, teachers have the power to ameliorate unwanted emotions or transform their emotional responses to stressors. However, teachers have to become aware of their emotions and recognize the affects it has on their health and emotional wellbeing. In the next section, I discuss the constant flux of teacher's identity in relation to power, agency and passivity.

8 Emotional Labor and Teacher Burnout

The dichotomy between emotion rules and actually lived experiences can be connected to emotional labor and teacher burnout (Hoschild, 1979). Through the lens of Michel Foucault (1982), emotional labor and teacher burnout persist when teachers struggle with understanding and constructing their emotional responses based on the emotion rules governed by society. When a teacher has power or gains power or authority over her own emotional experiences in the classroom, she experiences satisfaction, confidence and authority (Kemper & Collins, 1990). When teachers blame themselves for the lack or loss of power and agency over how they teach, emotions such as sadness, shame, guilt and depression emerge. When teachers blame administrators or policy makers for their loss of power and agency over how they teach, they become angry and shift into a mode that urges others to recognize their power (Kemper & Collins, 1990). In the two latter instances, teachers may become stuck on emotions that negatively affect their own emotional health and wellbeing as well as the health and wellbeing of their students.

As I reflected on my free-write, I realized that I experienced emotional labor. I tried to enact the strategies that I learned in the teacher education program without contextualizing the emotional experiences that I was facing due to the conflict between what was learned and what was being experienced. Decontextualizing the emotions teachers may experience in the classroom can lead to emotional labor. For example, without trying to understand the underlying causes of their emotions, a teacher might try to manage or hide emotions of anger, anxiety and vulnerability and express empathy, calmness and kindness due to the emotional rules. If a teacher experiences and expresses anger or frustration, they may become stuck on feeling guilty for expressing these emotions. Consequently, many teachers are not provided with strategies or time to reflect on and explore the causes behind stress emotions. Teachers are told how they should act without contextualizing and investigating the individual, school and societal based structures that influence the teaching and learning environment.

9 Theorizing the Underlying Causes of Stress Emotions

In my free-write I highlight stress emotions such as anger, fear, guilt and anxiety. I attribute experiencing these emotions to conflicts between my values and what was expected of me as a teacher. I also attribute these emotions to experiencing a lack of power and agency in my own practice. Michalinos Zembylas (2003) suggests that teachers' identities are constantly changing in a context embedded in power relations, ideology and culture. As Zembylas theorizes the constant flux in teacher identities, he acknowledges that the construction of teacher identity is influenced by emotions and is dependent on power and agency, which are embedded in teaching and learning practices. Questions of what knowledge and whose knowledge is valued emerges as teachers become aware that the standardized way of knowing may not work for them or their students. Therefore, I believe it is important to discuss how power and agency in the classroom influence the emotions preservice teachers may experience as they enter teaching and learning spaces. I do this through exploring the values and emotional experiences preservice teachers have in terms of teaching and learning math, investigating the origins of these values and discussing how they might navigate the emotions they may experience when challenges to these values emerge.

Zembylas (2003) defines power and agency as forming identities and providing the condition of its trajectory. However, I include passivity into this construction because a teacher's identities are constantly interacting with their own identities and identities of others, such as students, colleagues, administrators, policy makers, etc. As teachers form the trajectory of their identities they are also 'becoming like the other by being in with' (Tobin & Roth, 2006). Similarly, to Tobin (2012), I believe that passivity occurs in a dialectical relationship between power and agency and is a necessary ingredient in teaching and learning spaces.

Agency in teaching and learning is goal oriented and intentional. Agency can unfold when teachers become more aware of the emotions being enacted during interactions and consciously make efforts to not get stuck on unwanted emotions. Agency can also unfold as teachers become more aware of the political and social aspects that are embedded in teaching and learning and how it affects their emotional responses. At the same time, even though a teacher may be aware of the emotions being enacted as she engages with others, she may not have complete control over where the interaction may go. Tobin (2012) argues that passivity also affords learning even when there is no goal of learning and when they are unaware of what they learned. As agency and passivity are enacted 'all participants have opportunities to create emotional experiences that are positively valenced and contribute to receptivity to learn and possibly expand agency as well' (Tobin, 2012, p. 5).

The use of heuristics with preservice teachers affords passivity and agency in the exploration of emotions and emotional responses. As preservice teachers and I read the characteristics we enact agency as we choose which are salient to our practice and make changes. Simultaneously, as we read through characteristics we are passively influenced by the other characteristics and may return to them at a later time based on connected experiences. For example, when I first read the mindfulness heuristic in 2014, I did not focus on the characteristics that had to do with breathing patterns. Monitoring breathing patterns was not something that I found important in teaching and learning. However, now as I interact in challenging situations, I have become more aware of my breathing and realize that there is a connection between the emotions I am experiencing, how I respond to these emotions and my breathing patterns.

10 A Critical Approach to Exploring Teachers' Emotions

Throughout my current research, I collaborated with my preservice teachers at Brooklyn College to investigate some of the emotions that are embedded into teaching and learning spaces. During our exploration, preservice teachers and I focused on how our own values were entangled in the interactions we have with children, administrators, parents, societal and political members. We also explored what happens when our values and what was actually happening in the classroom or school do not align with the norm and how that effects our emotional wellness. In this section, I explain my understandings of the role of a teacher-educator | researcher. Additionally, I emphasize the difference between conducting research in my classroom and engaging in teacher | research by sharing a brief summary of my past and present experiences.

I approach this research with preservice teachers as a teacher-educator | researcher. I use the Sheffer stroke (|) to highlight the dialectical relationship between a teacher and researcher (Tobin, 2012). As a researcher, I collaboratively attempt to make meaning of what was happening and why using theory grounded in practice and practice emerging from theory. I use the word collaboratively because as a teacher-educator meaning resides in my interactions with my students, research squad and the environment. The idea of teacher as researcher stems from Stenhouse (1981) and has emerged into a dialectical relationship between the two constructs. Based on my experiences, I described the role of a teacher-educator | researcher as a teacher-educator who collaborates with students, other teachers and researchers to explore critical issues, such as emotions in connection to teaching and learning the content (Tobin, 2014), positivistic views that are embedded in teaching and learning experiences (Kincheloe & Tobin, 2009), gender (Corbett, 2016), race (Alexakos et al., 2016) and power (Zembylas, 2013) that are present and impact everyday teaching and learning experiences.

My description of a teacher-educator | researcher materialized from Alexakos' (2015) work on *Being a Teacher | Researcher*. Alexakos' description includes the works of Stenhouse, Dewey and Cochran-Smith and Lytle and extends their ideas into a critical approach that investigates what constitutes knowledge from a sociocultural lens. Therefore, a teacher-educator | researcher may go beyond investigating why preservice teachers are effective in teaching a content, and collaboratively explore the inequities in the educational system that affects the emotional experiences many teachers face.

Through participating in teacher-educator | research during the Spring 2015 and Spring 2016 semesters at Brooklyn College, I realized that my current research interest was framed from my own experiences as an elementary school teacher and the experiences preservice teachers shared during the course. More specifically, each semester I noticed that teachers' past emotional experiences with teaching and learning mathematics impacted the way they engaged with the content and others in the college classroom. I also noticed that my past experiences with exploring my emotions impacted the way I responded to the preservice teachers. Beginning with a research interest that emerged from my experiences as a teacher expanded the focus of my research and promoted inclusive and collaborative explorations that were salient to the experiences of participants. Additionally, as the research progressed, I saw the benefits of having a more expansive approach that included the experiences of the teacher-educator and preservice teachers and focused on critical issues that impacted the way they interacted in the world.

Exploring critical issues with preservice teachers encouraged them to become more aware of how accountability pressures affect their ability to be creative, build relationships with their students and reflect on their emotions. After exploring emotions in my Spring 2015 semester, math pedagogy course, Cassandra, a preservice teacher wrote:

> Cassandra: We are not artificial machine-based organisms, we're individuals with strengths and weaknesses and I'm speaking not only for the children, this goes for teachers as well. I want to adopt a style of teaching that is free spirited and open minded because I feel education needs more of that. I feel as though, I'm learning about all these philosophers of education like Dewey, Piaget, Montessori, etc. and I agree with them about how "Education is not a preparation for life; education is life itself." (Dewey). Yet there is disconnect with the ideal of education and teaching and the real-world view which includes standards and grades and pressures. Very nervous, and I barely can reconstruct the whole lesson in my head.

Cassandra's reflection connects to some of the struggles I experienced as a beginning teacher. Many of the teaching strategies and theories I learned in teacher education courses made sense in theory, but often times were very difficult to implement in the classroom. Stress emotions would then surface because I was in constant conflict with what was expected and what I learned. Dialectically, what I learned was also separated from my emotional responses. My description of a teacher-educator | researcher materialized from Alexakos' (2015) work on *Being a Teacher | Researcher*. Alexakos' (2015) description includes the works of Stenhouse, Dewey and Cochran-Smith and Lytle and extends their ideas into a critical approach that investigates what constitutes knowledge from a sociocultural lens. Therefore, a teacher-educator | researcher may go beyond investigating why preservice teachers are effective in teaching a content, and collaboratively explore the inequities in the educational system that affects the emotional experiences many teachers face.

Cassandra's reflection also illuminates the importance of empowering teachers to become critical researchers that study, analyze and expose insidious intentions and disconnect theory and practice (Kincheloe & Tobin, 2006). Through exploring and investigating insidious intentions, teachers can begin to think about possible strategies for navigating the emotional responses to challenges they may face in the classroom.

Exploring critical issues, such as emotions, also encourages preservice teachers to become more aware of how their past experiences influence their interactions in teaching and learning spaces. During the Spring 2015 semester, Carol, a preservice teacher, wrote the following as she reflected on a math lesson presentation she conducted at the end of the semester.

> Carol: Usually students will reveal their misunderstandings through their facial expressions. Some may have confusing looks on their face or move around in their seats. In my experience, a lot of teachers did not recognize my facial expressions because I would nod my head and pretend that I understood the material that was taught. I was a passive learner and rarely voiced out when I was confused or facing an obstacle. Therefore, I wanted to help out those who struggled to voice out their misunderstandings. In my culture, encouraging and praising others are rarely seen so I did not develop a sense of encouraging and praising others. As I gained more experience with children, I realized that they need encouragement and praise as a motivation or reward from the adults. The power of affirmation from teachers motivates children to learn eagerly, question without a doubt and feel the classroom as a safe learning environment.

Through exploring past experiences, while suppressing her emotions, Carol began to develop agency and power in changing the emotional experiences her students would receive. Alexakos (2015) suggests as teacher | researchers, we not only need to explore these power relationships but also need to create and develop interventions for more successful, equitable and socially just interactions. The relationship between passivity, agency, power, teaching, learning and emotions interact dialectically within micro-, meso- and macro-interactions that teachers are often times expected to manage. On the micro or classroom level, teachers and students learn about their own and each other's social, emotional and cognitive strengths and areas for growth in order to form relationships between themselves and others that are conducive to teaching and learning. Administration also permeates the micro-level based on formal observations of teachers; implementation of the chosen curriculum for the school and management of the students.

On the meso-level there are many structures that intersect. For example, as teachers learn about children, they also have to learn about the beliefs and expectations families and guardians have for their children and of them as teachers. Community influences and household income of families that live in the neighborhood also play a role in how teachers and children interact in the learning environment. Carol Gestwicki (2015) highlights incidences of drug use, violence, unemployment, and economic hardships some of the families may experience within their communities. As teachers work within these communities, they must find ways to explore and navigate the emotions that families and students enter the classroom with. On the macro level, the resources a school receives based on teacher implementation of the set curriculum and student achievement on standardized tests permeate the teaching and learning environment.

Within all of these levels, the emphasis on understanding the negotiations of teacher self through an exploration of emotions can lead to transformative practices in the self-care and emotional wellbeing of teachers. However, many times teachers' emotions are not explored due to the focus on producing knowledge that aligns with the norm. Therefore, emotional experiences become an insidious thorn that affects the teaching and learning environment but are rarely addressed.

11 Stress Emotions Are Not Explored in Teacher Education Courses

As I investigate why stress emotions are not explored in teacher education courses, I refer to my multiple readings of an article published by Joe Kincheloe and Kenneth Tobin (2009), "The much-exaggerated death of positivism." I reread this article at different points throughout my emotional journey to really develop an understanding of how positivism insidiously influences what is taught in teacher education programs. The insidious influence is clearly defined in this quote. "Positivism is so embedded into Western culture, academia and the world of education in particular that they are often invisible to researchers and those who consume their research" (Kincheloe & Tobin, 2009, p. 514). As a teacher, doctoral candidate, and beginning researcher, I have been the consumer and merchandiser of positivistic structures. More specifically, positivistic structures have been embedded in my education from birth through adulthood. In turn, I have shared these positivistic structures with the students that I interacted with in the classroom and the preservice teachers I had interacted with on the college level.

Through engaging in teacher | research in which I investigate how the world influences emotions and emotional responses, and interactions with Tobin and Alexakos on the hazardous effects of positivism, I have come to understand positivism as an ontological stance that privileges a reality that is separate from the knower. These ideas stem from Aristotle's conceptual framework, who believed that reality must be objective for it to be recognized as true. Truth was only discovered if it could be generalized from proven facts. Aristotle's work highlighted patterns or regularities that existed for people to discover. Once a researcher was able to identify, explain and predict the patterns and organizational principles of reality, then they would be able to generalize it to others. Auguste Comte (1880) elaborated on Aristotle's framework of positivism by claiming that human thought culture developed within three stages.

At the lowest stage of thought, researchers believed in supernatural agencies to explain the realities of the world. In the middle stage, researchers begin to shift from the supernatural and view elements of the lived world as the causes for the patterns that occur within reality. At the highest stage, which was viewed as the positivistic stage, researchers discovered the actual laws of what is happening and why through reason and observation.

Under Comte's positivistic influences, a researcher is fully evolved when they shift away from speculation to certainty and precision like the discrete answers found in mathematics. Even today, a core principle embedded in the mathematics common core standards for grades pre-kindergarten through twelve is 'attend to precision'. On the other hand, Comte viewed sociology, or the study of human interactions, as a most difficult subject to apply positivistic views, due to the spontaneous nature of individuals. He writes: "Such uncertainty in a subject so closely related to all others, produces great confusions in men's minds and affect their perceptions" (Comte, 1880, p. 20). Therefore, Comte believed that through using the scientific method, patterns of acceptable human behavior could be observed, measured and generalized for all to follow, leading to a socially and morally just world. Aristotle and Comte's work began the ideologies of positivism that influence the way most educational research is done today. These ideologies include tightly defined variables, testing hypotheses based on preconceived patterns, discrediting differences and assuming that research could be done separately from lived experiences and values (Tobin, 2012). I specifically extend these ideologies to the way emotions are viewed in teaching and learning environments.

11.1 *The Appropriation of Emotions*

From birth, children are taught what their culture defines as appropriate emotional responses to situations. Simultaneously, through interacting in teaching and learning spaces, culture produced permeates spaces outside of the teaching and learning space. More specifically, cultural processes do not possess a standardized meaning across people, spaces and time (Sewell, 2005); especially across diverse social, economic, gender, racial and cultural groups (Alexakos, 2015). However, within the cognitive view, emotional responses were defined by the intentions and judgment associated with them. All diversity, spontaneity and affect were removed from the idea of emotional responses. Emotional responses became an intellectual aspect of being, privileging the mind over the body. Through this intellectual aspect of being, emotional responses were socially constructed as acceptable and unacceptable. Acceptable and unacceptable emotional responses differed across cultures. However, for the purpose of this research I focus on Western culture, which integrates many different cultures, but privileges the norm. These norms turn into emotion rules that are suggested and implied in teacher education programs.

Through positivism emotions could not just be labeled as good or bad without any rationality. Therefore, emotions were attached to morals. Turner and Stets (2006b) define moral emotions through a sociological lens. They begin with a definition of morality as the evaluative cultural code that specifies what is right or wrong, good or bad, acceptable or unacceptable. On the macro-level, societal values are imprinted on individuals through various forms of media and governing laws that are set and generalized by individuals with power. When individual emotions do not align with the normed values, moral emotions such as guilt, shame and humiliation are infringed by others and upon the self.

Positivistic views have been influencing what is taught in teacher education programs. However, in recent studies, researchers (Tobin, Powietrzynska, & Alexakos, 2015) are shedding light on the importance of acknowledging and exploring teachers' emotions and other critical issues in preservice teacher education courses. My research extends these ideas by engaging with teachers as they use self-reporting methods (heuristics and free-writes) that encourage them to critically reflect on their teaching and learning experiences.

12 Disrupting Positivistic Values and Sharing Heightened Awareness

Zembylas (2005) summarized the importance of encouraging teachers to reflect on the effects of their emotional experiences during teaching and learning, how these emotional experiences are historically, socially and politically constructed, and become reflexive agents of their own emotional responses to promote health and wellness. Emotions are central to human interactions and embedded into notions of power, agency and passivity. The insidious nature of positivism becomes dangerous as it marginalizes people who are not emotionally, socially and cognitively aligned to what is predefined as normal through 'objective' truths (norm). Therefore, it is important to understand the way dominant power constantly operates to shape the outcomes of educational research and include diverse voices that often go unnoticed (Kincheloe & Tobin, 2006).

As a teacher-educator | researcher, I work with preservice teachers to develop a collaborative understanding that the emotions we experience do not define who we are. Effective teaching and learning environments include emotionally and physically healthy teachers who are aware of their emotions, without trying to suppress them based on societal rules. The key is to not get stuck on emotions that overwhelm and negatively affect a teacher's emotional and physical wellbeing.

My approach is embedded in mindfulness practices. Powietrzynska (2015) suggests that mindfulness practices empower teachers to change their relationships between their reflective thoughts and actions. John Dewey (1897) describes reflective thinking as the power and agency to not accept things at face value. More specifically, a reflective teacher-educator | researcher investigates why they think the way they think and how that affects the way they teach from a sociocultural lens. Changing the relationships between thoughts and actions affords reflexivity. Through reflexivity a teacher-educator | researcher traces the history of the emergence of their place within a societal structure as they critically reflect on their own emotions, values and ideas of knowledge that are framed by the social world (Bourdieu, 1992). Within mindfulness practices and reflexivity, a teacher | researcher is aware of the systemic forces that mediate their social and cultural world and acts as agents to explore and change hidden forces and processes.

Overall, I do not write this chapter to focus on a deficit perspective of teacher education programs or schools in general. As I stated earlier, I am currently a teacher-educator and instructional coach within this school system. I write this chapter to nuance my teaching journey and bring a critical lens to the importance of placing value on teachers' stress emotions in teaching and learning spaces. I believe teachers need to have understandings of the content they are teaching, and pay attention to the areas of strength, areas for growth and interests of their students. However, this does not summarize teaching. I believe it is as important to bring awareness to the emotional affects many teachers face daily that often times go undetected within a process of standardization and accountability. As a teacher-educator, I attempt to expand the roles of preservice teachers and encourage them to participate in exploring all aspects of education that are inclusive of their own emotional responses to the systems embedded in teaching and learning spaces.

Engaging in teacher-educator | research can be challenging due to limited time and space for teachers to investigate what is happening in their own classroom. Standardized educational reforms, such as the *No Child Left Behind Act*, have compelled teachers and teacher-educators to focus most of their time on teaching math and reading skills in order to prepare their students for a test (Ravitch, 2016). However, preservice teachers are anxiously aware of the effects of these requirements before they enter the classroom and are given little to no support on exploring interventions to ameliorate their anxieties. Yasmin, a preservice teacher writes,

> Yasmin: In my experience, educators tend to lose sight of the child as a whole person and look at them as just a report card receiving student; and this is not to blame educators, but to assess the system. In our modern-day society, administrators and parents alike are more concerned with test scores and state exams, but we mustn't forget the social, emotional, physical and self-help skills development that goes into becoming a successful and contributing individual.

As I began my career as a teacher educator, I struggled with balancing course time between exploring the math content, how to teach the math content and preservice teachers' emotional responses to the mandates and accountability pressures that they would experience as they taught mathematics in the early childhood classroom. However, reflecting back on my own struggles in the classroom encouraged me to rethink how I dichotomized learning the content with the exploration of emotions. I realized that the math content was embedded in the issues teachers were facing, such as their emotional experiences and responses to teaching and learning the content, equity of resources and support within the school system, or their preconceptions based on students' race, gender or culture as they enacted the standardized curriculum. Strict demands on curricula and material requirement take away a teacher's autonomy and authority in the classroom as they are no longer able to collaboratively teach with their students based on needs and interests. Consequently, when teachers are constantly held accountable to teach standardized materials that do not align with what is actually happening in their classrooms, this induces experiences of confusion, anxiety and doubt about their own competence (Jeffrey & Woods, 1996).

Throughout my journey, I have developed an understanding that content knowledge is not the only requisite for teachers to actively engage with students while teaching a subject. Teachers also need to be aware of the effects their values, emotions and previous experience have on how they learn and teach the subject. I argue for teacher-educators to engage in researching critical issues in their content college courses. Researching critical issues encourages the exploration of many undiscussed and unnoticed challenges that beginning teachers face as they enter the classroom. These challenges can often times impact a teacher's emotions and emotional responses which can be detrimental to their mental and physical wellbeing (Llena & Tobin, 2014).

Through incorporating the use of heuristics, free-writes and class discussions into the math pedagogy course, during the spring 2015 and spring 2016 semesters, preservice teachers had the opportunity to expand on the characteristics that are salient to them based on their past and current experiences. During the spring 2015 semester a preservice teacher wrote the following response after reflecting on her lesson presentation and receiving peer feedback based on characteristics she thought were salient to her practice presentation.

> Eucharia: I choose these characteristics from the teaching heuristic to know the level of performance whenever, I stand in front of a class to teach or present a lesson. I have noticed a change in my tone of voice because I am always nervous but did not know what to do. Again, I wanted to know if other people would notice these characteristics when I am teaching. Having my peer give me feedback based on these characteristics was helpful.

Eucharia's free-write illuminates what she learned about herself from others as she engaged in the lesson. Eucharia was able to choose the characteristic that she wanted to focus on based on challenges she experienced. She was able to receive feedback from her peers and make changes to her practice based on what was noticed.

During the spring 2016 semester, after engaging in weekly investigations on strategies teachers use to express empathy to themselves and others when stressors are present a preservice teacher wrote the following free-write response at the end of the semester.

> Olga: Class discussions helped me understand that having empathy for myself is not a weakness, it will help me get the right answer when the emotional/ psychological state of mind is right.

Olga's free-write response illuminated a shift in thinking. Due to the impact of positivistic structures the experience and expression of emotions can be seen as a weakness. However, through our class discussion she realized the importance of paying attention to her emotions. She also became more aware of how being stuck on emotions can impact her cognitive and physical practices.

As teacher-educators participate in exploring critical issues, they may simultaneously develop a more conscious awareness of their emotions, values and power struggles. Within this conscious awareness, teacher-educators and

preservice teachers are encouraged to think critically about the world in which they teach and learn. Questions may include:
- What overarching structures within our world influence how we experience and respond to emotional experiences? How does this impact the way we interact in teaching and learning spaces?
- How do our values and emotional responses conflict with what is expected in teaching and learning spaces?

While becoming more consciously aware of nuances within teaching and learning, teacher-educators and preservice teachers can begin to make changes to their practices that may benefit their mental and physiological wellbeing as well as the educational system as a whole.

References

Alexakos, K. (2015). *Being a teacher| researcher: A primer on doing authentic inquiry research on teaching and learning*. Sense Publishers.

Alexakos, K., Pride, L. D., Amat, A., Tsetsakos, P., Lee, K. J., Paylor-Smith, C., Zapata, C., Wright, S., & Smith, T. (2016). Mindfulness and discussing "thorny" issues in the classroom. *Cultural Studies of Science Education, 11*(3), 741–769. https://doi.org/10.1007/s11422-015-9718-0

American Federation of Teachers. (2015). *Quality of worklife survey*. American Federation of Teachers. www.aft.org/sites/default/files/worklifesurveyresults2015.pdf

Bourdieu, P., & Wacquant, L. J. (1992). *An invitation to reflexive sociology*. University of Chicago Press.

Comte, A. (1957). *A general view of positivism*. R. Speller.

Corbett, K. (2016). Gender, identity and culture in learning physics. *Cultural Studies of Science Education, 11*, 371–378.

Davidson, R. (2012). *The emotional life of your brain: How its unique patterns affect the way you think, feel, and live-and how you can change them*. Hudson Street Press.

Dewey, J. (1897). My pedagogic creed. *School Journal, 54*(3), 77–80.

Frazzetto, G. (2013). *Joy, guilt, anger, love: What neuroscience can – and can't – tell us about how we feel*. Penguin Books.

Foucault, M. (1982). The subject and power. *Critical Inquiry, 8*, 777–795.

Gestwicki, C. (2016). *Home, school & community relations*. Cengage Learning.

Gold, Y., & Roth, R. A. (1993). *Teachers managing stress and preventing burnout: the professional health solution*. Falmer Press.

Hochschild, A. (1979). Emotion Work, Feeling rules, and social structure. *American Journal of Sociology, 85*, 551–575.

Hochschild, A. R. (2003). *The managed heart: commercialization of human feeling.* University of California Press.

Jaggar, A. M. (1989). Love and knowledge: Emotion in feminist epistemology. *Inquiry, 32*(2), 151–176.

Jeffrey, B., & Woods, P. (1996). Feeling deprofessionalised: The social construction of emotions during an OFSTED inspection. *Cambridge Journal of Education, 26*(3), 325–343.

Kemper, T. D., & Collins, R. (1990). Dimensions of microinteraction. *American Journal of Sociology, 96*(1), 32–68.

Kincheloe, J. L., & Tobin, K. (2009). The much-exaggerated death of positivism. *Cultural Studies of Science Education, 4*, 513–528.

Kyriacou, C. (2001). Teacher stress: Directions for future research. *Educational Review, 53*(1), 27–35.

Lemke, J. L. (1990). *Talking science: Language, learning, and values.* Ablex Publishing.

McLean, L., Abry, T., Taylor, M., Jimenez, M., & Granger, K. (2017). Teachers' mental health and perceptions of school climate across the transition from training to teaching. *Teaching and Teacher Education, 65*, 230–240.

Powietrzynska, M. (2015). Heuristics for mindfulness in education and beyond. In C. Milne, K. Tobin, & D. DeGennaro (Eds.), *Sociocultural studies and implications for science education* (pp. 59–80). Springer.

Powietrzynska, M., & Gangji, A. K. H. (2016). "I understand why people need to ease their emotions": Exploring mindfulness and emotions in a conceptual physics classroom of an elementary teacher education program. *Cultural Studies of Science Education, 11*, 693–712.

Ravitch, D. (2010). *The death and life of the great American school system: how testing and choice are undermining education.* Basic Books.

Ryan, S. V., Nathaniel, P., Pendergast, L. L., Saeki, E., Segool, N., & Schwing, S. (2017). Leaving the teaching profession: The role of teacher stress and educational accountability policies on turnover intent. *Teaching and Teacher Education, 66*, 1–11.

Roeser, R. W. (2013). Mindfulness and human development: A commentary on the special issue. *Research in Human Development, 10*(3), 273–283.

Sewell, W. H., Jr. (2005). The concept(s) of culture. In G. M. Spiegel (Ed.), *Practicing history: New directions in historical writing after the linguistic turn* (pp. 76–95). Routledge.

Shott, S. (1979). Emotion and social life: A symbolic interactionist analysis. *American Journal of Sociology, 84*, 1317–1334.

Stenhouse, L. (1981). What counts as research? *British Journal of Educational Studies, 29*(2), 103–114.

Tobin, K. (2009). Tuning into others' voices: Radical listening, learning from difference, and escaping oppression. *Cultural Studies of Science Education, 4*, 505–511. doi:10.1007/s11422-009-9218-1

Tobin, K. (2012). Sociocultural perspectives on science education. In B. J. Fraser, K. Tobin, & C. J. McRobbie (Eds.), *Second international handbook of science education* (pp. 3–17). Springer.

Tobin, K., & Kincheloe, J. (2006). Doing educational research in a complex world: Preface. In K. Tobin & J. L. Kincheloe (Eds.), *Doing educational research* (pp. 3–13). Sense Publishers.

Tobin, K., King, D., Henderson, S., Bellocchi, A., & Ritchie, S. M. (2016). Expression of emotions and physiological changes during teaching. *Cultural Studies of Science Education, 11*, 669–692.

Tobin, K., & Llena, R. (2014). Emotions as mediators of science education in an urban high school. In K. Tobin & A. Shady (Eds.), *Transforming urban education* (pp. 205–223). Sense Publishers.

Tobin, K., Powietrzynska, M., & Alexakos, K. (2015). Mindfulness and wellness: Central components of a science of learning. *Innovación Educativa, 15*(67).

Tobin, K., Ritchie, S. M., Oakley, J. L., Mergard, V., & Hudson, P. (2013). Relationships between emotional climate and the fluency of classroom interactions. *Learning Environments Research, 16*(1), 71–89.

Tobin, K., & Roth, W.-M. (2006). *Teaching to learn: A view from the field.* Sense Publishers.

Turner, J. H., & Stets, J. E. (2006a). Sociological theories of human emotions. *Annual Review of Sociology, 32*, 25–52.

Turner, J. H., & Stets, J. E. (2006b). Moral emotions. In J. E. Stets & J. H. Turner (Eds.), *Handbook of the sociology of emotions* (pp. 544–566). Springer Science.

Zembylas, M. (2002). "Structures of feeling" in curriculum and teaching: Theorizing the emotional rules. *Educational Theory, 52*(2), 187–208.

Zembylas, M. (2003). Emotions and teacher identity: A poststructural perspective. *Teachers and Teaching, 9*(3), 213–238.

Zembylas, M. (2005). Beyond teacher cognition and teacher beliefs: The value of the ethnography of emotions in teaching. *International Journal of Qualitative Studies in Education, 18*, 465–487.

Zembylas, M. (2013). Mobilizing 'implicit activisms' in schools through practices of critical emotional reflexivity. *Teaching Education, 24*(1), 84–96.

CHAPTER 4

Living through a Pandemic

Exploring Emotions and Experiences of Living in the Time of the COVID-19 Pandemic through Narratives

Anna Malyukova, Fatima Alexander, Mary Bullen, Maria Cadme, Xiao Ling He, Sara E. Johnson, Jenna Sclafani, Suellen Taragano and Tara Toye

Abstract

In this chapter, I look at the experiences and complexities of living through the COVID-19 pandemic in the spring of 2020. Specifically, I explore the experiences of myself ("the instructor") and students in my graduate class in one of the City University of New York (CUNY) colleges. These graduate students were early childhood teachers, who had to quickly adapt to remote teaching in addition to dealing with individual challenges in their own lives. I address the COVID-19 pandemic as a historical event that transforms numerous structures on multiple levels for each individual involved in the study. Through graduate students' narratives, as well as my own, I aim to demonstrate what our emotions and experiences were during this global pandemic.

Keywords

COVID-19 pandemic – early childhood educators – narrative – emotions in teaching

1 Vignette: Not Myself

I pressed the "End Meeting" button on my Zoom window and covered my eyes with the palms of my hands. I wanted to not be seen. I wanted to hide my face from the scorching computer screen.

Finally, I let go.

I allowed myself to feel.

 | DOI:10.1163/9789004527348_004

I felt so many different things.

It was overwhelming.

"I am not myself," she said during our meeting.

"Not myself ..." I repeated silently, my hands rubbing my forehead ...

"Am I myself?" I wondered.

I realized, sitting in my chair in front of my computer, where I sit most of my time during the day, that these words said to me by my student after a class in Zoom made me wonder if I have been myself in these last weeks.

"I want to do the things I like to do, but somehow I can't do them," she shared.

Is this what it means to "be yourself" – to do the things that we like? We all had to adjust to a new world, and many of us can't do the things that we like, things that make us who we are. When she cried, I cried too, and I saw myself cry on the computer screen. That felt strange too. In the moment of isolation and struggle, the two of us found ourselves united, crying together – instructor and student – both trying to figure out – who we are now.

2 Events

The COVID-19 pandemic is a global event. We have witnessed it change the world on multiple levels. Entire regions and countries – have gone on complete or partial shutdowns and lockdowns with limited or no cross-border crossings allowed. But an event like the COVID-19 pandemic also shapes our lives on an individual level, as each family and individual has to adapt to the new reality.In this chapter I explore how the pandemic affected those who lived through it on three levels – macro (the world), mesa (in our case, New York City), and micro (the individual). As the pandemic continues, where this transformation will lead us is not clear, but we can already say that life as we knew it will stay in the past.

3 Macro Level – The World

'John Hopkins' coronavirus map' came up as the top search on my Google page. As the pandemic began, I searched it numerous times a day.

My eyes searched for numbers – breath shallow and short with each new update.

The World map showed increasing numbers that were hard to visualize.

The U.S. map had New York State at the top of the list for many months.

I watched the news feverishly every day … until I could not do it anymore.

Going home to visit my birthplace, Russia, didn't seem feasible any more.

We were in lockdown as a country. We were "sheltered in place" in our apartments.

"What is happening to us?" I wondered.

William Sewell (2005) writes about historical events and how historical events should be understood as happenings that transform structures. Structures, according to Sewell, can be conceptualized as multiple, overlapping, and transposable. Different clusters or systems of cultural meanings inform different realms of institutional practices (2005). Even on the personal level, structures are multiple. Each of us belongs to a family, ethnic group, city, country and each of these systems represents its own structure. In turn, structures will overlap with each other (like the structure of the city one lives in and the structure of one's family). Structures could be transposed, or moved, to a new place of "existence," just as a musical piece is transposed when we change the musical key. Sewell (2005) argues that events constitute what historians call "turning points." Events change the structures that govern human conduct. This global pandemic presented such a "turning point" for us as a collective, as everyday happenings transformed multiple structures in our lives. With structures like work, schools, restaurants, gyms, and recreational facilities, among other things, being closed and no longer holding the function in society that they normally do – institutional practices were changing swiftly. Human conduct and contact were changed drastically. Each of us had to figure out what our human conduct looked like now on a more local scale – meso level.

4 Meso Level – New York City

> As we read [in class] together in April, the university's hospital, New York-Presbyterian, was filled with victims of the pandemic. Across the city, hundreds of them were dying every day. So many elements of our civilization

> had shut down: churches, schools, and universities; libraries, bookstores, research institutes, and museums; opera companies, concert organizations, and movie houses; theatre and dance groups; galleries, studios, and local arts groups of all kinds (not to mention local bars). Who knew what would perish and what would come back? (David Denby, 2020, p. 62)

In the time of the pandemic, multiple structures began to overlap in a more visible way, as many of us noticed new intersections between home life, work life, and academic life. As an instructor at one of the colleges in City University of New York (CUNY), I, too, witnessed how many of the structures in my life changed rapidly. Working from home, teaching from home via video conferencing platforms like Zoom, became a new reality. For many, such as myself and my students, these structures were suddenly all confined into the same physical space – our homes. My college students, as early childhood educators, had to adjust their lives overnight as they had to begin teaching their students remotely. With high demands from parents, administrators, and society as a whole, teachers like my students were putting in longer hours of work, while still trying to manage other structures in their lives, like being a parent, a child to an elderly parent, or a spouse to an essential worker.

In April of 2020, I asked my students to share with me how their lives had been changing now that we were living through a pandemic. Many shared that they witnessed such "turning points" in their everyday happenings, as multiple structures were transformed.

> Tara: I was upset that my dance studio decided to close even before schools closed. I was upset when school finally closed, and I was not going to be able to interact with my students. I was upset when my fiancé's work schedule was completely changed indefinitely in the hospital.

In Tara's example, we see how different systems of cultural meanings – being a dance teacher, an educator, a partner – changed quickly, and how each system, in turn, informed and transformed different spheres of her everyday life. She could no longer be a dance teacher, had to adjust to being an educator in remote learning, had to *not* see her fiancé as often because he was now considered an "essential worker."

There are many aspects of our lives that were affected by a pandemic on a meso level. In the next few paragraphs, I address how our lives were changing in various ways such as teaching through a pandemic for early childhood educators and how young students were affected by the new type of a learning environment – remote learning. I address how adults (in their own words) were adjusting to the new normal and how the role of community was changing as well. I look at my own experience of being an instructor, and I address some positive things brought up by the pandemic as well.

4.1 *Teaching through the Pandemic*

> Laws and curricula can be changed but it is the teachers who do the teaching after all. (Alexakos, 2012, p. 41)

Many of my students work with children between 2 and 9 years of age. In just an interval of two weeks, they had to adjust to the new concept of remote teaching. Once the teaching began, their lives were changed as well, because being an educator suddenly looked and felt quite different. Teaching young students is typically hands-on, which now became impossible with remote learning. My students shared that they quickly realized how important it was to make the necessary adjustment for remote learning in order for it to be meaningful to students.

> Jenna: For children who have a hard time engaging in online learning – the right teacher will make all the difference!

Jenna's statement suggests that other teachers may have also felt that the pressure was on them *now* more than ever to be the kind of educator that makes a difference in the learning process, despite the challenges in the multiple levels of their own lives created by the pandemic. Many stepped up to the challenge and were enthusiastic to face it.

> Tara: I was proud of myself for quickly learning how to make interactive PowerPoints to support my students, how to teach through Zoom or Google Meet every day and ensure my students were actually understanding the content and I was proud of myself for actually leaving my bed in the morning to be there for my students through the "school day."

Both teachers, Jenna and Tara, state clearly their own role in their students' learning and talk about taking personal responsibility in making this new method of learning meaningful. It is clear to me that we often assume an individual responsibility to "make things work" without considering other structures, often larger structures, that inform courses of action in historically unfolding circumstances. Since larger structures like the educational system and our working environment have been changed for all and each of us, it was important to understand that we did not necessarily have the personal choice of "making things work," despite our best efforts to do so.

I felt such pressure acutely when teaching my college students. If I was not doing my best, I felt personally responsible, knowing full well that the current health, economic, and personal crises were not allowing me to fulfill my potential. Teachers' desires to do their best for students, while balancing the difficulties of remote teaching with the emotional upheaval in all of our lives, is not always enough. A lack of confidence in one's remote teaching and learning practices, an area of study given short shrift prior to 2020, added to the mix.

The approach to teaching was dramatically different now that we were all in front of electronic screens for long stretches of time without the ability to see each other in person, talk to each other freely (as we typically mute ourselves on a Zoom call when others are speaking), or even simply move around in one another's space. It seemed to me that this new approach was not ideal for learning, for interaction, for meaningful engagement. Was it just about the type of curriculum (in-class versus remote) or was there something else at play? Ken Tobin (2014) states that it is not easy to answer the question, "which approach to curriculum is best?", as the question itself reveals an oversimplified understanding of the problem that implies causal relationships among sets of variables. In my example, teachers do play a role in students' experiences in both classroom and remote learning environments, but it is not a simple causal relationship of variables – i.e., teachers' efforts lead to students' success (both "efforts" and "success" are problematic here and are simply used as an example). Tobin adds that to consider curriculum quality independently of context is a reductive approach to understanding social life, where important things, like social interactions or human emotions, could be easily overlooked.

In the case of teaching through a pandemic and adjusting to remote teaching, there are multiple elements of social life (like social class, employment status, family status, ethnicity, and race) that are important to consider when trying to understand what can be done to make learning during a pandemic meaningful. While it is important for each of us to take responsibility for becoming an educator that, as Jenna said, "makes a difference," it is often not possible given the circumstances, as students and teachers alike are dealing with changes in multiple structures of their lives. As I went through my education, I was so keenly taught that I am in control of the impact that I have in the classroom (both as a student and now as a teacher), that I often consider only my own efforts instead of looking at how systemic issues interact and shape our lives. No surprise that I, as well as my student who shared similar sentiments, may begin to feel like I am not capable of being who I want and who I need to be for my students, and, therefore, I feel like I "am not myself."

4.2 *Young Students in the Time of a Pandemic*

> Something else was becoming clear to me, and it had much to do with the golden rule I had been told about in childhood but had not often thought of in my own classroom as a teacher: I must not do to a child that which I would not have done to me. (Paley, 1990, p. 91)

Being an educator to young children involves active engagement with the students that includes movement, play, interaction, eye and body contact, and emotional attunement. Young children are even less capable of sitting in front of a screen for a long period of time than are older students and adults. Vivian Paley (1990) writes about young children and how important play is for them. She argues that play is the primary reality in preschool and kindergarten, and with play often comes storytelling. Paley also states that early play may well be the prototype for imaginative endeavors throughout our lives. This highlights the importance of play and use of stories in a classroom environment that often sets the stage for imaginative work, for example scientific thinking, later in children's and adult's lives. Lev Vygotsky (1981), as well, emphasizes the role of play in young children, stating that the influence of play on a child's development is enormous. In the time of living through a pandemic and learning and teaching through a pandemic, virtual Zoom and Google "classrooms" became the environments in which children were learning, and, in this new environment, play, imagination, and storytelling all had to adjust and be reinvented.

The students in my graduate class encountered new challenges teaching young children in the time of a pandemic.

> Maria: Many factors occurred, such as parents focusing on their elder children who are in DOE [Department of Education], families continuing to work from home, and families stopping [remote learning] because the child is not interested in Virtual Learning.

> Fatima: I teach 3-year-olds, I have been working with my team to send families resources and activities to do with their children. Some parents have been unresponsive during this time, which is understandable.

> Suellen: It has been rough [for the children] at first to focus and to participate … The virtual teaching has taken away the personal touch that children in early childhood dearly need.

Others shared more negative opinions about the new reality.

> Xiao Ling: I want to educate children and provide more learning experiences than just posting worksheets and short videos. The pandemic has prohibited and ruined my teaching and children's learning.
>
> Fatima: I have had a few Zoom meetings and have noticed that the children who were always bubbly and happy have reverted to being shy and will often leave the Zoom meeting.

Through these depictions, we see how these early childhood teachers struggled with not only simply reaching every student to join in the remote learning, but also engaging with them through a new digital platform, instead of in a physical classroom. Paley (1990) discusses the importance of including all students in classroom activities and her own responsibility as a teacher to reach *every* student. Although it does not speak to a parents' decision not to engage in remote learning, it does apply to those students who are present in a virtual classroom but seem disengaged. In a film by Armstrong and Dawson, Paley says: "If … (a) preschool activity cannot include all the children in the classroom in some way, then the activity has to be reexamined or the way one is doing the activity has to be reexamined" (2004). Both Maria and Fatima in the examples above, shared their concerns about students' participation in virtual learning. As teachers relied more on parents to engage with their children as students, and, at the same time, as parents often became more involved with their older children's learning, younger students were not prioritized to continue formal learning specifically *because* it was done virtually, which seemed to be understood by both parents and teachers as ineffectual for many young learners.

The idea that some parents were more focused on their older children resonates with Paley's statement about "reaching" every child, which, as suggested by my students, is harder to accomplish with younger children through digital platforms, and is therefore perhaps deemed less worthy of a parent's efforts. How can we create engaging virtual experiences for young children, focused on play and interaction, through Zoom? A lack of physical engagement changes the teaching dynamic and makes it harder for all. Moreover, what do we do, as educators, about children who are not attending virtual classrooms?

All teachers who shared with me their experiences of teaching young children through the pandemic pointed out the need for more developmentally-appropriate practices. As Xiao Ling says, not just worksheets and video, but the kinds of virtual experiences that involve active engagement on the part of students. Where Zoom is great for controlling background noise – simply click a button and the classroom is quiet – children are muted both in the classroom, but also symbolically. Fatima shared that some of her students were no longer "bubbly and happy." This points to a serious problem of teaching young children through Zoom, where a lack of engagement is a reflection of an emotional state. Children and teachers need engagement with each other to develop relationships and to have fun. Paley (1990) sees relationships in a classroom as important, arguing that children need to have a friend in a learning environment. Learning is a social process where students and teachers interact with each other in a variety of ways that promote learning from each other and with each other. For young children, as Paley highlights, friendships become incredibly relevant in a learning environment. A Zoom classroom is not ideal for establishing friendships within a class of 20 2-year-olds. At least not the same kinds of friendship we are used to.

4.3 *Adults Adjusting*

> They [Parisians] were also aware that they were participating in a momentous event, whose outcome could determine their future as individuals and as a nation .... (Sewell, 2005, p. 254)

Most of us who were living through the pandemic in the spring of 2020 quickly realized that we were living through a major historical moment. Sewell, in the quote above, writes about Parisians living through the taking of the Bastille, which led to the invention of the modern revolution. The COVID-19 pandemic had the potential to become an event of the same kind of magnitude in human history.

The COVID-19 pandemic disproportionately affected people of color, with minority communities averaging much larger numbers of cases than white communities (Fernandez, Bosman, Harmon, et al., 2020). Due to the long-term effects of existing racial inequality, many people of color did not have health insurance and did not seek immediate medical attention because of financial strains caused by long-standing systemic racism, thus finding themselves in more danger and at greater risk during the pandemic. This same long-term systemic racial and social oppression of minorities often presents itself through serious underlying health conditions, making people of color more susceptible to the virus and having more serious and lasting effects in their bodies' response to the virus. During the first wave of the pandemic, following the killing of George Floyd by a police officer in Minnesota, demonstrations for social justice in the form of racial and sexual equality and the rights of transgender people of color, took place in May and June of 2020 across the United States and around the world. Once police brutality, in the case of George Floyd's killing, among others, took place, it seemed like it was the last drop that made the cup of suffering run over. Combined with record unemployment numbers, and many people who suddenly had nothing to do but watch the news and worry about the state of the world and their place in it, what emerged was a historic social uprising. These events, stemmed from years of racial inequality and police brutality, created additional emotional turmoil that made it that much harder for both teachers and students to focus and engage on learning during this time.

No matter what profession we were, we had to adjust to the new world and assume a new role, and our inner force may have led us to such transformation. Anna Stetsenko (2017) writes that human agency is not something we simply have or do not have, but something that is developed within a unified community and with the help of cultural mediations and tools of its social practices. She argues that "the collective cultural practices and their mediations are not inherently constraining and hegemonic but have both an oppressive and a liberational power, the latter consisting in these practices' potential to open up ways for human agency to be developed" (p. 248). In the case of living through the COVID-19 pandemic, our collective cultural practices had the potential, as Stetsenko says, to be not only oppressive, but also liberating. As social practices were changing drastically, as a consequence of a global crisis, we saw instances of practices that were oppressive – such as racial slurs being propelled by the highest political figures in the United States toward Asian communities, because the virus purportedly originated in China – but also liberating practices – such as thousands gathering together to oppose police brutality and stand up for racial and sexual justice across the globe. These were instances of how adults, as well as youth, were adjusting to the new historical events that happened during the COVID-19 pandemic – a new wave of a fight for social justice that relates to how COVID-19 ravaged poor and minority communities more than any other. And although the focus of social fights was on police reform, COVID-19 and police brutality shone a bright light on racial inequality in our country. Teachers and students alike felt a lot of strong emotions elicited by the COVID-19 pandemic and the issues that were exacerbated by the health crisis. As educators, we needed to acknowledge these strong emotions that had entered our classrooms before we could focus on anything else.

4.4 *Adults as Students*

When it came to the experiences of being learners themselves in the time of a pandemic, students in my classroom held a multitude of diverse views.

> Tara: I am the type of student that needs to be in a classroom, and learns best when a teacher is physically standing in front of me.

> Suellen: I do miss coming to a class and getting hands-on instruction rather than the Zoom Classroom.

> Xiao Ling: I want to have a normal student life [rather] than just meeting each other on Zoom. I want to go to class so that I can feel physically present in the classroom environment.

> Fatima: Learning in a pandemic for me has been difficult. I have been trying to finish up my thesis but honestly feel discouraged, unmotivated, stressed, depressed at times.

> Mary: I tried to read my assigned books and articles, but I found myself drifting off and wondering, as I heard many ambulances' sirens blazing, as they passed by every few minutes. I wondered, who was the next victim of this faceless monster that caused so much pain and havoc on families, friends, coworkers, professors, students and regular people in New York City, New York State, and the entire world, simultaneously.

The students who shared their views on learning through a pandemic gave similar views on how their own learning was constrained by not being in a physical classroom. Considering that most of them are teachers, specifically teachers to young children, it is revealing how they viewed their own remote learning as much more challenging now that we could not meet in a classroom. The Zoom experience was emotionally strenuous for Tara, Sullen, and Xiao Ling while Mary and Fatima emphasized general lack of interest and motivation to do their own studying, because of the uncertainty caused by the pandemic. I did not get any positive responses from the students about *learning* through a pandemic (some positive effects of living through a pandemic are addressed later). However, it is unclear whether it was because no one saw any benefits, or because only those who felt the struggle chose to share.

4.5 *Child's Eye of Community*

Another aspect of human interaction on a meso level is the role of community and how this, too, has changed in the times of pandemic. One of my graduate students, Jenna, shared with me her thoughts on the role of community, specifically how the role of community was changing in the eyes of young children.

> Jenna: The structure of our 'community' is changing so fast. We [students and teachers] used to physically talk to community workers because we would see them and visit them often – cops, bus drivers, firefighters,

> postal workers. I wonder what those community workers will look like now? … Will we have a new curriculum topic now of 'essential workers?'

During the pandemic, many people suddenly found themselves working from home, "glued" to their seats in front of computer screens, but there were also people who continued to work in their jobs as before – such as medical professionals, grocery workers, food delivery workers, transportation, warehouse, and delivery workers, among others – risking their lives to make everyone else's lives better. Jenna's comment raised a very important point about the role of community and the role of workers, especially those who we began to call 'essential workers' during the spring of 2020.

Neighborhoods all over New York City erupted with applause every day at 7 p.m. to say "thank you!" to those who worked "on the front lines." When we first heard of this show of appreciation on March 27th, my 10-year-old daughter and I opened our window at 7 p.m. and clapped our hands, shouting "thank you!" With every passing day more and more people joined the clapping, as cheering sounds spread through New York City streets to acknowledge and express gratitude to the essential workers. In July, some twelve weeks later, we still clapped every night, and we had drums, trumpets, pots and pans, and shakers, joining together to express our recognition and regard. This social practice became a new ritual that brought our immediate community a little closer, as we became more united in our everyday practice of coming together, even if just for a few minutes. Every day we looked to find each other out the windows, proud and joyous to share a moment like this with each other. (This did not happen in every neighborhood in New York City, but my daughter and I were grateful that it happened in ours). It was nice to feel proud of our neighbors when we previously passed them without a blink. It was a moment to reassess who is essential, who matters, who is really brave. It also made us, my daughter and I, think about how those often considered "unskilled," and therefore less wealthy, are just as important as wealthy "skilled" workers in keeping our communities moving forward.

In my daughter's eyes, and in the eyes of other children, the role of community may have been changing even more so than in adults' eyes. Alexakos et al. (2012) share about the role of the community, in their case the science classroom, and how students seek knowledge and skills from each other in order to participate in solidarity-building classroom interactions. In our daily ritual of clapping together, the activity became a solidarity-building community interaction, where my daughter learned from and was positively influenced by the community around her. Randall Collins (2005) writes about solidarity, which, according to him, is the symbolically mediated emotional energy that generates social membership and group structure.

4.6 *Teaching through a Pandemic* (*Instructor's Point of View*)

My own experiences of teaching through a pandemic seemed to be more positive than I anticipated. I did spend a lot of time "stuck" in front of a computer, either in Zoom classes, prepping for classes, or grading students' work, which brought about fatigue and exhaustion. However, I also felt that I had a lot more flexibility now that remote learning was the new way of teaching students. The first few weeks were spent more on sharing our thoughts about the events occurring on a global and local scale, rather than on instructing and lecturing, which, again, showed the importance of shared experiences during this time of structural transformation. I wanted to have an opportunity to talk with my students and let them express their feelings and thoughts. Together we each shared what we felt was the hardest part of our lives in that moment, but also tried to look for some silver lining. It was not easy. One student told me there was no silver lining in sight, because of everything that was happening to her. Several of her family members were sick, and she was homeschooling her own child while working – teaching – from home. This was hard to manage. She was trying to do her school work, but there was never time, and she felt unmotivated. She insisted there was nothing good.

Several days later, I received an email from her to let me know that she thought about it more and finally found something positive. I felt very happy at that moment. As an instructor, I should probably aim for my students' academic success, which I do, of course, but at that moment, it seemed to me that I helped another human being, not just a student, and somehow that felt more meaningful, reaffirming the role of the classroom as a complex community.

4.7 *Positive Effects of a Pandemic*

Like in Plato's allegory of the cave, many of us may find ourselves content living in the world as we know it, watching mere shadows of life while we stay shackled inside the cave of what we "know" – spending our lives watching the shadows pass us by (Plato, 1955). After I first read Plato's allegory of the cave, I thought about the prisoners and how hard it is for them to leave the only world they know because change, and the fear of the unknown, can be frightening. Just as how the prisoner feels once they are finally led out of the cave and are instantly blinded by the sunlight, change can feel difficult to get through. But change also has the potential of being good for us. In life, as in Plato's allegory of the cave, with time people begin to see things more clearly and adjust to their new reality, just as one eventually adjusts to the bright sunshine after emerging from the darkness of the cave. I searched for moments of clarity in our new reality, as time went by and we began to adjust to the new normal.

Sewell (2005) adds a more positive note, as he writes about historical events as moments of creativity. He argues that, "the uncertainty of structural relations

[that] characterize events can stimulate bursts of collective cultural creativity" (Sewell, 2005, p. 229). Tobin (2014), too, writes about the importance of examining events, stating that Sewell's event-oriented inquiry opens up promising possibilities for inquiry. Research about a pandemic and about social life in the times of a pandemic will eventually be substantial, as it presents a unique opportunity to study human behavior and conduct. Tobin also compares an event to a "rupture of a coherence trajectory – a spike in the curve" (Tobin, 2014, p. 140). Such a spike presents a moment that offers a chance to study human life in the most unusual and unique circumstance, offering us new understanding and insight into who we are as a species.

Systems and practices, as Sewell (2005) argues, are complementary concepts, where each presupposes the other. Culture, according to Sewell, is the dialectical relationship between systems and practices. As researchers we need to look for patterns of thin coherence – patterns in cultural practices that do not apply broadly to the social world but are full of contradictions and that are consistent with a reproduction | transformation relationship (Tobin, 2018). Sewell writes that thin coherence is at stake due to the unstable and varying application made of it in practice. Sewell also argues that the role of historical culture under examination is very important to consider. The historical nature of the global pandemic was setting the stage for instances of contradictions, which presented ample opportunities for inquiry. These are positive outcomes of a very dramatic event and if we pay attention and use this moment to look for such insight it can bring about knowledge about ourselves and awareness about our own potential.

On an individual level, there were plenty of positive moments, not necessarily related to being in the classroom, and my students shared those with me as well. Their words demonstrate both our resilience and perseverance, as well as our ability to cherish what we have but may take for granted.

> Maria: I was able to take on a project over the past 2 weeks to create a video with content from each staff member in my school. I get to spend [time] with my children. We have more time together than we could have ever imagined. We are loving it!

> Sara: I would say that the COVID-19 pandemic has provided me with an unprecedented opportunity to reconnect with my family. I have found a restorative peacefulness in the constant togetherness. Though the learning curve was steep, I have learned a tremendous amount about teaching remotely. This new knowledge has inspired me to explore alternate modes of interaction with my students in a remote capacity, some of which have been extremely joyful. I have strengthened my practice of

presence and gratitude and have reevaluated my priorities, both personally and professionally.

Tara: This pandemic has made me realize the importance of family and being there for each other. I have been providing groceries and other necessities for my grandparents and my family.

5 Micro Level: The Individual

Each time my heart is broken it makes me feel more adventurous. (Frank O'Hara, from *Meditations in an Emergency*, 1967, p. 38)

5.1 *Emotions*

A lot of what has been discussed above is saturated with strong emotions. These emotions were felt on multiple levels: macro, meso, and micro. In this section I explore the role of emotions, specifically emotions of individuals who participated in the study, and how ignoring emotions can be dangerous.

Historical events are characterized by heightened emotion. Sewell states that, "Emotion not only is an important sign of dislocations and rearticulations, but also shapes the very course of events" (2005 p. 249). He also writes this about emotions and social scientists:

> Most social scientists avoid emotions like the plague. They seem to fear that if they take emotions seriously as an object of study, they will be tainted by the irrationality, volatility, subjectivity, and ineffability that we associate with the term – that their own lucidity and scientific objectivity will be brought into question. (Sewell, 2005, p. 248)

In the case of the global pandemic, emotions were intensified and hard to ignore on all levels. Collectively, our society went through waves of emotions – fear, worry, anger, and even joy, as we strived to find humor in our new reality. Individually, we experienced shifting emotions daily. We often dealt with these emotions privately and silently. Our emotions often guided our actions, whether we were aware of them or not, and also guided our practices, and shaped multiple systems in our lives. Overall, emotions played an important role in our practices and well-being. Ignoring emotions, as I noticed in myself, led to worsening health and overall well-being. When I felt grief, fear, sadness, or worry, I could not just turn a blind eye to it, to pretend that it was not there, or to feel guilty for feeling this way. I needed to accept these emotions, feel them, be patient with myself, and wait for them to pass. In a pandemic we were all going through this "event" together and could relate to one another, which gave us an opportunity to become aware and acknowledge such emotions. Emotions are always present in one's life, one's classroom, one's teaching, but in a time of a pandemic a lot of us experienced these emotions being heightened – making it harder to ignore them. What I learned through my own personal journey, was that it is important to recognize emotions as they come and go, knowing that everything passes.

Venerable Pramote Pamojjo, a highly respected and appreciated Dhamma teacher, writes about recognizing that nothing in life is permanent, be it happiness or sorrow (Koffman, 2012). Mindfulness, in Pamojjo's teaching, is the awareness of physical or mental phenomena, specifically awareness of what the body is doing in real time. Such awareness eventually leads to moments of insight and wisdom that eventually bring us to the end of suffering. "True wisdom cannot arise unless the mind is in its proper place. Temporary peace and calmness can arise, but not wisdom that leads to the end of suffering" (Koffman, 2012, p. 45). My personal goal was to find that proper place and state of mind, where I could learn to recognize emotions rising and falling, where the nimble mind – thoughts moving freely and quickly – was a good place to be, where I learned to surrender and just be, hoping that true wisdom would arise.

5.2 *Not Myself – Current Self*

In the beginning of this piece, I reflected back on a moment when my student, Jenna, and I shared a feeling of "not being ourselves." This was echoed by other graduate students in my class on the new normal.

> Tara: I did not feel like myself. I was not used to staying home for such a long period of time. I love my family, but we were always so busy that I never got to see them every day for a long period of time. I was used to working a lot, making extra money, and being active. I found it very hard to adjust to this kind of simple, stay at home life.
>
> Suellen: Just to say I'm running to the store or to get coffee has been taken away. I am a very independent person and feel my independence has been taken away.
>
> Fatima: I sometimes spend so much time on the computer and phone that by the end of the day I have a headache and must tackle my son's work before 10 pm.

I also asked my student, Jenna, who was on the Zoom call with me that started this chapter, to reflect back on that Zoom conversation.

> Jenna: The biggest feeling I had in that moment was guilt because I felt like I had let you down by letting myself down … And then I felt guilty for crying to you … that wasn't me … I'm sort of realizing that so much of these changes are about grief. I had to grieve for our classroom space, my classmates …

I thought about my own emotions in that moment as well. I was grieving, too. I was grieving for the ordinary life that was gone, for the routine that I was used to, for not being with students in a physical classroom, for not being able to get a cup of coffee from a coffee shop, for not driving home in the dark streets of New York City after teaching, among other things. However, in the moment of me typing this, five months since the pandemic reached American shores, I know that the grieving is gone, at least that moment's grieving. Pamojjo's teachings remind me to become aware of my emotions, to not pass judgment, but simply notice them rise and eventually fall. On a macro level, our world continues to change and now (summer of 2020) the COVID-19 pandemic is no longer at the top of the news. Other historical events, such as social and racial inequality, police brutality, and justice for all, have replaced the urgency of a global health crisis, at least for now. On a meso level, New York City has moved on as well, where we are no longer the hot spot for new cases, at least at this moment. On a micro level, I still find myself adjusting to the "bright sunlight" of change. This adjustment is not permanent and knowing this gives me a peace of mind. Regardless of how I feel right now, I see myself telling my future grandchildren about the days of living through a global pandemic in the spring of 2020.

References

Alexakos, K., Jones, J., & Rodriguez, V. (2011). Fictive kinship as it mediates learning, resiliency, perseverance, and social learning of inner-city high school students of color in a college physics class. *Cultural Studies of Science Education*, *6*(4), 847–870. https://doi.org/10.1007/s11422-011-9317-7

Alexakos, K., & Pierwola, A. (2013). Learning at the 'boundaries': radical listening, creationism, and learning from the 'other.' *Cultural Studies of Science Education, 8*(1), 39–49. https://doi.org/10.1007/s11422-012-9470-7

Armstrong, D., & Dawson, M. G. (2004). *Vivian Paley and the boy who could tell stories* [Film]. Ball State University.

Collins, R. (2005). *Interaction ritual chains*. Princeton University Press.

Denby, D. (2020, August 29). The lockdown lessons of "Crime and Punishment." *The New Yorker.* https://www.newyorker.com/magazine/2020/06/29/the-lockdown-lessons-of-crime-and-punishment

Fernandez, M., Bosman, J., Harmon, A., Ivory, D., & Smith, M. (2020, December 9). The virus is devastating the U.S., and leaving an uneven toll. *The New York Times.* https://www.nytimes.com/2020/12/04/us/covid-united-states-surge.html?referringSource=articleShare

O'Hara, F. (1996). *Meditations in an emergency* (2nd ed.). Grove Press.

Paley, V. G. (1990). *The boy who would be a helicopter*. Harvard University Press.

Pamojjo, P., Koffman, J. P., & Kittisobhaṇo B. K. (2012). *To see the truth: The teachings of venerable Pramote Pamojjo*. Suan Santidham.

Plato. (1955). *The republic.* Penguin Books.

Sewell, W. H. Jr. (2005). *Logics of history: Social theory and social transformation.* University of Chicago Press.

Stetsenko, A. (2016). *The transformative mind: Expanding Vygotsky's approach to development and education*. Cambridge University Press. https://doi.org/10.1017/9780511843044

Tobin, K. (2014). *Using collaborative inquiry to better understand teaching and learning.* Springer. https://doi.org/10.1007/978-94-007-4360-1_8

Tobin, K. (2018). Methodological bricolage. In S. M. Ritchie & K. Tobin (Eds.), *Eventful learning: Learner emotions* (pp. 31–55). Brill | Sense.

Vygotsky, L. S., Cole, M., John-Steiner, V., Scribner, S., & Souberman, E. (1978). *Mind in society: The development of higher psychological processes* (rev. ed.). Harvard University Press.

CHAPTER 5

Reflections from an In(discreet) Body

Carolyne Ali-Khan

Abstract

Whose bodies are treated as if they are valuable, and whose are valued less? In this chapter I draw from autoethnography to examine the worth of a body. I invite readers on a personal journey as I delve into how the experiences of class, age, race, gender, pleasure and pain in my life, have been structurally connected to a broader social and political truths. I present my body as a site of knowledge about complex and contested understandings. Throughout this work I suggest that we all can (and should) carefully examine the journeys of our bodies and use this knowledge to imagine a more equitable world.

Keywords

body – autoethnography – critical ontology – BLM – COVID-19 – biracial identity – pleasure – vulnerability

1 Differential Vulnerability

Discussing "the differential distribution of vulnerability" Judith Butler (2010) remarked, "whose lives are worth grieving and whose are not? Whose lives are presumed from the start, to be grievable and if lost would be grieved and whose lives are from the start understood as already lost and so ungrievable?" (Butler, cited in Bell, 2010, p. 147).

In 2020 Judith Butler's insights seem more relevant than ever. COVID-19, Breonna Taylor, George Floyd, #Metoo, Black and Trans Lives Matter have each brought into public view what it means to belong to a population whose lives are treated as if they were from the onset "already lost." As I try to understand how to move forward with this knowledge, I am struck by how the movements of the collective and the individual are always inextricably intertwined. I am also once again reminded of the centrality of the body to hierarchies of privilege and vulnerability.

 | DOI:10.1163/9789004527348_005

In what follows I use moments in my life to suggest that we foreground the body as a site of knowledge in order to understand questions of in/equality. I begin with some reflections on this historic moment as it pertains to thinking about the body. I then move on to share a few key autoethnographic moments. I use autoethnography to examine how across five decades, one body (mine) has been central to and indicative of broader political questions of equity. My aim is to move past the longstanding Cartesian mind-body divide to present for analysis insights gleaned from corporeal and somatic knowledge. Specifically, I connect my (biracial, female, immigrant) lived experiences of age, race, class, gender, through pleasure and pain, to broader sociological contexts. I present my body as a site of knowledge about a complex and contested understandings. Throughout this work I suggest that we all can (and should) carefully examine the journeys of our own bodies and then use this knowledge to imagine a more equitable world.

2 The Nightmare of History

> *The macabre image of refrigerated makeshift truck morgues haunted my dreams, until the sound of begging broke through, "I can't breathe!"* (Diary notes, summer 2020)

Sheltering in place in 2020, I felt haunted. The violence of the pandemic, the violence of misogyny, and the violence of racism together left me (and continues to leave me) deeply unsettled. The news – ever more graphic and horrific – permeated my waking and sleeping thoughts. As I struggled to make sense of what was happening I also tried to understand how to think about my own body in the midst of this. As an academician I turned to theory for help. Two voices stood out: Michael Foucault (1977) cautioned me to think about the ways that biopower seeps into my flesh as I accept the ways my body is policed and controlled. Joe Kincheloe (2003) reminded me to frame my somatic experiences in the context of a critical ontology and the "civic web of the political domain, the biotic web of the natural world, the social web of human life, and the epistemological web of knowledge production" (p. 48). I realized that my anxiety was pushing me to consider three main questions that I now thread through this chapter: How is harm distributed? How has my body has been shaped and regulated in ways that are harmful to me and others? And what knowledge emerges when I give my body serious political and epistemic consideration?

2.1 *From the Knowledge of Bodies…*

One of the most powerful recent examples of bodies that have demanded to be taken seriously lies in the widespread protests for racial justice. BLM marches and activism across the country have shed a light on the pattern of racial violence and harm that is inflicted on the Black body (Thomas, 2019) – a harm that Black communities know all too well. BLM has further used knowledge from deep within the body i.e., "I can't breathe" to mobilize resistance and action. The movement has built on refrains from the AIDS activism of the 1990s where the theme of "Silence = Death" used by Act Up (in the AIDS epidemic) morphed into "White Silence is White Violence" thirty years later. It has underscored how erasure and marginalization (e.g., "silence") is systemic. Breaking this silence requires collective recognition of individual corporeal experience (e.g., if I use my non-Black body to protest the lack of justice afforded Breonna Taylor, I work to break the silence of Whiteness and police violence). BLM continues to highlight how systemic racism kills in the U.S., in ways that are visible (e.g., direct police or White Supremacist violence) or less visible but equally damaging (e.g., inequitable life expectancy, inequitable education, redlining, poverty, discrimination in incarceration, health disparities). It also highlights how the ideologies of colorblindness and race neutrality (e.g., studying race = studying only non-White populations) have protected White people from examining their own race and their complicity in systems of oppression.

BLM is not the only recent social movement to hinge on exposing the body and corporeal vulnerability. #Metoo exposed the horror and systemic nature of sexual violence, rampant even in the otherwise protected spaces of largely White middle-class life (e.g., Zarkov & Davis, 2018). Trans Lives Matter has similarly brought into view the added levels of systemic harm inflicted on queer and trans bodies (e.g., Adams, 2020). In addition, COVID-19 continues to ravage the country and expose health disparities. A recent study of 17 million people (Wu, 2020) has exposed how poor and working-class people are trapped in economic situations that put them in public spaces where they are exposed to higher risk of illness, with less access to healthy food, medical care and stress reduction – and a correspondingly higher likelihood of death.

3 Living through Race, Age, Class and Gender

These inequalities push me to question the journeys that all of our bodies make. I turn now to moments in the journey of my body, to examine a few instances in which my corporeal tale has led me to social and political insights.

3.1 *Race and Liminality*

My body walks in liminal racial space. Although I am protected from the specific form of hate that is manifested on the Black body, my White privilege is never quite assured. My biracial heritage (German and Pakistani) and the ability of my skin to brown quickly places me in a slippery racial category. I am sometimes Brown, sometimes White, and sometimes Asian. These racial designations are usually affixed *to* me, rarely *by* me, and are contingent on who is seeing (or not seeing) me.

Multiple factors influence how I am racially perceived: politics, history, geography, class and gender have, sometimes with great speed, changed my race in the eyes of others and highlighted or minimalized the impact of race in my life. As I have bounced through these evolutions, the story of my racialized body has been one of multiple reinventions. Here are some examples: In England – where I am from – I am generally considered Asian (as the Indian subcontinent is Asia). As a brown working-class child in London, "Paki" or "N…" (interchangeably)[1] were the slurs hurled at me. I believe that the elementary school peers who would surround me to use those words did not explicitly know the sordid history of their slurs, but they clearly understood that those syllables had the power to convey hate. When I moved to Pakistan as a teenager, these taunts were replaced by "Get out Britisher!" which ironically redefined me as White through the legacy of colonial history. When I moved to the U.S. in my mid-twenties my racial identity surprisingly shifted again, now to become an asset. In the cosmopolitan environment of New York City in the years before 9/11, I inhabited and enjoyed an intersectional meld of age-race-class-gender privilege. I floated between White (with many of the privileges that entails) and "Exotic" (as a brown skinned woman with a heritage from a place many could not find on a map). When 9/11 happened my "visible identity" (Alcoff, 2005) again changed suddenly and overnight I found myself transported to my new signifier-home of Arab/Terrorist – a category that I have drifted in and out of in the years since. Now, living in the U.S. South, I seem to somewhat erratically be perceived as alternately White, Other, PoC (person of color), Latinx (to which I have no ethnic or cultural connection) and Arab/Muslim.

What is salient here is that for the most part my racial/ethnic categorization has been assumed and thereby often has been out of my control. As it is often true for those who occupy the category of "other" – e.g., women, African Americans, Trans folk, PoC, my otherness has often been weaponized. In the more painful of these moments race has been not only affixed to me by others, but has been a deficit, a shameful category, a visible marker of my being unworthy of normal social benefits and not welcome at the table of those who sit outside of race and who are able to be "just human" in the world.

But this is only part of my story; the complexity of race is that it is a distinction that carries the weight of both pain and pleasure. As a biracial person, my whiteness, like my brownness mix together in a layered swirl. On the one hand my brown skin has been my place of deep shame. This was particularly true in my childhood where I chaffed against my "otherness" and (full of guilt at my thoughts) I responded by spending countless hours scheming ways to one day pass as a White person (Ali-Khan, 2009). Yet my race has also become a site of comfort and connection. At this point in my life I enjoy my liminal brownness. I laugh at it and in it. I use the color of my skin to try to bond and find resonance with those both like and unlike me. I recognize my body as the signifier of political categories and from this space I to try to understand those whose racial oppression far outweighs mine, using the knowledge broadcast through the color of my skin to connect to others. In short, my body is a source of complex knowledge, both of vulnerability *and* of connectivity and joy.

Adding to the dissonance of racial pain/joy, my mirror shows me a woman infused with the lineages of both oppressor and oppressed. The milky brownness of my skin is a space from which I contemplate the complexity of being connected to very different historical lineages. My Germanic white parentage genetically threads me back to the deeply discomforting reality of Nazi history. As a child I heard my family whispering of Nazi relatives and quickly silencing these conversations as I walked into the room, and I have a clear memory of a swastika snatched from sight. Yet my Pakistani/Indian brownness also connects me to the oppression of colonialism. Through these lineages my skin reminds me of history as (to borrow from James Joyce) a nightmare from which I am trying to awaken (1920/1986). But here again this is not where knowledge ends. As brown and white pigments meld together in my biracial body, I am aware that my skin is also a testament to the joy of sexual desire for that exotic other (Germanic White and Indian Brown) which allowed me to be born in the first place. It is a visible reminder that I exist as the embodiment of a swirling mix of racial pain and racial desire. These insights, even when they are dissonant, are important in that they continually push me away from thinking of the world as one with easy answers, while they simultaneously remind me that my body (like all bodies) is a site of complex historical knowledge.

3.2 *Living in an Age*

The age of a body, like its race, class, and gender greatly impact the way it is understood and treated. I believe that we can learn a lot about how hierarchies operate in our society by examining the category of age and by understanding how age has operated in our lives. To offer one example, I vividly remember the frustration of age in adolescence, as I chaffed against my lack of power. As soon as I turned seventeen, I claimed the agency I had and moved to the other side of the world from my family. I immediately became politically active (Ali-Khan, 2009). In recent contexts the youth who have led the movements for environmental stewardship and gun control have claimed their knowledge and exercised their agency in ways that are far more significant. As I reflect on recent youth activism, personal memories and my professional experiences working with youth (in two decades of high school teaching) I am drawn to questions about whose bodies are considered worth hearing. The work of Nancy Lesko is instructive. Lesko (2012) powerfully historicizes and challenges the popular argument that youth are less rational than adults and should therefore be subject to a broad range of segregating, paternalistic, and dehumanizing policies. Through this lens I am able to see how my body, like the bodies of most youth, was essentialized and how age is often broadly used as a rationale to "other" and dismiss.

We seem to be at peace with the idea that segregation and marginalization based on age is just, and that those at the edges of "the prime of life" have little of value to contribute to the social whole. This appears as significant for an aging population as it is for youth. The lack of public outcry at the frighteningly high rates of COVID-19 deaths in those over 70 and the willingness of many (particularly on the political right) to accept the concept of herd immunity as a viable solution to COVID-19 terrifyingly suggests that the elderly are considered disposable. (The irony here is that we all hope to belong to this population eventually). I have come to believe that ageism (be it against youth or the elderly) is directly connected to capitalism and more specifically the production of capital. I see correlations between those who are deemed worthy of and being listened to and those who are not, as parallel to those who are able to produce the most (or any) income. Poor people, people of color, children, and the elderly are (for the most part) not major players in the consumption and circulation of capital (although their labor may produce it) and consequentially they are dismissed and marginalized as literally worth less. I believe that here again our bodies have much to tell us. If we each examine the manifestations of ageism in the chronological arc of our own lives, I think we might learn much about the dark hierarchy of human worth in capitalist society.

3.3 *Being a Classy Body*

In *How You Say It*, Katherine Kinzler (2020) dissects the ways that markers of social class and belonging are signified through language. My mother intuitively understood this, and in tragically comic moments akin to those in the film *My Fair Lady* she worked to rid me of my inner London cockney accent (which was a clear marker of my belonging to the working-class). Although she had little success, a shift in geography eventually did the work for her. When my family left London to move to Pakistan I was (with my thick accent) simply not understood by my English-speaking Pakistani relatives. I had no choice but to develop a place-neutral accent. Many years later and having settled in the U.S., both my language (the words I use) and my language practices (the ways I use them) position me as belonging less to a national origin than to a social class. As a professor my "ways with words" (Heath, 1983) broadcast my class status. I am ashamed to admit that I find comfort in both this linguistic cultural capital and in the perhaps delusional idea that the ability to name the world might be a way to be safe in it.

Marxists would argue that class is the overarching category that structures somatic experience, and I have found some truth to this. In many ways becoming increasingly educated later in life (I began my master's degree in my mid-thirties and my doctorate in my forties) layered onto my body an almost palpable protective coat of class privilege. My shift from working-class to middle-class was not just an economic shift but a somatic one, as I moved away from what the labor of my body could do (as an au pair, waitress, and bartender) to what the labor of my voice could do as a university professor. (I use the term "voice" here in both of its meanings, as a string of sounds that my body produces, and a metaphor for opinions.) As I "progressed" from manual working-class labor to a more disembodied middle-class labor my worth increased. This trajectory followed clear class lines, as in capitalist society the physically laboring body has long been devalued over the intellectual and logocentric body. (As an aside here, I find it interesting that there is an academic convention of assuming that a disembodied objectivity is possible and desirable and signifying this by rejecting the use of "I" in professional writing – thereby removing even this last vestige of corporeality.)

Inscriptions of class are broadcast not only through how our bodies speak and labor but equally through how they dress to face the world. As a teacher educator I am deeply concerned about the policing of class through "appropriate" dress, as I believe it is indicative of the ways that neoliberalism operates through social mores in schools. We live in a time where – despite the sizable evidence of this folly – money is still equated with knowledge. Teachers are encouraged to believe that in order to be taken seriously as professionals they should dress as if they belong to corporate America on casual Friday. Their bodies become billboards for capitalism as they quietly broadcast the idea that knowledge belongs to the (White) middle class.

In response I choose to quietly weaponize my body by refusing to comply. I dress both professionally and personally at the borders of good taste and I talk about why this might matter as we discuss professionalism in my teacher education classes. Choosing this quiet rebellion is a bodily pleasure that is both sensual and directly and deliberately political. I am encouraged by queer theorists and the recent sex positive movements that insist that pleasure is not peripheral to the human experience and the construction of meaning. In my attire I try to challenge the reified class bias of what "professional" means in

K-12 teaching and teacher education settings, to refuse to be a brain on a stem, and to deeply and publicly enjoy being a body. I recognize that this is in many ways a minor act of playing at the margins of political debate, but it allows me to feel as if I can literally address issues of gender and social class as I teach. It is my hope that by speaking with my body I can encourage others to begin to examine and reconnect their bodies to their teaching and to a broader body politic.

3.4 *Grappling with Girl*

Like many women, my body also tells a story that is a cautionary tale. As a teen I was overweight, always the wrong ethnicity or nationality, not graceful or good at sports, and a bit strange. I sank to the bottom of adolescent social hierarchies. I am hardly the first to note that women in the U.S. are still raised in a society that incessantly pressures them to conform to corporatized ideals of beauty, to be hyper-critical of their bodies and to engage in body dysmorphia. Beginning in childhood, girls (and increasingly boys) are constantly sent the message that they must squeeze themselves into an "ideal" body and to alter and "enhance" parts of their bodies. Attempts to comply often come at great physical and emotional cost. In many ways the story of my body is typical as it exemplifies the ways that success is structured for women and the means by which patriarchy inscribes itself into the flesh.

To the detriment of my health, as a young woman I succumbed to a patriarchal line of reasoning that demands domination over all things (in particular the body). I lifted weights, swallowed pills, threw-up and starved. I developed the kind of female body that is celebrated, and I used that to access the warmth and affection that should be afforded to everyone. My adult body became an object of desire and with this commodification came a level of social connectedness that as a child I could never have imagined. Suddenly my physical existence afforded me access to both social worlds and individual relationships where I was not shunned but welcomed. The price of this access was harm to both my physical body and my mental health. Self-hatred and shame were my normal. Looking back, I can see how my willingness to traffic myself speaks to the limited avenues for success that young women have. I simply did what I believed I had to, even if it hurt.

This quest to be desirable brought me love that I cashed in on (socially, sexually and economically). I shaped my sense of self around it and became confident in using my body to forge social connections. I believed that I could fashion a flirtatious yet authentically gregarious personality around the truth of my bones, if just I stayed boney enough (the reasoning here, typical of eating disorders, is that one can never be too thin). Even now, comfortably in middle age, I do not know how much of my gregariousness and desire for physical affection and physical contact is the result of those earlier convoluted conversations between my flesh and the way it has been responded to. What I draw from all of this, is an understanding of the dialogical way that body, self and society inform each other. These conversations are complex, and I believe they merit serious consideration as we each seek to distill meaning from our own corporeal life stories.

4 Mythology, Pain and Pleasure

4.1 *The Mythological Body and Stuff We Don't Say*

Americans like to think of the U.S. as a meritocracy, "the land of opportunity," a body-blind society in which the willingness to work hard matters, and the bodies we come in do not. It follows that public dialogue that points out how a body's age, class, gender and race influence social, political and economic access, (e.g., BLM, #Metoo, etc.) have been demonized as divisive, un-American and taboo. The current conversations that are occurring nationwide about structural racism, misogyny, and homo/transphobia expose meritocracy for what it is: not a reality but a cherished lie. The truth is that we are not all given equal access to opportunity and the good life, the bodies we are in matter. This makes any study of the significance of our bodies directly political as such thinking calls into question the veracity (literally the meat and bones) of meritocratic thinking.

Within the body-blind taboo there exist subcategories of *things we simply do not talk about in polite society*, aka topics which are deemed as too personal (physiological or psychological) and therefore separate from the social, economic, and professional. In my own life this dichotomous thinking has been deeply problematic and simply unsustainable as the experiences of my body in pleasure or pain have ruptured across social boundaries. Each example of this in my life has called into question the assumption that it is reasonable to believe that we can or should neatly compartmentalize human experience and that we can or should believe that our individual bodily experiences do not have pedagogical, political, social and epistemic value – not just to ourselves but also to the collectives to which we belong.

4.2 *Pain*

Pain and discomfort do not have a place in our national narrative of ruggedly strong individualism and achievement, so discussions of them are rare. Given the ubiquity and perhaps inevitability of pain to the human condition (particularly as life expectancy increases), it seems reasonable to question why pain is such a taboo topic. One answer perhaps lies in the inexpressibility of pain. Eileen Scary (1987) argues that as a society we have discursive trouble expressing and understanding pain. But clearly this needs to be challenged. Barbara Ehrenreich (2018) points out the absurdity of treating the body as if it were a perpetually fixable product with an ever-expanding shelf life (much as we might wish this to be true).

As a case in point, I write this trying to navigate the discomfort/pain that is a result of my deteriorating and misaligned bones. I wrestle with a voice in my head that insists that because my ability to sit and work in normal chunks of time is compromised, I am of less ontological worth than my colleagues. Although I believe that this type of thinking is in part a direct result of a Calvinist ethic which correlates endless productivity (and the absurd idea of continuous improvement) to human worth, my intellectual understanding does little to mitigate the shame I feel. This shame drives me to question: What if we were to listen to our bodies as they journey through pain? What if we connected pain to knowledge of the human condition, and to the economic and political conditions in which our bodies live? Is it possible that public discussions about the ubiquity of the body in pain might (through some public outcry) lead to more humane professional protections – particularly for those in the working class whose bodies are deemed replaceable, whose bodies are so often abused, and whose labor is already considered dispensable? I think it is time to publicly address these questions.

Bodily pain in my life has also taken the form of multiple and unrelated incidents of sexual assault and multiple unrelated incidents of domestic violence. This is not the product of bad luck, as these experiences are not confined to me alone, they are widespread and systemic (WHO, n.d.). The shame and isolation from these types of violence created more pain and cycles of self-harm in my life. I have tried to use this somatic history to facilitate change by first examining these acts of violence and trauma that they caused, and then sharing this in my teaching. I have found that my college students have repeatedly responded by sharing and seeking help for their similar stories (Ali-Khan, 2016). I would like to believe that as a society we have turned a corner with regard to this, that the recent activism of women, Black, Queer and Trans bodies (who have used their pain to mobilize movements), has exposed political power of the body in pain, calling into question the shame of a society that harbors so many hidden and therefore "ungrievable" bodies. Confronting this I believe that our bodies can teach us to speak out. We can name suffering and its causes and by doing so work to heal ourselves and our communities. A refusal to be shamed by pain might help us move toward creation of spaces for safety and healing.

4.3 *Pleasure*

If we as a nation are squeamish about pain, it is rivaled only by our reluctance to share the ways that our bodies respond to pleasure. As an educator I find it sad that the word "pleasure" is rarely used in academic spaces and is, conversely, so easily dismissed therein. Even sex educators have to fight to try and move away from the medicalized spaces of reproduction-harm-and risk, to instead teach from a framework that is pleasure based (e.g., deFur, 2012). Their fight is instructive as it sheds light on broader puritanical bifurcations that separate pure minds from filthy bodies and are operationalized in brain-on-stem school policies and practices (e.g., dress codes and bathroom policies). As Martha Stoddard Holmes and Diane Freeman (2003) note, there is a long history to the idea that commitment to life of the mind (in teaching in particular) necessitates a denial of any physicality. Even canonical literature has been washed clean of sex and sexuality (White & Ali-Khan, 2020). Teachers are expected to perform intellectual labor in genderless and sexless bodies. They are instructed by administrators to give children "side hugs" so as to limit physical contact. And the idea that a teacher might notice, be attracted to or even dream about a student is considered deeply dangerous (e.g., Rubin, 1984; Kipnis, 2015). In the longstanding tradition of moral panic, even our thoughts about students' bodies are enough to render us unprofessional and impure (Johnson, 2004). The assumptions here are troubling in that they rest on a deep silencing of any discussions or teaching of *actual consent* and instead demonize even the most benign forms of physical connection.

My personal truth – crystalized by the life-draining misery of the COVID-zoom – is that teaching is meaningful to a large extent because it is physically pleasurable and that this pleasure is significant to rather than incidental to the life of my mind. (I write this in the midst of the COVID-19 lockdown and I am struggling with disembodiment.) Here are some examples of embodied and pleasurable teaching that I hope to return to and may resonate with fellow educators: I enjoy and am energized by physical proximity of students both in classroom and office spaces. I take pleasure in sharing space. I feel a rush of somatic connection when holding eye contact while connecting about intellectual ideas. I enjoy responding to cadence, reading micro-expressions, reacting to shifts in movement as I teach. I respond enthusiastically to the physical presence of students, complimenting them on their tattoos, the ways they lean in to listen, their new haircuts and their laughter. I am happy to hug. I have been moved to tears with students.

These are enactments of a form of love, that dirty little secret in education that makes what we do emotional and meaningful. Garber (in Alexander, 2003) suggests that it is the "very potential for loving, for falling in love that makes education possible" (p. 163). I believe that the ways that we individually and collectively use our bodies, physically and lovingly in the classroom is not peripheral to the teaching-learning experience, it is – for many of us – central to it. I am angered by the suggestion (implicit in so much educational policy) that to be fully and pleasurably physically present with students is to be perverted, sexually deviant or exploitative. Such thinking is inhumane, and it does not protect us to pretend to be dead.

5 Coming Together

In 1927 Meridel Le Sueur observed that we can know the world formally from newspapers or we can know it equally through our bones (Le Sueur & Hedges, 1927/1990). I believe this remains an important insight. Recent events and this writing journey have nudged me toward a deeper understanding of the body's centrality to political, social, and epistemic questions. Although my sins of omission here are telling (in all of the categories I did not touch upon as salient to my life as a straight, able-bodied, cis-gendered woman), the central point remains: my body is shaped by the power relations of the day, and all of our bodies have much to tell us.

I have come to believe that the experiences of our bodies are not isolated and discrete; rather, they deeply connect us to each other in ways that are in line with Foucault's insights on the connectedness of biopower and Kincheloe's vision of a web of somatic interconnectivity. As Donna Haraway describes in talking about the importance of the body to social life, "we make with, and we become with each other" (Franklin, 2017, p. 57). Furthermore, when we join together, the sum of our bodies' knowledge has a formidable collective power. I have some suggestions on how we can do this: We can work toward understanding biopower by examining the social knowledge that is contained in the stories of our own bodies (as I have tried to do here). We can use our knowledge to join those who engage in radical hope and critical healing (e.g., Desai, 2020). We can refuse to be domesticated, tamed and silenced and instead speak out about how race, age, gender/gender identity and other corporeal/social positions have led us to be treated better or worse than other populations. We can be brazen in our shamelessness and act out with our voices and our bodies – exposing the politics of pleasure and pain. We can think about how our bodies have been conduits and conversely receptacles for both love and hate. We can use our bodies to stand with those like and unlike us as they fight for equality.

I hope that we all journey into exploring the knowledge that our bodies contain and that we act on these understandings. I hope our explorations help us to see and to speak out against the structures that permit harm and self-harm, and to see and respond to the unequal distribution of vulnerability. I believe that taking our bodies seriously as sites of political knowledge can help us to better care for both ourselves and each other. I think this is an important journey, particularly now.

Note

1 I reference the terms "Paki" and "N..." with caution here as these are words of pain and it is not pain that I wish to carry forward. But these are words that have been used violently against me, and to silence that story (even if I am the one silencing it) is to negate it and relegate it to shame. I believe that power for evil contained in these epithets of hate comes not from them being used for academic purposes (or in pop culture) but from their use by White people against Black people and people of color.

References

Adams, F. (2020, August 8). Black and trans lives matter: The link between policing, anti-blackness and anti-transness. *En-Gender!* https://eprints.keele.ac.uk/8535/

Alcoff, L. M. (2005). *Visible identities: Race, gender, and the self.* Oxford University Press.

Alexander, J. (2003). A 'sisterly camaraderie' and other queer friendships: Gay teaching and interacting with straight students. In D. P. Freeman & M. S. Holmes (Eds.), *The teacher's body embodiment authority and identity in the Academy* (pp. 161–177). SUNY Press.

Ali-Khan, C. (2009). On being us and them: A voice from the edge. In Ö. Sensoy & C. D. Stonebanks (Eds.), *Muslim voices in school: Narratives of identity and pluralism* (pp. 151–168). Sense Publishers.

Ali-Khan, C. (2016). Dirty secrets and silent conversations: Exploring radical listening through embodied autoethnographic teaching. *International Journal of Critical Pedagogy, 7*(3), 13–33.

Bell, V. (2010). New scenes of vulnerability, agency and plurality: An interview with Judith Butler. *Theory and Society, 27*(1), 130–152. https://doi.org/10.1177/0263276409350371

Berger, J. (1972). *Ways of seeing.* Penguin.

deFur, K. (2012). Getting to the good stuff: Adopting a pleasure framework for sexuality education. *American Journal of Sexuality Education, 7*(2), 146–159. https://doi.org/10.1080/15546128.2012.680864

Desai, S. R. (2020). Remembering and honoring the dead: Dia de los Muertos, Black Lives Matter and radical healing. *Race, Ethnicity & Education, 23*(6), 767–783. https://doi.org/10.1080/13613324.2020.1798391

Ehrenreich, B. (2018). *Natural causes: An epidemic of wellness, the certainty of dying, and killing ourselves to live longer*. Twelve.

Foucault, M. (1977). *Discipline and punish*. Pantheon.

Franklin, S. (2017). Staying with the Manifesto: An interview with Donna Haraway. *Theory, Culture & Society, 34*(4), 49–63.

Freeman, D. P., & Stoddard Holmes, M. (2003). Introduction. In D. P. Freeman & M. S. Holmes (Eds.), *The teacher's body embodiment authority and identity in the Academy* (pp. 1–33). SUNY Press.

Heath, S. B. (1983). *Ways with words*. Cambridge University Press.

Johnson, T. S. (2004). "It's pointless to deny that that dynamic that is there": Sexual tensions in secondary classrooms. *English Education, 37*(1), 2–5.

Joyce, J. (1986). *Ulysses*. Random House. (Original work published 1920)

Kincheloe, J. L. (2003). Critical ontology: Visions of selfhood and curriculum. *JCT: Journal of Curriculum Theorizing, 19*(1), 47–64.

Kinzler, K. D. (2020). *How you say it: Why you talk the way you do – And what it says about you*. Houghton Mifflin.

Kipnis, L. (2015). My Title IX inquisition. *Chronicle of Higher Education, 61*(38), B6.

Lesko, N. (2012). *Age your age: The cultural construction of adolescence*. Routledge.

Le Sueur, M., & Hedges, E. (1927/1990). *Ripening: Selected work*. Feminist Press at CUNY.

Rubin, G. (1984). Thinking sex: Notes for a radical theory of the politics of sexuality. In P. Nardi & B. Schneider (Eds.), *Social perspectives in lesbian and gay studies: A reader* (pp. 100–133). Routledge.

Scary, E. (1987). *The body in pain: The making and unmaking of the world*. Oxford University Press.

Thomas, D. (2019). Black Lives Matter as resistance to systemic anti-Black violence. *Journal of Critical Thought and Praxis, 8*(1), 30–45.

White, J. W., & Ali-Khan, C. (2020). Sex and sexuality in the English language arts classroom. *English Education, 52*(4), 282–309.

World Health Organization. (2017, November 29). *Violence against women*. World Health Organization. Retrieved November 12, 2020, from https://www.who.int/news-room/fact-sheets/detail/violence-against-women

Wu, J. (2020, July 13). Study of 17 million identifies crucial risk factors for coronavirus deaths. *The New York Times*. https://www.nytimes.com/2020/07/08/health/coronavirus-risk-factors.html

Zarkov, D., & Davis, K. (2018). Ambiguities and dilemmas around #Metoo: #for how long and #whereto? *European Journal of Women's Studies, 25*(1), 3–9. https://doi.org/10.1177/1350506817749436

CHAPTER 6

Restoring the Balance

The Sacred Union of Our Divine Feminine and Masculine Energies

Sister Tibebwa

Abstract

This is a deeply personal journey into restoring the balance of my own masculine and feminine energies in one body. It is written from my experiences and the lessons held therein. As a personal narrative it is only my truth, not necessarily "the" truth, it is told in my way and shared from my heart as an offering to our collective wisdom. The terms Divine Feminine and Masculine energies are used to refer to eternal, archetypal energies that run through our bodies and are present in all things, including humans, both men and women. While writing and living this chapter I realized that it is in the place where both energies meet that we can access the most energy and find the sacred balance.

Keywords

divine feminine energies – divine masculine energies – tantra – sacred union – balance – self-contained – Kemet

1 Introduction (*Written in July 2020*)

To help the reader to understand this chapter, I would like to explain a few things first: I wrote this over the course of one year as unknowingly, I had to actually step into living the chapter first before I could give birth to it (full explanation is included). This has meant that it turned out to be a deeply personal journey into restoring the balance of my own masculine and feminine energies. It is written from my experiences and the lessons held therein. As a personal narrative it is only my truth, not necessarily "the" truth. It is told in my way and shared from my heart as an offering to our collective wisdom. I pray it is received as such.

Please understand that when I use the terms the Divine Feminine (DF) and the Divine Masculine (DM), or Feminine and Masculine energy, I am referring

 | DOI:10.1163/9789004527348_006

to energies that run through our bodies. They are eternal, archetypal energies that are present in all things. Most famously referred to as the "Anima" and "Animus" (*l.*), by Carl Jung (Jung, 1917). Regardless whether we are in a male or female body, we still have the presence of both masculine and feminine energies. Often people run more of one energy and less of another, and the percentage ratio needs to find the balance differs from person to person. It is important to note that just because we may be in a female body it doesn't mean we only run female energy. Many women are very much daughters of their Father and run mostly male energy, and many men can very strongly run feminine energy. It is widely held that the quality of Feminine energy is magnetic, lunar and flows inward while the Masculine is electric, solar, and flows outwards. The Masculine energy usually manifests as stillness, focus, discipline, logic, clarity and will. Whereas the Feminine manifests as flow, intuition, surrender, receptiveness, creativity and flexibility.

When we run these energies through our being, we can notice that as we step into our DM, into our heads, we use our rational self, our logical self, the "I Am" (how we describe ourselves, the "I am … this" and "I am … that"), the mental self, the conscious spiritual part of ourselves. When we step into our DF, into our bodies, we use our creative self, our emotional self, our nurturing self, our communicative self, into the intuitive rooted part of ourselves.

2 Finding Balance Within (*Written in August 2020*)

My interest in restoring the balance between the DF and the DM in one body, deepened as my Tantric calling intensified. I realized in many tantric traditions, women are encouraged to be ultra-feminine and men are encouraged to be ultra-masculine, so that together in relationships they can find the sacred union and balance. This combination of ultra-men and ultra-women, ultra-masculine and ultra-feminine, creates a polarity and a battery effect, so that when they come together in unity and in relationship, they generate the maximum amount of energy, and can use that generated energy for creation and manifestation. However, I still find myself outside this definition, and then my interest heightens after my initiation into the traditions of the Ancient Afrikan teachings of Kemet (Imani, 2008). Following these teachings, I realized that there is masculine and feminine in all things, including within one body. This notion resonates deeply with me, as I am neither an ultra-woman nor an ultra-man. I actually dwell within a beautiful and tiny woman's body, but traditionally I run mostly strong, powerful masculine energy. This means that I was unwilling to deny either of these energies that are so much an integral part of me. Also, as a fully celibate being, I am most interested in finding the balance of the feminine and masculine energies within myself, rather than in relationship with another (The Three Initiates, 1908).

2.1 *The Laws of Tehuti*

The eternal African Avatar Tehuti (*md.*) (Thoth/Hermes Trismegistus (*g.*)) gave us the Laws of Tehuti better known as The Seven Hermetic Principles. To further understand the significance of these ancient teachings, it is important to note that according to Gill (2011), the esteemed fathers of learning, such as Herodotus 484–425 B.C.E. (Father of History), Strabo 63 B.C.E.–ca. 24 (Father of Geography), Hippocrates 460–377 B.C.E. (Father of Medicine), Plato 428–347 B.C.E. (Father of Philosophy) and Pythagoras 580–500 B.C.E. (Father of Mathematics), all talked in their writings of Hermes Trismegistus, who is described as coming to Ancient Egypt from the stars some 27,000 years B.C.E., bringing the wisdom and knowledge of all the ages and holding in his hand the Caduceus, a symbol of medicine, and of a whole healthy being (Gill, 2011). Although all seven are vital truths that provide us with keys for understanding our universe, for the purpose of this chapter, I focus on two laws in particular:

- Principle of Gender: Gender is in everything, everything has its masculine and feminine principals, gender manifests on all planes, and,
- Principle of Polarity: Everything is dual, everything has its pairs of opposites; like and unlike are the same in essence, opposites are identical in nature, but different in degree; extremes meet; all truths are but half-truths. All paradoxes may be reconciled.

3 The Longing for Balance and Life in the DM (*Written in October 2019*)

The state of Ma'at (*md.*), or Balance, is the key for me as a Gemini; these twins inside me each seem to have an equal voice, and can both put up a convincing argument for their often-opposite views. Generally causing lengthy internal debates and self-reasoning about some projected important future event, which can then lead to the onset of a depressing and crushing paralysis, especially when I have to decide on what is "best" or "right" thing to do.

Although with my children, keeping the balance usually means a balance of time for schoolwork/play, movement/quiet time, reading/playing on screens, self-care/hanging with friends, healthy food/deserts, inside/outside, etc. I slowly realized that this is really about balancing their physical and mental states, and although I have always tried to encourage this in my family, I still could not find the solution or key to balance my own two very different sides.

In my 20s, through becoming a Rastafarian and also an Ethiopian Orthodox Christian and submitting myself to Father God (or the DM), I found that keeping strict spiritual disciplines and ascetic laws was an effective way to keep the internal discussions down to a minimum. I used a strict code of right and wrong, good and evil, Father God and Satan the Enemy of Life, the spirit and flesh, etc. to overcome my bodily desires with fasting, prayer, prostrating, abstaining, ritual and repetition, lengthy work in humble service and deep spiritual contemplation. With relief, I realized that these practices keep the inner debates to a minimum, the paralysis at bay, and my body moving forward by providing me with direction. I eagerly learned how to subdue my body and soar to high spiritual heights. Willingly, I hid my light in the cupboard, to be able to receive the greatest spiritual rewards from my Father, God. Through the deepest trials of endurance, I found inner strength as an obedient daughter, sitting at the feet of my Eternal Father, a humble servant of the Most High God. I reveled in my DM energy, finding relief in the simplicity of hard work, focus, discipline and will-power. Yet the more I strive for the spiritual heights and fight the constant spiritual battle on the side of light, the less my life works out and the harder and harder I have to fight …

And then the Divine Mother calls for me, and I realize there is so much more. I sense that my body holds a truth that longs to be heard and the balance of her voice is deeply needed.

4 Stepping into the Quest for Restoration of Balance (*Written in December 2019*)

I have to explain that I started composing this chapter when a good brother of mine in September 2019, asked me to write for his book on wellness and well-being. I thought "Oh, yes! I can easily and quickly write on Balance (on Ma'at within), on perfectly balancing the Masculine and Feminine energies within one body!" I haughtily thought to myself that I have the balance down now that I have reached 50 years of age, and that I have finally managed to balance both energies well and can quite evenly express both sides of myself. Outwardly, I supposedly managed to keep a relatively seamless balance, by learning to totally accept that I can often feel opposing ways about the same thing, but that I don't actually have to choose which one is right. So, in Oct. 2019, believing that it would be quick and easy to write just one chapter. I quickly scribbled the first piece on the Tube, while traveling in London, strangely running out of time as I reached my stop, as soon as I finished the DM part! … And then the Universe laughed out loud and said "Oh yeah, so you think you know it all? How balanced are you really?" And then turned things upside down on me. Plunging me into my own shadow world of questioning my very essence. I quickly realized that I was being catapulted directly into the chapter, and thereby unfolding a year of actually living inside this quest for Balance.

5 Awakening the DF (*Written in December 2019*)

Through the world of Tantric yoga, five years ago, I seemed to find my opposite calling in the Divine Feminine, becoming an accomplished celibate tantric teacher I ostentatiously learned to listen to my body and her infinite wisdom, and devotedly I taught the same. However, through living this chapter, I now have to ask myself do I really listen to my body? Or do I just treat her as a vehicle, like my beloved car? Caring a lot about her inside engine workings and her smooth running, so that she can keep me safe and do what I want her to do. So, I fast and eat good healthy food, I don't drink or do drugs, I religiously exercise her and wash her when she's dirty. I regularly service her, but care less about how good she looks, and never do I treat her gently, or tenderly. I often push her to her limits and even take her for granted that she is always going to do what I want her to do. I get amazed when she breaks down, gets weak or sick and no longer obeys my will. And I am totally shocked at how quickly and how deeply low I plunge into the shadow world …

6 Mothering and Menopause (*Written in November 2019*)

I felt blindsided when the rupture came through my beloved son. Mothering is the main archetype of the DF that I have worked with, having been a mother to many over the past 26 years, I really thought I had it down. Yet, to help me learn, questions arose about my powers of Motherhood, in relation to my closest child, who is now a man. Quickly, my strong healthy body fell into sickness and pain as I agonized over how best to repair the rupture with my son. Due to this added stress, the ME-NO-PAUSE hormone fluctuation suddenly kicked in, with an abundance of fire-energy shooting up my body from the Earth in hot flushes both day and night, making my favorite time of rest and contact with my real home (the dream world) fraught and disturbed. I decided to try to totally embrace my DF side, by surrendering, slowing down and turning inwards. I made a concerted effort to stay at home and reduce all outside interaction as much as possible. Spending my time with my younger children and working with the Earth, planting seeds, tending my trees, baking sourdough bread, making artistic projects, sorting out my home, resting more if I want to, eating good foods, and indulging in extra pleasurable treats etc. I wanted to try to fully experience and embody my DF side. However, it seemed the more I dropped into that receptive, open vulnerable space, the more I got lower and lower in energy and confidence and the more I got sick (again) and wanted to do less and less, stopping all my Yogic practices, running, journaling and even interacting much at all. I found myself less and less interested in this earthly realm and more and more longing to go home to the life between lives. As I tried to use self-pleasure and self-generation of my sexual energy to build my general energy level, the less interested or responsive I was, the shallower and hollower my practice became. Through the act of letting go and surrendering, the more I was drawn into focusing on my eternal side and the less interested I became in my bodily vehicle. I felt deeply the longings of my spirit/soul to transcend the body and it was only the grounding love of my children that held me in place. As I delved deeper into my shadow world, I searched myself to see what I was trying to avoid or run away from in the body? I quickly saw the negative self-talk around not doing and being able to tick off as being done! I felt the crushing weight of the ever-growing lists of tasks that needed to be done to keep the vast raft of responsibilities that fall on my shoulders as Queen of a large Queendom. It felt harder and harder to be inspired by the incredible creative downloads that I regularly receive, of amazing works that the Holy Spirit/Cosmic Consciousness/Universe asks me to do. The self-debate would start over whether these incredible works were really mine to do, or whether these downloads are just habitual impulses from a system that has learned to derive self-worth from "doing" rather than from "being"! So, I kept trying to be true to the promise I had made to myself to sit still in my DF and receive, rather than abiding in my DM and going and doing these huge new exciting works. Over time I realized that as much as I love to stay at home, rest, relax, vibe with the youths, the animals, the earth and plants, and receive these DF creative downloads, there are major benefits in going out and following these DF signs. I felt the spark of energy flowing through me again and used my DM energy of focus, discipline and will. Slowly I realized that I felt more energized in those few days than I had for all the past few months!

But then the debate began again … I ask myself; Is this because I am feeding my addiction to doing? Is it because my Ego needs to feel important and do something? Is it because I fear going deeper into the nothingness and darkness of receptivity of the DF? Or is it because the fertile, receptive, magnetic and creative ground of a body/soul/spirit at rest in the dark shadow side of the DF, actually needs the activity, discipline, focus and electric impulse of the DM? Deep down I knew that both are necessary to generate the friction and energy that is created when these two seemingly opposing forces meet together, which in turn manifests the electro-magnetic impulse to create, attract and manifest, which then restores the balance of our own Feminine and Masculine energies. Once again we can see that the very same act can be seen through so many different lenses, and that the curse/blessing of a Gemini, of seeing the same thing in several different ways at the same time has once again paralyzed me, so I decided to go back into the DF mode of sitting and waiting, in the knowledge that I will receive all that is truly mine and that all the rest is just a distraction …

7 Plandemic[1] (*Written in April 2020*)

Over half my life spent running on DM Energy being strong, being disciplined, being focused, providing safe protected spaces for my children as a single mother, and for many, many other people. I realize I have lived my life being serious, analyzing, prioritizing, critically thinking, being celibate, ascetic, spiritual and supporting and helping in my closet while hiding my light under a bushel, constantly serving as an obedient daughter of The Most High Father. Then this crazy COVID-19 world pandemic put me (and most of the world), even deeper into our DF. This is a time, like none I have ever experienced before, where total surrender is required, we have to stop doing, start being, stop planning, start accepting, stop preparing, start flowing, stop thinking, start feeling, stop working, start pleasuring, and stop taking, start receiving. We got told to sit down and surrender, to be quiet and receive and go within to find the strength and the love to overcome the fear.

8 Reveling in the DF (*Written in August 2020*)

Through diving deeper into my feminine side, and working with the Mama Gena School of Womanly Arts (Thomashauer, 2016), I further learned and experienced that we must embrace our dark side as much as our light. This enables us to be able to hold space for all our emotions, no matter how uncomfortable we feel, thereby learning to love ourselves in the shadows as much as in the light. So when, once again through the vehicle of motherhood, rupture between mother and (the same) son found me, and yet again I went deep into the underworld, and was tested severely physically, emotionally and spiritually. This time, I managed to delve deep down under the apparent sadness and found the fear that lurked therein. Instead of using the spiritual practices of detachment and prayer, that I had learned through all those years of serving the DM, to come out of this deep dark place, I used my new-found skills of serving the DF, of actually sitting still in the midst of the fire. Allowing myself to feel, allowing myself to crumble and fold, to cry and rant, to tremble and then cry some more, allowing myself to break open and finally surrender and then still cry even more. All the while adding in the turn on and trying to keep my focus on pleasure (DF) through the pain.

It was through my bi-monthly discipline (DM) of holding international focused intentions for the new and full moon (DF), that I was again reconnected with life. While connecting my heart (DF) to all the heartbeats of the planet in the focused intention, on the August new moon, I realized in that heartbeat, that all I needed to do is kneel down and pray using my (DM) spiritual discipline, and to hold on to life with my rock-solid faith. That no matter how the future looks in this crazy pandemic, I know through experience that my Divine Father and Mother have me and my loved ones, and all of life in their hands. Knowing that They have always held me and will always do so, empowered me in that instant to get up and live life fully again in this body with all of the shadow and light. I reminded myself that my soul has actually chosen to manifest on Earth at this time. Through this experience I learned to trust my body as the DF and her emotions, that she knows how far, how deep and for how long she needs to fall, and that she has the innate wisdom to heal herself, when she is ready, by calling in the DM and restoring the balance. I once again realized that it was actually through the interplay of the disciplines of the DM and the opening of the DF, that my balance was restored and I was able to rejoin life on Earth.

9 The Differences between the Divine Feminine and Masculine

9.1 *The Divine Masculine* (*Written in May* 2020)

As my journey unfolds and I am focusing more and more on discerning the subtleties of both energies, it seems to me that often they speak different languages … I realize that my experience of the DM internally is in the energy of the eternal "I AM," manifesting in the archetype of Heru (*md.*) (Horus (*g.*)), the boy/hero – king – sacrifice model. He helps me to manifest the state of pure consciousness, of stillness, of clarity, of will and discipline, logic, rationality, and thinking. As the Hawk I fly high in the sky, seeing things from an eternal perspective, keeping my focus outwards, scanning the horizons for possible dangers, putting up protections and preparations, making sure that my domain and all who dwell therein are secure and well-protected. As I soar overhead, I search the future for all possible outcomes, wisely studying each option and then often deciding on the outcome that is best for all concerned. The hero can see things with perspective and detachment and always strives to do the right "thing" from a soul or eternal life perspective. Endeavoring to decide on what would be the "right thing" for all involved and for the long term, not just for the moment.

It is important to recognize that it is our DM that has kept us alive. He has protected us and he has given us the strength and courage to protect our families, encouraging us to use the gift of clarity through detachment, to enable us to see and hear things clearly, through accessing his power of will we acquire the ability to get up and do things, and through his power of discipline we are able to work (even when we might not want to) and to move forward in our lives. Through his outward focus he gives us the gift of giving. Through his gift of persistence, he gives us faith, and through his gift of focus we experience true presence. His power lies in his ability to think, to see all angles, to use clarity and logic, intellect and reasoning, to detach to be able to objectively make decisions, to study and understand the past to plan and protect the future. This power is seated in his brain. Although he himself is stillness, we can access him through movement, regular exercise, walking, running, solitary sports, reasoning with like-minded people, reading high vibrational books, listening to motivational music and words, intellectual works, fasting and praying, high level yogic practices and breath work, mantras, etc. We can also access him through pursuing any spiritual pathway that teaches detachment and discipline.

9.2 *The Divine Feminine* (*Written in June 2020*)

We can hear the whisperings of the DF within our bodies, which are made of the same elements as the Earth. When we listen carefully, we realize that within our physical shell, we can have many different voices, including those of the heart, the gut, the yoni(*s.*), the womb, the breasts (reproductive organs) and then of course, we have all of our six senses. Reflecting this myriad of potentially different feelings, my experience of the DF is multi-faceted, like a cut diamond whose sparkle is created by the reflections of her facets. In turn this is reflected in the myriad names and faces of the goddess throughout the world. All these manifestations of the DF can be experienced through the archetype of the Kemetic Goddess Auset (*md.*) (Isis (*g.*), Pattini (*s.*)). The voices of our body can tell us differing stories, but they are all unanimously concerned with the here and now, and many seem only interested in personal desires and needs. Through her inward focus she gives us the gift of receiving. It is the DF who has encouraged us to be receptive to her bubbling fountain of creation, grounding us to find our way home, opening us up to be able to feel the depths and the heights of life on Earth, connecting us to our hearts and all the emotions held therein so that we can learn to love more fully and deeply, encouraging us to submit to the circular nature of the giving and receiving of nurturing, enabling us to be vulnerable enough to receive the gifts of life, keeping us flexible to be able to bend with the storms of life and fluid enough to flow gracefully with the changes of life. Empowering us to surrender and let go, freeing us to be able to flow in all directions without limitations. Her power lies in subjectively feeling things, and we can experience her wisdom through actually feeling them, through sensing them, through tasting them, through smelling them, through seeing them, through hearing them, and through intuiting them. She wants us only to experience them in the present moment. Although she herself is creativity and movement, we access her through quietness, stillness, meditation, dreaming, gardening, reconnecting with the soil, singing, rest, journaling, yoga, nurturing, playfulness, joy, beauty, sewing, bathing, stargazing, etc. We also access her through pleasure, and through learning to please our senses. Her obvious power lies in the emotions, seated directly in the heart.

10 Father Earth and Mother Sky (*Written in June 2020*)

Through learning inner wisdom from the ancient Afrikan teachings of Kemet (Egypt/Nile Valley), we observe that the goddess Nut (*md.*) is Mother Sky and that the god Geb (*md.*), is Father Earth! This would appear to be opposite of the usual acceptance of Mother Earth (Shakti (*s.*)) and Father Sky (Shiva (*s.*)), until we remember the Hermetic Law of Polarity, where all opposites reconcile and the Law of Gender where we see the two genders or energies present in both the Ether and the Earth.

When we explore this concept more deeply, and try to search out what is feminine within the stillness of the Ether, we see that she can be found in the lightness, airiness and playfulness of the feminine spirit. Like the element of the Air (Interestingly "Ruach" meaning "breath" or "wind" in Hebrew is always referred to in the feminine, and can often be used to refer to the Holy Spirit!) she is ever moving, always creating, destroying and recreating life in a never-ending cycle. And what of the masculine held within the Earth? Where is his spirit to be found? In the stillness of the deepest caves, in the heights and majestic power of the mountains, in the hardness of rocks and the solidity of the mineral world and even sometimes in strength and endurance of the most ancient of trees. Like the element of the Earth, he remains solid and stable, a strong foundation on which to build safe protected spaces.

10.1 *The Interaction and Play between the Two Energies* (*Written in July 2020*)

After all these months of delving deeply into the experiences of stepping into the DF and the DM energies separately, I realized how important it might be to study the interplay between the two, as it is the friction between the two polarities that causes the creative life force. What happens when the DF energy of fertile intuition meets the DM energy of focus and direction? How does the interaction between stillness and movement feel? Where do the mind and body directives meet? How about the balance of logic and emotions? How do we look both outward and inward? When does the future interact with the present moment? Where is the edge between detachment and fully feeling? The place where the Path of Will meets the Path of Surrender?

After so long of being in my DM, and especially now, with all the online work I have been doing with the Mama Gena's School of Womanly Arts, combined with this very feminine experience of the COVID-19 shut-down, I finally feel rooted enough in my DF, to be able to fully explore the interplay between the two and somehow instinctively I know that it is here I will find the key to balancing them within one being.

11 Yin/Yang (*Written in July 2020*)

When I meditate on the Yin and Yang once again I am reminded of the Hermetic Laws of Gender and Polarity. The workings of these laws can be seen not only in the fact that in the Chinese teachings the feminine Yin is considered to be stillness, and the masculine Yang to be action, showing us that all paradoxes can be reconciled, but also in the fact that when we look at the Yin and the Yang and we see that although in shape and form they are equal and that they fit perfectly into each other in balance of the black and white, yet there is a point of light held within the dark and a point of dark held within the light. I finally understand that this symbol demonstrates that although the DM and the DF are somehow separate and equally balanced, they also simultaneously each hold a seed of the other within themselves. Inside the masculine is the feminine and inside the feminine is the masculine, again showing us that all things contain both.

As I meditated further, I realized that one of the key archetypes of the DF, and a vital part of being feminine is working with the Sekhmet(*md.*) energy, the Kali (*s.*) energy, the Warrioress energy, that lioness protector energy that enables us as mothers to be fierce protectors of our young, we as nurturers and defenders of the weak to stand up and protect those in our care, and again we, as warrioresses, are able to stand against injustices with all of our power. It seemed to me that this must be the part of the Masculine held within the Feminine, the light held within the darkness, the Yang within the Yin.

I also observed that when I am deep in my DM, looking at life from Heru the hawk's perspective, seeing things from that eternal angle and trying to decide what is the "right" thing to do, I realize that I am usually making decisions based on what is right for all concerned, what would bring about the greatest good for all involved, rather than from what might be the expected DM influence of wanting to protect only what is mine. So again, here we see that deep within the Masculine sphere of providing safe protected spaces, there is a deep need to nurture and care for the all, rather than just the narrow perspective of me and mine. There is also the giving, caring part of the DM that only really wants to make the DF happy. Here again, it seems to me, that this is the part of the Feminine held within the Masculine, the darkness held within the light, the Yin within the Yang.

This phenomenon is also reflected in the realization that it is through the energy of its opposite, that we can actually access its counterpart. It is through stillness that we can access the DF, even though she herself is movement, and it is through movement that we can most easily access the DM, even though he himself is stillness. All these are examples of the seeds of the masculine within the feminine and the feminine within the masculine.

12 Healing through the Balance of Sacred Union (*Written in July 2020*)

12.1 *The Caduceus*

Remembering the studies I had done 2 years ago, in preparation for teaching Ta-Nut-Ra, an Afrikan Tantric pathway, I realized that the Caduceus or the Staff of Hermes/Tehuti/Thoth itself is a perfect symbol of the healing that takes place when we fully restore the balance between our Feminine and Masculine energies. Thereby, becoming a clear vessel for the ascension of Kundalini (*s.*)/ Umbilini (*xh.*)/Sekhem (*md.*) creative life-force energy, which in turn gives us access to cosmic consciousness and divine bliss.

This potent healing symbol consists of a central golden rod called the Djed(*md.*) Pillar or Sushumna(*s*). It is associated with the element of Earth and represents the spinal column. The black entwining serpent on the left ascending counter clockwise is called the Lunar Snake/Ida (*s.*), is associated with the element of Water and represents female energy. The gold entwining serpent on the right descending clockwise is called the Solar Snake/Pingala (*s.*), is associated with Fire and represents male energy. Each of the serpents encircles the Sushumna three and a half times which adds up to seven, the number of energy centers/chakras (*s.*)/arushat (*md.*) in our human bodies. (Please note the caduceus is three dimensional not two, as it is usually seen drawn on a paper or carved on a flat surface!) These snakes are the conduits that carry the energies of the earth up through the body so that they can unite with the etheric energies brought down from above, bringing the physical and spiritual realms together, and allowing access to cosmic consciousness. The wings of the caduceus are associated with the element of the Air and represent that unification with the entire cosmos and give us the freedom to explore it. The round ball at the top of the staff symbolizes both the prima material (*g.*), (the first matter), the pure diamond body and the pineal gland, associated with the 3rd Eye and is considered to be our metaphysical connection between the spiritual and physical worlds. Together these symbols that create the Caduceus, express the importance of the restoration of balance of the masculine and feminine energies, to enable the opening of a clear connection to higher cosmic intelligence, and show us how to use that energy as a personal power and healing source, enabling us to achieve our full potential.

13 The Play of E-Motion (*Written in July 2020*)

We can also see the eternal interplay of these two fundamental energies, in the realm of our emotions, which although they are the domain of the DF, they are often a product of our thoughts, which of course is the domain of our DM. It is usually the stories of our "I Am" that cause the depth of our feelings. The thought is the electrical activation force, which sparks emotional, magnetic, creative force. To fully process these e-motions, (as the English word implies), we must use motion, which helps us to access these powerful energies. It is only through acting out our emotions safely, that we can allow them to pass through us, and not lock them deeper into our being. So, the DF needs the DM to provide the safe held space and presence, for her to use her movement to unleash the creative force of her emotions for the health, growth and wellbeing of the entire body, mind, spirit and soul.

14 Surfing the Waves (*Written in June and July 2020*)

I finally understood that somehow the restoration of balance, involved reaching a point of balance – which is not actually a point, nor is it a circle, nor is it even a line, it's actually a wave – a wave of balance between the two energies.

It undulates and moves like a wave, it is never static always shifting and changing, and moving back in on itself in curves like waves of the ocean. It is by surfing that wave between the two energies we can build the maximum amount of energy and life force, which can then be absorbed into our being. This is similar to the practice of Yoga Nidra, when we surf the Theta brain wave state (the state between waking and sleeping), to download cosmic consciousness, enter deep meditation, receive creative impulses, heal ourselves and others and manifest desires. It's in that same way that the more we surf the wave between the Feminine and Masculine energies or consciously go to that place between them, the more generation of electro-magnetic energy there is to be used for healing and manifestation.

The Chinese Taoist teachings also seem to corroborate this understanding of the wave energy being created by the interplay of pulses of feminine (rising/expanding) and masculine (falling/contracting) energy. In his book, *The Secret Teachings of Chinese Energetic Medicine*, Jerry Johnson (2014) explains that:

> When describing sound energy resonances, the pulse is described as the generating aspect of sound, arising from the energetic force of expansion and contraction. Energetically, the pulse is the fundamental field which simultaneously creates wave and form patterns. And a sound wave is represented in the rising (expanding) and falling (contracting) rhythm of an energetic pulse. The original pulse is always contained within the wave. (p. 195)

Bodi Avinasha (2016) in her book *The Ipsalu Formula: A Method for Tantra Bliss*, echoes the existence of a wave created by the interplay of the DF and the DM when she shows us that "All of creation consists of vibrations based on a sine wave, a simple oscillation between pressure and relaxation, between movement (Shakti) and stillness (Shiva), occurring in a vast spectrum of frequencies" (*p.* 88). It is further interesting to note that the lower ranges of these frequencies are signature vibrations for each emotion and for the human body. Whereas, the highest ranges of frequencies reach up to various dimensions of subtle energy and finally to pure consciousness. Thereby, reinforcing the theme that the DF is the body and the DM is the etheric consciousness, and somewhere in the interplay between them we will find the perfect balance.

15 Cosmic Cobra Breath (*Written in July 2020*)

I also realized that even in my daily Ipsalu Tantra Kriya Yoga Cosmic Cobra Breath practice, I use a balance of the Masculine and the Feminine to generate sexual earth energy, to be used through the breath, for spiritual transformation. This energy is generated in my own body by a series of contraction and relaxing exercises, and is created by the interplay between the opening and the closing, the movement and the stillness. Then with my breath I bring that creative earth energy up and bring her into my heavens and then from there, I bring down the heavenly stillness and clarity. Again with contraction and relaxation and breath, I bring him back down and use that interaction of the Feminine and Masculine energies as a personal, renewable, energy source, to facilitate creative projects, healing, expansion and rejuvenation. This ability to use the interplay of the DF and DM to generate an infinite power source, is also recognized by Christine Page (2008) in her book *2012 and the Galactic Center,* when she states that "When two opposite poles of existence, such as our own Masculine and Feminine natures, work together in perfect synergy and harmony, the result is a self-perpetuating flow of energy that has no end" (2008, p. 45).

16 The River (*I Have Written about This Theme Many Times over This Past Year*)

The final analogy I want to use to more fully convey what I have learned through stepping into this chapter, is one of a river. A river, which is often seen as reflecting the nature of the DF, is made up of the coming together of many tiny drops, all the time growing and gathering power as she joins with other droplets. As small streams begin to cut their path, joining up with others as their combined power grows, their pathway gets cut even deeper. Now joining the river, in coming together, the more the water amplifies, the deeper and stronger the banks of the river grow. When we study the river, we realize that she is actually using those banks to push up against, which creates an opposite reaction and as the wave is reflected back in towards the center, the river absorbs the power back into herself and flows forward more freely. As a creative volcano, the DF needs those banks to keep her moving forward towards her goal, as otherwise, she tends to stagnate when there are too many different ways she can go.

These banks are the DM, they are the self-discipline, the ability to look forward, the ability to stick to goals and plans, the ability to say no, the ability to delay gratification, even though we really want something now. They are the ability to stop and think, even though your body yearns for something. They are the ability to look at what is the highest good for all concerned in that situation. Those banks, with their focus, willpower and discipline allow the water to flow efficiently, quickly, powerfully and unstoppably. It's the banks themselves and the absorption of the energy generated in the push and pull of the waves that are created by the interaction of the two "opposing" forces, that allow her to gather momentum and achieve what she wants to achieve – which is always to go back to the Sea. Here it is important to remember the Yin and Yang and the wisdom of Kemet, where we see that although the water appears to be feminine, it can also be masculine, and as easily as the banks appear to be masculine they can also be feminine.

Somehow in that interplay of the feminine – let's say water – pushing up against the masculine banks – the earth, the reverse action happens of the water coming back unto herself and increasing her own power. I see that after downloading our creative impulses, and using the momentum and movement of our DF, it is then important to push up against our DM, and use the pressure of the discipline and the focus, to gather force back into ourselves to be able to go forward. Then in reverse, as a balance; when we are too much in our DM, relentlessly pushing forward and being too focused on future goals, we need the DF, to help us slow down, drop into our bodies and feel into the present moment, listen to our feelings and intuition, plugging into our joy and playfulness, which then creates a fertile ground for creating and manifesting. That is the time when we reach the delta state, where we don't need the banks anymore. It is the quiet times, the times for settling down, spreading outwards, meandering, contemplating, meditating, praying, being still, and just being present. The delta times are when there is not necessarily anywhere to go nor any particular direction, when the banks have long been broken down and eaten away and there is no need for discipline. It is those times where the river and the earth, through their eternal interplay become fertile together, where the river becomes fat and lazy, dissipating her energy into the earth to become fertile and creative, giving rise to the abundance of the delta!

Note

1 Planned Pandemic: plan (noun) – A detailed proposal for doing or achieving something; demic (adj) – Characteristic of or pertaining to a people or population.

References

Avinashaa, B. (2016). *Ipsalu method for Tantric bliss.* Ipsalu Publishing Company.

Gill, J. (2011). *Origins of the Caduceus: As told in the world's oldest language: Symbolism.* https://worldglobetrotters.com/wp-content/uploads/2020/05/caduceus.htm

Imani, P. (2008). *Afrikan yoga*. TamaRe House.
Johnson, J. A. (2014). *The secret teachings of Chinese energetic medicine, Volume 1*. The International Institute of Medical Qigong Publishing.
Jung, C. (1973). *The psychology of the unconscious*. Princeton University Press. (Original work published 1917)
Page, C. (2008). *2012 and the Galactic Center: The return of the Great Mother*. Bear & Company.
Three Initiates. (1908). *The Kybalion: Hermetic philosophy*. Yogi Publication Society.
Thomashauer, R. (2016). *Pussy: A reclamation*. Hay House.

Appendix: Teachers (in Chronological Order)

- K'edamawie Haile Selassie and Itegue Menen Asfaw (Whole Life Teachings)
- Nayano Burdine (Ipsalu Tantra Kriya Yoga)
- Yirser Ra Hotep (Kemetic Yoga Yogaskills Method)
- Jabari Ozaze (African Genesis Institute Historian)
- Pablo Imani (Pablo Imani Method Afrikan Yoga)
- Regena Thomashauer (Mama Gena's School of Womanly Arts)

CHAPTER 7

Generating Perspectives of Wellbeing in Aotearoa New Zealand

A Case for IronMāori

Tabitha McKenzie, Joanna Higgins, Suskya Goodall and Grant Zouch

Abstract

Nestled within the South Pacific Ocean, Aotearoa New Zealand is a bicultural nation shaped through a partnership between indigenous Māori and non-Māori peoples. Framed by a Māori worldview, we discuss perspectives of holistic wellbeing as characterized by models and frameworks. A case study of IronMāori, a series of multisport events initiated by Māori, is examined with regard to physical, emotional, mental, social and spiritual wellbeing. Through notions of third space and hybridity, we suggest IronMāori is both a series of wellbeing events and a transformative movement that acts as an educative opportunity for Māori and non-Māori of all ages. We argue that the power of IronMāori resides across multiple coexisting social and cultural fields, expanding possibilities for how we think about wellbeing, and how wellbeing is promoted through seemingly dichotomous structures with ever-present contradictions and thin coherences that lead to transformation of fields.

Keywords

holistic – wellbeing – IronMāori – transformation

•••

E tipu ai te pakiaka tangata, me whakatō he purapura wairua.
Whakahaukūtia te whenua ki te waiora pūmau kia puta ai ko te hauora.

[For the roots of humanity to grow well, spiritual seeds must first be sown.
Irrigate with the enduring waters of life, and wellbeing will result.]

 | DOI:10.1163/9789004527348_007

1 Orientation

The opening assertion highlights the importance of holistic perspectives of human wellbeing in our relatively small group of islands in the South Pacific Ocean. Aotearoa New Zealand's geographically remote location provides its population of five million people with a long coastline and a diverse range of natural features that instill a strong connection to the physical environment. The indigenous people of this land are known as Māori and indigenous fields of knowledge are generated through using Te Reo Māori, the Māori language. As de facto official and official languages, English and Te Reo Māori respectively underpin the bicultural nation of Aotearoa New Zealand. Aotearoa is a Māori term for our country that translates as the "land of the long white cloud" and will be used hereafter in conjunction with the term New Zealand. Te Reo Māori is necessary to generate nuanced perspectives of holistic wellbeing and in weaving a narrative of wellbeing in this land. Respecting a Māori worldview and associated fields of knowledge calls for the embodiment of Te Reo Māori in the text. Consequently, and for the purpose of this chapter, the representation of indigenous deities, frameworks, quotes and wellbeing-related vocabulary will be in Te Reo Māori, an essential element of exploring and generating wellbeing perspectives in Aotearoa New Zealand.

"Size, strength, vigor and longevity" characterized pre-colonial descriptions of Māori (Moewaka Barnes & McCreanor, 2019, p. 20). Prior to the arrival of European explorers such as James Cook in 1769, Māori experienced relatively long life-spans for the time based on collective structures of health and wellbeing within tribes and autonomous sub-tribes underpinned by a connection to the land. The relationship of Māori to the land is encapsulated in the notion of Papatūānuku, the Earth Mother, who is considered to be the ancestral mother of all Māori. For different tribes, their land is foundational to their interactions with others, their tribal histories, and confirms their identity through reference to geographical features such as mountains, rivers and lakes (Royal, 2005). Within a Māori worldview the wellbeing of indigenous communities is considered as "existing within a web of relationships and obligations" (Pitama et al., 2002, p. 22) that accentuate notions of interconnection, interdependence and balance (Royal, 2005). Relationships are known as whanaungatanga and have their roots in the family group, sub-tribes and tribes.

According to Royal (2003), "the cultural milieu is rooted both in the temporal world and the transcendent world, this brings a person into an intimate relationship with the gods and his universe" (p. 23). Epistemologically, the indigenous view of reality is based on genealogy. For Māori, knowledge flows from the beginning of time through to Papatūānuku and Ranginui, the

Sky Father, through their offspring and on to their descendants, including the current generation. Māori exist within a natural world where the future is not a discrete concept, but rather "an extension of the past" (Walker, 1997, p. 175). Māori reality consists of "the present, the immediate past and the past until the beginning of creation" (p. 175). "The Māori approach to life is holistic. There is no sharp division between culture, society and their institutions" (Royal, 2003, p. 33). In meetings, gatherings and formal welcoming ceremonies people choose to share their tribal affiliations and genealogy to introduce themselves and establish identity and heritage links with others who are present. Walker (1997) points out that Europeans tend to "do exactly the opposite: they look to the future in relation to the past. It is a different cultural orientation, which is fundamental" (p. 175). Genealogy, then, is what connects Māori "to one another, to past and the future generations, and to the world around them" (Pitama, Ririnui & Mikaere, 2002, p. 22).

Rongoā Māori are traditional Māori healing practices "designed to promote mental, physical and spiritual wellbeing ... based on [such] beliefs, which go back to the time before the spread of Western 'scientific' bio-medicine" (Dussault & Erasmus, 1996, p. 325). Māori health was based on five categories of healing: rituals, prayers, remedies derived from plant material for application and digestion, massage, and water. In relation to the pre-colonial period, McClintock (2018) observed "Māori had robust constructs, values, and beliefs that worked for people healthy and strong of physical stature" (p. 72). These categories of healing have shaped current wellbeing frameworks.

From a Māori worldview, wellbeing has been characterized by holistic models (Durie, 1998; Pere & Nicholson, 1991). A commonly referenced framework based on the notion of wellbeing is that of Te Whare Tapa Whā (Durie, 1994), originally depicted as four walls of a meeting house. The model includes four aspects of wellbeing that are necessary to ensure strength and symmetry: taha tinana (physical wellbeing); taha whānau (social wellbeing); taha hinengaro (emotional wellbeing); and taha wairua (spiritual wellbeing).

An alternative holistic model is that of Te Wheke (Pere & Nicholson, 1991), which is depicted as an octopus, defining individual and collective wellbeing. The body of the octopus is used as a metaphor for the interconnected dimensions of wellbeing: the family is portrayed as the head; wellbeing as the eyes; and the eight tentacles as related dimensions of health. These eight dimensions are hinengaro (the mind), taha tinana (physical wellbeing), whanaungatanga (extended family), mauri (life force in people and objects), mana ake (unique identity of individuals and family), hā ā-koro mā, ā-kui mā (breath of life from forebears), whatumanawa (the open and healthy expression of emotion), waiora (total wellbeing for the individual and family), and wairuatanga

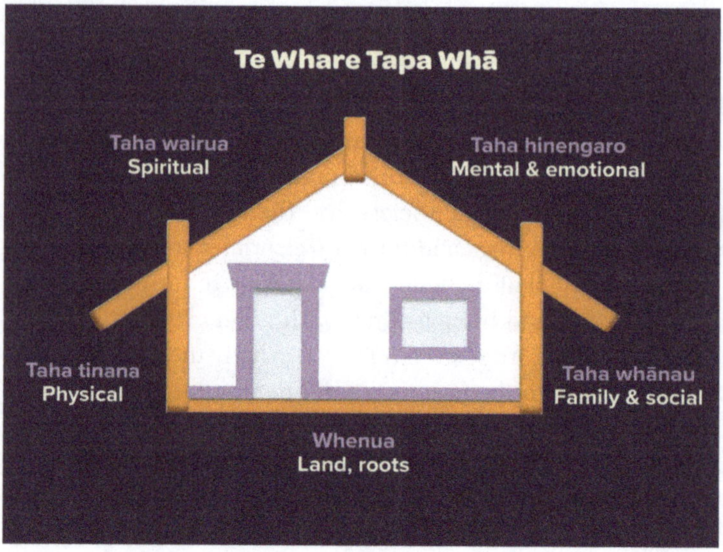

FIGURE 7.1 Te Whare Tapa Whā model of wellbeing (image developed by the Mental Health Foundation of New Zealand)

(spirituality) (Pere & Nicholson, 1991). In all these models, wellbeing is considered holistically with shared community responsibility from birth to death.

When Europeans arrived by ship, they interacted with Māori and impacted the land. Ahuriri-Driscoll (2019) noted that over a period of almost one hundred years there were "waves of contact with explorers, sealers, whalers, traders, missionaries, [and] British Crown representatives who would proclaim British sovereignty over 'New Zealand' via a treaty of cessation (the Treaty of Waitangi) and then annexation, and finally, settlers" (p. 190). The European colonization of Aotearoa New Zealand had begun, and the cultural landscape changed irreparably for Māori, the first people of the land.

2 Historical Context of Māori Health and Wellbeing

Colonization significantly influenced the physical, emotional, social and spiritual wellbeing of Māori and disrupted the political, economic, cultural and social structures to the extent that "a hundred years ago the Māori people of Aotearoa New Zealand were commonly thought of as a 'dying race'" (Lange, 1999, p. VII). In the initial period of European contact, Māori life expectancy was estimated to be between 28 and 30 years, which dropped to between 23 and 25 years by 1891 (Lange, 1999). From an estimated 100,000 when Europeans arrived, the 1896 census data showed that the Māori population had dropped to around 40,000. This was in stark contrast to the number of non-Māori in 1896, which had grown to almost 700,000 (Statistics New Zealand, 2013). Disease, warfare and disconnection from the land were central to the initial decline in the Māori population. As immunity to introduced diseases increased, "Health conditions improved and the downward trend of population figures was reversed" (Lange, 1999, p. VII). However, a Western perspective dominated health and wellbeing discourse throughout the 20th century.

Traditional Māori health and wellbeing knowledge and practices were sidelined, and in some cases lost, through the process of colonization. Ahuriri-Driscoll and Boulton (2019) explain that "In colonial settings such as New Zealand, traditional health systems were frequently outlawed by authorities, which in turn led to the large-scale adoption of introduced approaches and a monopolistic situation in which medical doctors had the sole right to practise medicine" (p. 58). Political measures supported this suppression. In 1907, the Tohunga Suppression Act was passed and was only repealed in 1964. The preamble stated:

> WHEREAS designing persons, commonly known as tohungas, practice on the superstition and credulity of the Māori people by pretending to possess supernatural powers in the treatment and cure of disease, the foretelling of future events, and otherwise, and thereby induce Māori to neglect their proper occupations and gather into meetings where their substance is consumed and their minds are unsettled, to the injury of themselves and to the evil example of the Māori people generally. (New Zealand Legal Information Institute)

Unsurprisingly, the field of Māori health and wellbeing was slighted and ignored within historical narratives of Aotearoa New Zealand. Until the 1990s, narratives focused on Eurocentric aspects of "anthropological, epidemiological or demographic" (Bryder & Dow, 2001, p. 3) importance, largely ignoring the critical connection with the first people of the land.

Māori health and wellbeing is intrinsically connected to the land. Māori suffered displacement in various ways, such as, "legislation, confiscation, and force, … actions [that] dispossessed Māori people of their land, denied their self-determination and undermined their culture" (Ahuriri-Driscoll & Boulton, 2019, p. 190). Connections between Māori and the land were further disrupted as the Māori population became increasingly urbanized, at times impacting their identity, links to the Māori worldview and the erosion of intergenerational ties. The latter part of the 20th century saw the access to and depletion of traditional food sources (e.g., seafood) and primary resources as well as the proliferation of introduced pests and pollution.

Additionally, a series of colonial policies and practices almost annihilated the use of Māori language in Aotearoa New Zealand, sparking further disconnection from pre-colonial notions of wellbeing. Māori narratives tell of a basket of knowledge bequeathed from the highest heavens containing Te Reo Māori, the language (Macfarlane et al., 2019). From early stages of colonization, speaking Te Reo Māori was officially discouraged and suppressed in schools within a Pākehā-dominated world (Ministry for Culture & Heritage, 2020). McKenzie (2014) notes that:

> In 1867, the Native Schools Act made English the language of instruction within these schools. Māori children who attended schools were often actively discouraged from speaking Māori and were told to "leave te reo (the language) at the school gate." (p. 15)

In the century following the Native Schools Act, Te Reo Māori as a language of communication severely declined (Simon et al., 2001). This deterioration was to such an extent that The Ministry of Māori Development (2003) warned, "Māori would be a language without native speakers once the contemporary generation of Māori speaking adults had passed on" (p. 11). As a people of oral narratives and traditions, suppressing a gifted basket of knowledge impacted Māori cultural development, identification and wellbeing.

The narrative of Māori disadvantage in areas of health and wellbeing continues to the present day. Durie (2004) comments that:

> Many Indigenous peoples, young and old, appear to be trapped in risk-laden lifestyles and do not have recourse to the codes of living that may have protected their grandparents from harm. Risks are especially high where poverty is greatest, where risk-taking behaviour is the norm within a family or community, and among youthful populations. (p. 183)

From a point of cultural languishing under the unrelenting impacts of colonization, we consider inspiring health and wellbeing initiatives to promote the ongoing wellbeing of Māori. Since the 1970s, initiatives have been instigated by the government, non-government organizations, communities and tribes. We have selected the multisport event, IronMāori, to illustrate perspectives of wellbeing from a Māori worldview.

3 The Case of IronMāori

The "masterminds" behind IronMāori were Heather Te Au Skipworth (referred to hereafter as Te Au Skipworth) and her husband Wayne, Missy Mackey and her husband George, and Lee Grace. Te Au Skipworth and Grace are the current trustees of Te Tīmatanga Ararau Trust, the entity set up to manage the affairs and finances of the IronMāori organization. In 2009, IronMāori started with a triathlon that had a 300-strong field. The event was in Napier, an east coast city on the North Island of New Zealand. Two years after the first event, numbers increased fivefold to 1550, and by 2019 the number of competitors in IronMāori events had swelled to upwards of 6000. Although the event was originally aimed at Māori, IronMāori is open to people of all origins and cultures. Events are now held throughout Aotearoa New Zealand, on the Gold Coast of Australia, and include participants from a range of nationalities. IronMāori also caters for all age groups, from children and young people through to adults and elders. The desire to be inclusive of both younger and older competitors demonstrates the importance of IronMāori as a life-span wellbeing movement.

Though the original IronMāori event was a standard swim-cycle-run triathlon, these days other formats such as duathlons (run-bike-run) and aquathlons (swim-run) are also adopted. Some events have a specific theme, e.g., The Amazing Women's Duathlon, and the Kaumātua Aquathlon for elders, while others celebrate the tribal areas in which they are held. Distances vary slightly from event to event, as do the activities on offer. Participants can enter as individuals or as part of a team. Teams are encouraged to cross the finish line together, where family members are often waiting to hang medals around the necks of their champions.

As Durie et al. (2012) observed, IronMāori is "not necessarily about winning the race" (p. 24). It's bigger than that. It's about family and relationships: It's about the connection we have with the land that surrounds and sustains us; it's about the relationship we have with ourselves and with the people with whom we interact. "Once you come to an IronMāori event," says Te Au Skipworth, "you become part of the IronMāori family, so whether you're Māori or not, you'll always be an IronMāori" (Tūwharetoa Māori Trust Board, 2018, 06:28).

IronMāori came about as a response to issues of ill health amongst the Māori population and aims to "promote good health … through being active and having a nutritional lifestyle" (Marae, 2012, 00.38). It has prompted people like Wainuiōmata (a suburb of Wellington) mother of four, Monica Stretch, to re-examine their lifestyles. Monica recalls, "At the time, I was drinking hard and smoking hard. But we all decided we wanted to turn something negative into something positive" (Catherall, 2017). However, as intimated above, the rationale runs deeper than just attaining personal fitness goals. "A lot of people think IronMāori is about achieving their goal and then going on to do another triathlon and another triathlon," says Te Au Skipworth, "but really it's about getting that sense of achievement and then transferring that mindset to any part of your life" (Tūwharetoa Māori Trust Board, 2018, 05:14). "It's not really the event; IronMāori is a journey" (Marae, 2012, 04:54). The goals of IronMāori are to:

1. Run events that provide the inspiration and incentive for participants to reach for and attain positive lifestyle changes.
2. Run events that embody the Trust's values and concepts of hospitality, positive relationships, face-to-face interactions, and Māori sovereignty and self-determination.
3. Encourage healthy food choices, regular exercise, being smoke free, and alcohol and drug-free lifestyles. (Pohatu, 2015)

A salient objective of the Trust is to ensure that any changes for individuals are permanent and permeate through to the individual's family. Consequently, the movement impacts the wellbeing of people from all ages and stages of life.

4 Holistic Wellbeing

Although the training, events and nutrition are often seen as primarily physical experiences, a holistic approach provides insight into supporting elements of mental, emotional, spiritual and social wellbeing. The IronMāori movement transcends purely physical notions of health and wellbeing. Naturally, building physical strength and fitness in the individual and group training sessions is foundational to the movement's emergence and growth. Nutrition features as one of the lifestyle changes participants have been inspired to make. From takeaways to healthy dinners with the odd treat or shared healthy food after workouts (Catherall, 2017), participation in this movement has improved people's health in many ways.

Reflecting on her own first Iron Man participation, Te Au Skipworth recalls, "You never forget it. It took me 14 hours. It's a long time to be out there, thinking and in your own head" (Strang, 2016). The mental and emotional element of Te Au Skipworth's Iron Man experience allowed her to contemplate something different, something daring, something new; IronMāori. Similarly, when she thinks of her life coach clients, Te Au Skipworth explains the importance of mental wellbeing in changing mindset and influencing physical weight. "It's about getting that sense of achievement and then transferring that mindset to any part of your life" (Tūwharetoa Māori Trust Board, 2018, 05:23). New mindsets expand ways of thinking and develop new conceptions and practices of wellbeing, generating possibilities for a healthy life.

With positive reciprocal relationships as a core value, the IronMāori movement inspires ripples of social connectedness. Te Aka Māori-English Dictionary describes whanaungatanga as "relationship through shared experiences and working together which provides people with a sense of belonging" (Moorfield, 2003) with kin, family and friends. Supporting the development of social wellbeing, as outlined above in the Te Whare Tapa Whā framework, taha whānau is integral to the emergence, growth and strength of this indigenous movement. For some, whanaungatanga lies in connecting with others through a sense of camaraderie on the IronMāori journey. As 72-year-old Robert Campbell noted, "It's exciting to be part of this whānau (family), there's lots of support. I really enjoy the classes and the company" (Stuff, 2016). Additionally, participant Monica Stretch could not swim so a fellow IronMāori participant taught her.

Social connections between tribes, sub-tribes, and family underpin a Māori worldview and are fundamental in the IronMāori environment. The concept of whanaungatanga also lies in strengthening ties within family, sub-tribes and tribes, whether it is participating in the events together or advocating for a loved one. Stretch shares the joy of connections as part of her IronMāori journey: "All of my family were there watching. My husband loved coming and watching IronMāori and seeing everyone getting together" (Strang, 2016). Furthermore, some participants link their connections with family and friends as an integral part of their motivation and legacy. Campbell, who has recently been cleared of Type 2 diabetes, claims: "I'm there to challenge myself and to inspire my children and mokos" (Stuff, 2016). Campbell's use of the word "mokos" is a reference to his grandchildren and his IronMāori participation serves as part of his legacy for future generations.

Whanaungatanga is a recurring theme throughout interviews of IronMāori participants. "We have our te reo (language) and our tikanga (customs and protocols), and if we're not healthy, we can't pass that on to our whānau (family)" (Marae, 2012, 04:20). Being part of a community coming together to enhance collective health and wellbeing provides positive emotions for participants and their supporters. "It was so incredible to be part of it. There's an amazing vibe, it's the whole whanaungatanga. I can't explain it but it becomes addictive because you're there as part of something" (Catherall, 2017). Uplifting Māori through enhancing collective health and wellbeing aligns to Te Au Skipworth's original intention of creating a team environment" (Strang, 2016). With various events across Aotearoa New Zealand, there are more opportunities to take part. For some, this may involve returning to their tribal land, reconnecting with their people, or, for others, making entirely new connections.

Along with mental, emotional and social wellbeing, spiritual wellbeing features as part of the IronMāori experience. In conceptualizing IronMāori, Te Au Skipworth's holistic motivation was about making a difference in people's lives, linking with Durie's concept of waiora, often seen as spiritual wellbeing. "That sense of achievement is what I wanted to pass on, so they [other IronMāori participants] can go off and be whatever they want to be in life" (Strang, 2016). According to Durie (2004), "waiora is linked more specifically to the natural world and includes a spiritual element connecting human wellness with cosmic, terrestrial and water environments" (p. 183). The air, water and earth are key elements of the events and associated activities in connection to spiritual wellbeing, while also underpinning holistic health. Pivoting from describing the orientation, history and IronMāori, we now move to critically exploring contradictions and coherences of wellbeing in this context.

5 Transformation

The genesis of IronMāori was born from Te Au Skipworth and friends' participation in Iron Man. The lack of Māori competitors at this Iron Man event combined with a concern for Māori health and wellbeing prompted them to generate an indigenous event both attractive and accessible to Māori. In this section we draw on William Sewell's (2005) theoretical notion of culture to consider IronMāori as cultural enactment in a social field. A social field "is constituted by structures, which are resources that afford cultural production and creation" (Tobin, 2012, pp. 5–6). Considering Iron Man as a social field, the sets of structures became resources in the production of the new field of IronMāori.

IronMāori is a space for the production of culture that generates multiple perspectives of wellbeing, encapsulated in multiple overlapping fields. In order to expand on our description of the event and movement and to show what is salient to the transformation of this wellbeing movement, we examine scenarios in which we illuminate key constructs that exemplify the transformative power of IronMāori. Building on Sewell's (2005) examination of historical events where he notes that "initially localized ruptures always have the potential of bringing about a cascading series of further ruptures that will result in structural transformations" (p. 228), we suggest that IronMāori has not really been "scrutinised as a theoretical category" (p. 225).

Previously we have discussed, through the words of Stretch, how she and her friends were immersed in heavy drinking and poor eating practices associated with challenging life circumstances. She related how participation in

IronMāori prompted shifts to wellbeing-focused goals that drove intentional changes in lifestyle and potentially different collective mindsets of wellbeing. The routine of heavy drinking and poor eating practices can be construed as an event. Events, according to Sewell (2005), can be thought of as "sequences of occurrences that result in transformations of structures. Such sequences begin with a rupture of some kind – that is, a surprising break with routine practice" (p. 227). In the example of Stretch, the break (or rupture) of routine prompted the transformation of structures shown through new wellbeing practices, such as sufficient sleep and healthy eating that enable participation in early morning training sessions.

Depending on where an IronMāori event is located, the host tribe tailor events based on their people's needs, including a range of age groups, various physical elements and local customs, protocols and tribal dialects. Simultaneously, these context-based divergent practices, when considered as a whole, contribute to what unifies people in the spirit of IronMāori. In considering each IronMāori event as a social field, structures emanating from tribe-based versions of the event become resources for action in events hosted by other tribes. Fields interpenetrate because they have no boundaries, therefore one field's structures become resources for action in other fields (Tobin & Ritchie, 2012). As seen in the different tribe-based IronMāori events, each new social field becomes a site for the production of practices with patterns of thin coherence and ever-present contradictions.

Individual events are nuanced for specific tribes yet retain the essence of IronMāori as patterns of thin coherence generated from the Māori worldview and principles of Māori ideology. At the same time, there are numerous ever-present contradictions as both an individual and collective event. The dialectical relationship between individual | collective (indicated by a Sheffer stroke) illustrates how each part informs and mediates the other to constitute the whole and in the case of IronMāori shows the transformation of event | movement.

Furthering this dialectical approach affords the application of multilectic lenses to reveal the complexity of relationships that may be simultaneously contradictory and coherent. Fellner (2014a) proposed the term multilectics to "value the intertwined relationship between multiple perspectives, lenses of perception, modes, meanings and voices" (p. 172). Moreover, IronMāori can be multilectically considered as an event | race | movement. The conception that IronMāori is composed of three potentially opposing constructs of an event, a race, and a movement is useful in showing complexities and polysemic and polyphonic characteristics of IronMāori.

6 Additional Thoughts

Holistic perspectives of wellbeing are generated and transformed throughout Aotearoa New Zealand. We have presented the case of IronMāori as an example of how an event | movement expanded opportunities for Māori and non-Māori to participate in a multisport event that is embedded within a Māori worldview. Prior to the arrival of Europeans to Aotearoa New Zealand, Māori had existing collective structures of health and wellbeing that meant as a people they were flourishing in areas such as language, health and wellbeing underpinned by a deep connection to the land. We argued that IronMāori is one example of cultural resurgence and transformation that provides opportunities for people, regardless of ethnicity, to embrace and use Māori language, customs and protocols.

Springboarding from an Iron Man event, we have shown how IronMāori has transformed to become a hybrid or interstitial space championing and enabling options of wellbeing as a way of life from birth to dying; "what the geographer Edward Soja might call a 'third space' or Homi Bhabha a space of 'hybridity'" (Fellner, 2014b, p. 1282). As Bhabha (1994) explains, "these 'in-between' spaces provide the terrain for elaborating strategies of selfhood – singular or communal – that initiate new signs of identity and innovative sites of collaboration" (p. 2). The power of IronMāori resides across multiple coexisting social and cultural fields, expanding possibilities for how we think about wellbeing, and how wellbeing is promoted through seemingly dichotomous structures with ever-present contradictions and thin coherences that lead to transformation of fields.

We envision the continued development and potential of Māori models and frameworks as embedded, practiced and lived across multiple fields and pathways. Intergenerational wellbeing structures and practices provide educative opportunities for the citizenry to individually | collectively flourish, now and into the future. The following whakataukī by Āpirana Ngata in 1949 captures the essence of how the founders through their experience of competing in Iron Man grew IronMāori to its current form as a multisport event and wellbeing movement.

> E tipu, e rea, mō ngā rā o tōu ao; ko tō ringa ki ngā rākau a te Pākehā hei ara mō te tinana, ko tō ngākau ki ngā taonga a ō tīpuna Māori hei tikitiki mō tō māhuna, ā, ko tō wairua ki te Atua, nāna nei ngā mea katoa.
>
> [Grow up, tender plant, to fulfil the needs of your world; your hand grasping the tools of the Pākehā for your physical needs, your heart centred on the treasures of your Māori ancestors as a plume for your head, and your soul to God who made all things.]

References

Ahuriri-Driscoll, A. (2019). Teaching but not preaching: Delivering compulsory Māori public health content in an undergraduate health science degree. *Pedagogy in Health Promotion, 5*(3), 190–198. https://doi.org/10.1177/2373379919863305

Ahuriri-Driscoll, A., & Boulton, A. (2019). Traditional healing and Indigenous wellbeing in Aotearoa New Zealand. In C. Fleming & M. Manning (Eds.), *Routledge handbook of indigenous wellbeing*. Routledge. https://doi.org/10.4324/9781351051262

Bhabha, H. (1994). *The location of culture*. Routledge.

Bryder, L., & Dow, D. A. (2001). Introduction: Māori health history, past present and future. *Health and History, 3*(1), 3–12.

Catherall, S. (2017, May 23). *How the Iron Māori event is changing lives*. Stuff. https://www.stuff.co.nz/life-style/well-good/inspire-me/92645709/how-the-iron-maori-event-is-changing-lives

Cram, F., Vette, M., Wilson, M., Vaithianathan, R., Maloney, T., & Baird, S. (2018). He awa whiria — braided rivers: Understanding the outcomes from Family Start for Māori. *Evaluation Matters — He Take Tō Te Aromatawai, 4*, 165–206. https://doi.org/10.18296/em.0033

Durie, M. (1994). *Te Whare Tapa Whā: Māori health model*. https://www.health.govt.nz/system/files/documents/pages/maori_health_moel_tewhare.pdf

Durie, M. (1999). Te Pae Māhutonga: A model for Māori health promotion. *Health Promotion Forum of New Zealand Newsletter, 49*. https://www.researchgate.net/publication/200830130_Te_Pae_Mahutonga_A_model_for_Maori_health_promotion

Durie, M. (2001, November 22). *Cultural competence and medical practice in New Zealand* [Paper presentation]. Australian and New Zealand Boards and Council Conference, Wellington, New Zealand.

Durie, M. (2004). An indigenous model of health promotion. *Health Promotion Journal of Australia, 15*(3), 181–185.

Durie, M., Hoskins, T., & Jones, A. (2012). Interview: Kaupapa Māori: Shifting the social. *New Zealand Journal of Educational Studies, 47*(2), 21–29.

Dussault, R., & Erasmus, G. (1996). *Report of the Royal Commission on Aboriginal Peoples*. Canada Royal Commission on Aboriginal Peoples, QSpace. http://hdl.handle.net/1974/6874

Fellner, G. (2014a). Broadening our lenses of perception to advance learning: An introduction to multilectics. *Teaching and Teacher Education, 37*, 169–182. http://doi.org/10.1016/j.tate.2013.04.015

Fellner, G. (2014b). Toward a broader dialectic: Joining Marxism with Mailer to forge a multilectics that advances teaching and learning. *International Journal of Qualitative Studies in Education, 27* (10), 1262–1284. https://doi.org/10.1080/09518398.2013.825346

Lange, R. (1999). *May the people live: A history of Māori health development 1990–1920*. Auckland University Press.

Macfarlane, A., Macfarlane, S., & Curtis, T. (2019). *Navigating Kaupapa Māori fields of knowledge*. Oxford University Press.

Marae. (2012, February 5). *Marae investigates: Māori of the year 2011* [Video]. YouTube. https://www.youtube.com/watch?v=QjXeC8Q_a9M

McClintock, K. (2018). Review of maea te toi ora: Māori health transformations. *Journal of Indigenous Wellbeing: Te Mauri-Pimatisiwin, 3*(1), 72–74.

McKenzie, T. (2014). *The challenges and opportunities of using mobile devices to attain Māori language proficiency* [Unpublished doctoral thesis]. Victoria University of Wellington.

Ministry for Culture and Heritage. (2020) *History of the Māori language*. https://nzhistory.govt.nz/culture/maori-language-week/history-of-the-maori-language

Ministry of Māori Development. (2003). *Te rautaki reo Māori: The Māori language strategy*. Te Puni Kōkiri.

Moewaka Barnes, H., & McCreanor, T. (2019). Colonisation, hauora and whenua in Aotearoa. *Journal of the Royal Society of New Zealand, 49*, 19–33. http://doi.org/10.1080/03036758.2019.1668439

Moorefield, J. C. (2003). *Te aka online Māori dictionary*. https://maoridictionary.co.nz

New Zealand Legal Information Institute. *Tohunga Suppression Act, 1907* (7 EDW VII 1907 No. 13). http://www.nzlii.org/nz/legis/hist_act/tsa19077ev1907n13353/

Pere, R. R., & Nicholson, N. (1991). *Te wheke: A celebration of infinite wisdom*. Ao Ako Global Learning.

Pitama, D., Ririnui, G., & Mikaere, A. (2002). Guardianship, custody and access: Māori perspectives and experiences. *Australian Indigenous Law Reporter, 7*(4), 80–89.

Pohatu, L. (2015). Iron Maori: *A Kaupapa Māori driven hauora initiative* [Unpublished doctoral dissertation]. University of Otago.

Royal, T. A. C. (2003). *The woven universe: Selected writings of Rev. Māori Marsden*. Printcraft.

Royal, T. A. C. (2005). *Pre-European society. Te ara: The encyclopedia of New Zealand*. http://www.TeAra.govt.nz/en/maori/page-2

Sewell, W. H., Jr. (2005). *Logics of history: Social theory and social transformation*. University of Chicago Press.

Simon, J., Smith, L. T., Cram, F., Hōhepa, M., McNaughton, S., & Stephenson, M. (2001). *A civilizing mission? Perceptions and representations of the New Zealand native schools system*. Auckland University Press.

Statistics New Zealand. (2013). *Results of a census of the colony of New Zealand taken for the night of 12th April 1896*. https://www3.stats.govt.nz/historic_publications/1896-census/1896-results-census/1896-results-census.html?_ga=2.113150212.1440165458.1592439358-918325131-1592439358

Strang, B. (2016, March 7) *Māori lives are being transformed thanks to work of IronMāori and Ironman NZ*. Stuff. https://www.stuff.co.nz/sport/other-sports/77592486/maori-lives-are-being-transformed-thanks-to-work-of-ironmaori-and-ironman-nz

Stuff. (2016, August 23) *IronMāori entrant says goodbye to diabetes, hello to better life.* https://www.stuff.co.nz/taranaki-daily-news/83464741/ironmaori-entrant-says-goodbye-to-diabetes-hello-to-better-life

Tobin, K. (2012). Sociocultural perspectives on science education. In B. Fraser, K. Tobin, & C. McRobbie (Eds.), *Second international handbook of science education* (SIHE Vol 24). Springer. https://doi.org/10.1007/978-1-4020-9041-7_1

Tobin, K., & Ritchie, S. M. (2012). Multi-method, multi-theoretical, multi-level research in the learning sciences. *Asia-Pacific Education Researcher, 21*(1), 117–129.

Treaty of Waitangi [English & Māori versions], February 6, 1840. https://archives.govt.nz/discover-our-stories/the-treaty-of-waitangi

Tūwharetoa Māori Trust Board. (2018, April 19). *IronMāori grass roots event - Lake Taupo* [Video]. YouTube. https://www.youtube.com/watch?v=ajMRXiHm4so

Walker, R. J. (1990). *Struggle without end: Ka whawhai tonu matou*. Penguin.

Walker, R. J. (1997). Māori identity and anthropology in New Zealand. *Mana, 3*(1), 169–178.

CHAPTER 8

An Afro-Caribbean Science Teacher's Quest for Healing

A Wellness Project

Theila Smith

Abstract

In this chapter, I present an autoethnographic account of my experiences as an Afro-Caribbean science teacher in one of New York City's public schools. Through event-oriented inquiry and narrative inquiry, I use hermeneutic phenomenology to investigate and explore my experiences. A central focus in these emergent and contingent narratives is the onslaught of emotions I encountered as a racialized "Other" in a majority White context. Emerging from my telling was the urge to embrace mindful breathing and other therapeutic techniques as a way to mitigate my emotions and set me on a path to wellness. A major implication of this chapter is the critical need for science teacher preparation and professional development programs to address wellness techniques and the emotional and physical wellbeing of teachers of color, Black teachers in particular, as a way to respond to their experienced stress and resulting health challenges, especially in racialized work settings.

Keywords

emotions – wellness – mindfulness – Afro-Caribbean – autoethnography

1 Identity, Emotions and Wellness

A salient part of undervalued teacher development is the teachers' emotions and wellbeing in performing their responsibilities inside and outside the classroom. I include responsibilities outside the classroom since teachers' professional duties do not just begin or end within the confines of the physical space. Powietrzynska, Tobin and Alexakos (2015) argue for mindfulness to be a prominent part of the curriculum in classrooms, science classrooms, in particular. Likewise, students are encouraged to develop a well-rounded repertoire

 | DOI:10.1163/9789004527348_008

of skills to mediate their world and lead productive lives. In helping students procure these skill sets, what are their teachers' roles in this process? How are teachers engaging with mindfulness to develop healthy minds and habits as professionals?

In teacher professional development, the focus is on performance targets similar to their students in mastering content knowledge. This emphasis is evident in the teacher performance targets in the Danielson Framework, teacher rating rubrics and calls for performance-based compensation (Cartel & Lochte, 2017).

Teachers' professional responsibilities extend beyond teaching and learning into the unseen labor of teacher duties that include committee work, sports and event-coordination, planning and preparation. In this chapter, I advocate for teachers' emotional wellbeing and overall wellness needs to be a priority in their professional development.

The foci of this chapter are grounded in the emotional state and wellness of teachers in science education, more specifically Black teachers in science classrooms. As teachers shape-shift to respond to the evolution of demands and duties of their positions, they experience varied emotional states that affect their mental and physical health (Tobin, Powietrzynska, & Alexakos, 2015). Mindfulness is a purposeful and in-the-moment construct that is sociocultural and multidimensional (Tobin, Powietrzynska, & Alexakos, 2015). The practice allows participants who engage in the exercise to be fully attentive to their affective and emotional states and learn to mediate these states. For the purpose of this chapter, the participants would be teachers, Black teachers specifically, engaging in this practice for their emotional, mental and physical health.

The four basic emotions often studied include fear, anger, sadness and happiness (Turner, 2009). The high intensity emotional energy that is experienced are borne out of feelings invoked and instigated during interactions. In the classroom the teacher and students may experience high-intensity fear and anger or low-intensity fear in the form of concern or apprehension and low-intensity anger in the form of irritation (Bellocchi et al., 2014). Our emotions and how we deal with them are not fixed; they are adaptable and dialogic, emergent and contingent in and from the interaction (Bakhtin et al., 1994).

Throughout this chapter, I describe the emotions I experienced in my interactions with students and colleagues in our shared spaces. I use the term "shared space" instead of the physical classroom because the emotion-derived experiences I have with my students are not held in suspension in some time warp only to be encountered in the physical space of the classroom. I experience them long after they have occurred. As teachers our professional lives are inextricably linked to our personal lives (Zembylas, 2002), and our teacher self is intertwined with our sense of self (Rivera Maulucci, 2013). Our sense of self and self-esteem are laid vulnerable to, and, therefore, mediated by our emotions (Zembylas, 2002). Lucy Avraamidou (2020) argues that the process of science identity development is emotionally arduous, especially for groups that are systemically underrepresented. Moreover, teacher identity is not stagnant or one-dimensional. Instead, in addition to being fluid and multidimensional, a person's science identity is forged and evolved within varied social and environmental contexts (Avraamidou, 2020).

In the social realm, our interactions with others mold our identity: how we view ourselves is in keeping with our interactions with others (Tobin & Llena, 2012). From a professional and environmental stance, a science teacher's identity is grounded in how we portray ourselves in our viewpoints, orientations, values, beliefs and knowledge of the subject matter and our actions within a particular context (Avraamidou, 2014). Identity, the process of becoming, is diachronic and is not constructed in a single given moment in time (Bakhtin et al., 1994). It is, rather, ceaseless in its mold across time, space and context.

My place and identity are strongly linked to being Afro-Caribbean, an immigrant in the US. As Stuart Hall (2019) has argued, identity is informed by our positioning: the way we are positioned and how we position ourselves in the stories of our histories. These different aspects of identity (for example, being an Afro-Caribbean woman and immigrant) have colored my experiences and have been critical in informing my emotions and professional life in and out of the classroom. My focus on my identity as an Afro-Caribbean woman in the US allows for a nuanced exploration of the cultural and racial components in the discussion on emotions and wellness.

With this chapter I intend to further expand on the existing literature in science teaching and learning that raises the criticality for teachers to have opportunities to learn how to engage with and ameliorate their emotions with the overall intent of improving their wellbeing through wellness practices such as mindfulness. Another implication of this study is to shed light on how the emphasis on emotions and wellness can help stem the attrition of teachers of color from the science education profession, especially Black teachers from diverse cultural backgrounds.

1.1 *Methodology*

I adopt a hermeneutic phenomenological framework for this study. As Konstantinos Alexakos (2015) argues, the hermeneutic phenomenological research framework encompasses "a bricolage of methods and methodologies in doing inquiry to explore" and unpack "our lived experiences" (p. 32). Our lived experiences, he continues, are informed by historically- and socially-situated contexts and the interactions we encounter in these places (Alexakos, 2015).

Autoethnography serves as a positive response to critiques of the traditional canon of what research is and should be. This methodology acknowledges and accommodates subjectivity, emotionality, and the researcher's influence on research, rather than hiding from these matters or assuming that they do not exist (Ellis, Adams & Turner, 2011). How best can I express the nuances of teaching? Autoethnography provides an answer to this question. It allows the researcher to share stories that readers can connect to and broaden their own understanding or gain insight. A strong critique of autoethnography is its ability to provide generalizability and validity in research. Critics of the methodology argue from a positivistic stance where the subject is separated from the research. However, as Ellis, Adams and Turner (2011) have countered, the reader provides validation as they read and connect with stories. These stories elicit more than relatability but provide continuity as they bring to light cultural practices that may be relevant to the wider society. Furthermore, to echo Tobin's (2000) position on generalizability in ethnographic studies, the purpose in my pursuit is interpretive and the aim is to find out what happened and why it happened from a perspective of one: my own lived experience.

Thus, in addition to the use of autoethnography account, I employ Tobin and Ritchie's methodology of event-oriented inquiry to allow for the emergent and contingent around "what is happening, why is it happening, and how changes might be made to afford positive, collective and individual changes" (Tobin, 2015, p. 3). Working with multiple forms of inquiry affords thicker descriptions of what is happening and broadens the scope on why it is happening. The interpretation I deduce from the what and why will be knowledge gained in the body of research on how to improve science teaching and learning.

On top of event-oriented inquiry, I also employ Jean Clandinin and Michael Connelly's (1996) narrative inquiry. Narrative inquiry allows for the researcher to paint a picture as we move from different frames. One frame is our "work in the field," then we move to our second frame, "… from the field to field text." Field texts are our recollections of what happened in the field. Sequentially, we move from the third frame of the recollections of what happened in the field to the final frame of moving "… from field text to research text" (p. 60). In moving to the third frame we are interpreting, analyzing and theorizing as researchers of what happened in the field. Moving between these frames is not a linear but cyclical process as these frames afford us, the researchers, a three-dimensional frame to look "inward, backward, and forward within a situated in place" (p. 49) across space and time (Clandinin & Connelly, 1996).

In the coming sections, I share narratives by describing particular events that occurred during the span of time I spent as one of few Black teachers and Afro-Caribbeans on staff at a middle school in one of the more affluent neighborhoods in Brooklyn, New York. In keeping with the adopted frameworks, I use autoethnography, event-oriented inquiry and narrative inquiry as methodologies to share my experiences. To draw on these inquiries, I include email correspondences and stories to capture significant events of my time at the school and shed light on the varying emotions I experienced and how I strove for wellness over the course of time. The identifiers in the emails and stories have been changed to maintain anonymity.

1.2 *Brief Pause*

> *Where does it hurt? In my inner soul, my inner being like ... What does it feel like? It feels like a fractioning of who I am: a loss of my self-confidence and self-worth and like feeling less than. Right. That's what feeling less than brings about: pain. Because you are experiencing this pain that you're going through, this, like onslaught of not being enough in the space you are. The pain of never being enough, right? Never being enough in the space and always trying to prove otherwise. [You feel as if you are an interloper] working hard to prove that you belong. In this space. In this space not only a teacher, but as a science teacher. Always proving that you are, proving that I am capable of doing it. I am doing it. And, also, trying to prove that I should be accepted. Right. So always like this. So that's what I wanted to convey, that this: trying to prove your worth all the time. So, I belong here, so I need to prove to you that I belong here, and I need other students to know that they need to prove to the world that they belong there too.*

Wow ... it is more difficult than I thought. The above epigraph was shared in one of the research squad meetings. I was encouraged to follow the feeling and say how I felt about my experiences and what I wanted to convey in this chapter. Initially, I had started writing the reflections that are to follow in the coming sections of the paper on a long bus ride from Virginia to Washington D.C. I was on my way back from a conference hosted by the Science Education, Equity, Diversity and Social Justice (SEEDS). I was amped from the conference and more motivated than ever to share these narratives. My story could offer insight for new teachers on how to mitigate their emotions and ensure their wellbeing, especially in contexts that are racialized and oppressive to their humanity. In the words of Hall (2019), I was excavating and unearthing the overlaid, hidden and suppressed. But sharing was not easy. I realized quickly that writing these reflections was more than letting the words flow. I was reminded of Leah Pride (2018) who shared quite candidly the jarring process of writing her dissertation and of how she cried and wrote and cried and wrote (Pride, personal communication, July 16, 2019). Her tears became the ink in her pen as she wrote about her experiences as a woman of color, a scientist and a science educator (Pride, 2018).

2 The Events That Led to Inquiry

In the coming sections, against the backdrop of varied encounters in different instances in my time as science teacher in a predominantly white teaching staff and student body, I discuss the need for attention on emotions and wellness for Black teachers and by extension their Black students. My experience becomes racialized through my embodiment of Blackness and Caribbean-ness in the white culture that undergirded the school environment.

2.1 *The Token Other*

The following is an email response I wrote to a former classmate from our Master of Arts in Teaching (MAT) degree program. I wrote and sent this email when I was in my first year of teaching.

> They had me come in to teach the last day of school to do my demo lesson, and they hired me. I heard they said they liked my spirit ... whatever that means. *But it has been hard Jay. I never realized working in the professional realm can be so emotionally draining. I love teaching the kids. Jay, I am one of three black women in the school and the only Caribbean nationality on the teaching staff. The two paras are of Caribbean descent. This was my biggest hurdle to get over. There were some days I felt lonely, and I didn't like the feeling. And one morning I cried in the shower when I realized how isolated I was feeling.* BUT I am coping and allowing myself to be open to change and stepping out of my comfort zone, timidly of course. Also, it is a great school, and the kids are amazing.

I felt tokenized. I felt I was a token hire and would spend the next four years proving to myself and everyone else that I was more than qualified for my job. Ironically, among the new hires that year when I joined the staff, I was hired after doing a panel interview, a demonstration lesson and a debrief and follow-up interview after the lesson on the last day of the school year. Another new hire that year, a young White woman, also a newly minted teacher, was invited to join the teaching staff after only one interview. No demo lessons. No follow-up interviews. And *I am the one who* felt like a token hire!

The feeling of having to prove myself was mired in how Black and other bodies of color and intellect are scrutinized in professional settings, education and the classroom notwithstanding. There is a hyper-visibility and invisibility that goes with being a Black body in a predominantly White space. My very presence was an intrusion that disrupted the normal that underpins the culture of whiteness in the classroom and larger school environment (Yancy, 2014).

It was important for me to have other Black teachers and Caribbean teachers for support. An affinity group to be exact. This having been an underlying tension throughout my experience in the US. I needed these spaces and opportunities. In my undergraduate and graduate studies, I had these spaces and friendships, and I drew on them as a source of strength to persist. Alexakos (2011) argues that fictive kinship groups (close personal friendships similar to familiar ties, like calling each other brother or sister) provide the positive emotional feedback and an environment that fosters successful coping skills, perseverance and resilience among the group members. Having the affinity group was not a singular experience. The support such kinships provided was an undercurrent in my experience throughout my undergraduate and graduate programs. I could depend on this community of Black women for emotional support and relief, especially considering the fact that these programs did not boast a large representation of Black women. Although we were small in numbers, our solidarity fortified our resilience and resolve to persevere. For me, to be working as a teacher and be one of very few Black people on staff rang loudly that the school was not my place. I felt a sense of loneliness that sapped my energy. I needed to remain resolute and not break under the gaze of others. However, to conjure up that inner strength day in and day out left me emotionally and mentally tired.

2.2 *The Myth of Meritocracy: Stinkin' Thinking*

The following excerpt is an email I sent two of my teaching colleagues following a book club meeting. We were reading Beverly Daniel Tatum's (1997) seminal book on the psychology of racism in schools, *Why are all the Black kids sitting together in the cafeteria? And other conversations about race*. In the meeting, I had spoken about two separate encounters with two Black students I taught. After being called out by a couple of the other teachers, I reflected on how I, as a Black teacher, engendered micro-aggression and micro-violence against other Black students.

> So, yesterday, I was all micro-aggressing: Calling Axel loud and telling a 12-year-old child to stop being who she is. I have to reread it myself (for

> obvious reasons), but the article talked about how black girls in schools are subjected to middle-class whiteness as the "correct way of being" And Much More. Signithia Fordham (1993) wrote a book about the concept as well.

Joyce Meyers is a preacher, author and founder of Joyce Meyer Ministries. She uses the phrase, "stinkin' thinking" quite often in her sermons on getting your mind right and living a God-fearing life. She would admonish the audience, including those tuning in on television or the internet, to change the way they thought in order to have a better life. I listened to Joyce Meyers religiously during my undergraduate years. She had a sermon series on "Excellence and Changing Your Mind." The ideas of digging deep and pushing on came from many of her sermons coupled with my own upbringing. Dig deep. Change your mind. Unfortunately, I brought these very shame-laden mantras into the classroom. My students of color, especially the Black girls in the room, would feel that pressure of pushing the envelope and challenging their thinking. The pressure on girls of color, Black girls, being one of the few in the room, afraid to make a mistake, would opt to remain silent and not participate because the pressure of getting the answer wrong is too great a burden to even attempt a response. Responding carries too great a responsibility should you get the answer incorrect and reflect poorly for an entire Black community.

These sentiments were not foreign to me. I felt this way in most of the science courses I took as an undergraduate student in the US. And, worse, my middle school Black students experienced it. The diversity committee, at the school, had launched an affinity group-type club called Pretty Brown Girls[1] for Black and Brown girls at school. In our first meeting, some of the eighth-grade girls, whom I had taught the previous year, shared how much they felt this burden of their actions, especially their academic performance, reflecting negatively on the Black community. These girls were 13 going on 14 years old. They had not even begun to realize their full potential and were already plagued by this deficit-oriented perspective. Upon hearing this I was shocked, angry and embarrassed. I was angry that the girls, so young, carried such a burden; I was embarrassed and angry at myself for also perpetuating this myth of meritocracy in my classroom. Frazetto (2013) describes anger as fear cloaked in armor. Anger is a spontaneous or a slow-seething defense that is there to protect the self from any offense or ill-will. The fear and anger arise when we need to defend ourselves against something or avoid it. However, when anger is reflected to oneself, we feel guilt. Guilt arises when we have brought harm to someone else; it is our moral compass. Guilt arouses shame. The shame of disgust with oneself, feeling inferior and unworthy (Frazetto, 2013). I was well aware that I had been unfair to my Black students, especially the Black girls. In the name of good intention, I was stricter and demanded more of them. They were not happy nor was I. Looking back, I feel I had created a miserable and unsafe class environment for the very students I had desired to support.

In their article on "Mindfulness and discussing "thorny" issues in the classroom," the authors in citing Zembylas' work on "grievability and vulnerability," caution that in being aware of our responsibilities as educators is that there are also shared responsibilities, although asymmetrical, in who is being victimized versus who is the victimizer (Alexakos et al., 2016, p. 746). Based on how we negotiate the self | other dialectic, there are multiple ontologies. What emerges from these multiple ways of enacting, one can be under duress, experiencing violence, from systematic oppression whilst simultaneously being an offender. For my students and I, the Black students especially, we occupied two sides of the same coin in this racialized stew of wanting to and pushing to be better to counter the narrative that Black women and girls are not as successful in science as their White peers.

Fortunately, I had the opportunity to apologize to some of these Black girls. Expressing my sincerest apology was the best way, I thought to make my students aware that this behavior is absolutely wrong, and they should be celebrated as who they are. In the name of high expectation, I had created an atmosphere where I pushed my students to strive for values that were not entirely their own instead of celebrating what they had to bring to the lesson. They were more than enough. Steele (2010), in his seminal work on stereotype threat, argued that for Black students, the need to prove or disprove the stereotype of having less cognitive abilities than their counterparts in class engage in what is described as "over-efforting." What the students aced was persistence: they persisted and tried twice as hard to disprove the negative label reinforcing the old adage "Black people have to work twice as hard to prove themselves as worthy." What Steele (2010) and his fellow researchers found was that when students were under stereotype threat, the pressure increased to disprove the negative stereotype about their intellectual abilities compared to their White classmates.

2.3 *Wellness and Teaching: "Something's Gotta Give"*

I was feeling this state of being out of control. No matter how much I would dig my heels in and persevere, I still felt unsatisfied with the progress I had made as a teacher and the general state of affairs of the Black children in the school community. I felt as if I were running in place without making any progress: I was running faster and faster but felt stuck in the same place. I was experiencing the Red Queen effect. This hearkens back to the famous story of Charles Lutwidge Dodgson's (pseudonym Lewis Carroll) (1865) *Adventures of Alice's*

Adventures in Wonderland's Red Queen Effect analogy used in biology textbooks to discuss the human fight against bacteria and viruses. Scientists are tackling a major battle where bacteria and viruses are evolving into stronger strains that are resisting our strongest synthetic drugs. This is how I felt: I was stuck.

We had come a long way as a school community. The administration was committed to overhauling the admission policies and disrupting long-standing inequalities in our school. But I felt like I still had to push. I was fighting an inner demon that was engulfing me. I saw the inequalities in performance in my classroom along racial lines. There were very few Black students in the general education classes where the higher performing students were grouped with one teacher compared to their greater numbers in the classes that were co-taught and had more students with Individualized Education Plans (IEPs), a characteristic of special education classes. I raise this point not to belittle the importance of coteaching and the need for some children to have a community that supports their academic growth. On the contrary, in the US, Black and Brown students are under-represented in gifted or honors programs, but are overly represented in special education classes compared to their White counterparts, a striking evidence of inequality in education (Ford, 2012).

In my second year, the school's administration had procured the services of a racial diversity training organization for a year-long diversity training with the staff. It was a grueling process. The following year, the school hired more staff members of color and committed to reshaping the admission policies and prepared plans to offer algebra regents to all students. Even with a more diverse staff and commitment to racial diversity, I still lacked a sense of wholly belonging.

I was working harder but I was crashing. I had over-committed to too many things. I was spending longer hours at school and my emotional, mental and physical health were in turmoil. The last two years of teaching at the school, I was rarely without a cold. Yet, out of those four academic years, I took two sick days: once when I had strep throat in my fourth (and to be the final year) and in my first year when I left half a day early because I was too ill to continue teaching and remain at work.

I felt like I was drowning …

> I was alone in the classroom; the building was deserted. The afterschool staff had left, and the custodian had already cleaned my side of the classroom. I could not breathe. That's how it felt. I was inhaling as deep as I could, trying to fill my lungs to its greatest capacity but instead, my chest felt tight like it would burst open. I could not breathe. My mind raced. Calm. Down. Breathe. I flung open both of the classroom's doors, pushed

up the two windows that could actually be opened and unhooked my brassiere. I needed to breathe. To fill my lungs with air. I was having my first panic attack. At the time, I did not know it. I was scared. What was going on? My family's health history was one riddled with all types of lifestyle-related illnesses, hypertension being the most common. Both my maternal and paternal grandfathers had passed away as a result of a heart attack. Was some family trait of poor heart health finally presenting itself?

I would have more of these episodes over the course of the first half of the school year. I was in my fourth year of teaching.

I had one on the way to a Professional Development in the Bronx. Because of this one, I had stopped taking the express train and rode the local line that had more stops and more chances of escaping to safety and fresh air if I needed to. The packed number 4 train during rush hour had stopped in between stations. A wave of panic overcame me as I could not breathe and felt like I was suffocating in the packed car. I remember craning my neck above much of the other people's heads to try to breathe in big gulps of air. As soon as the car had pulled into the station, I bolted for what felt like safety on dry land. I remember how helpless I felt. I texted my friend to share what had happened to me. He tried to reassure me that everything would be all right. I just felt helpless. I sat on one of the benches on the platform to collect myself. Once I felt like I could breathe normally, without strain, I got on the next train that was not as crowded. I sat there scared and feeling out of control. I sat in that car, breathing deeply, tears streaming down my face as the train rolled out of the station heading to the Bronx.

2.4 *Meditation and Yoga: "The Tipping Point"*[2]

As a student in the Adolescent Science Education program at Brooklyn College (CUNY), our advisor had challenged the way we thought about educating our students and cared for our health as educators through his use of mindfulness in the classroom and focus on coteaching experiences. In most of the graduate classes, we practiced several minutes of mindful breathing before class began. I used the word "challenge," as my Pentecostal Christian upbringing had cautioned me to avoid meditation and yoga practices which were perceived as conforming to Buddhism. In those early days of classes, I would join in the practice and quieten the admonitory inner thoughts that I was shunning the third commandment: *Thou shalt have no other gods before me*, Exodus 20:3, KJV.

Regardless of my religious reservations, I was aware that being mindful of my emotions, or even, my breathing was a skill to develop in my teaching practice. As part of the course requirement, we also attended the monthly

Urban Science Education Research Seminars (USER-S) at the Graduate Centre (CUNY). At those meetings, I would learn more about the importance of mindfulness in education. I vividly recall a speaker, at one of the seminars, had shared how he was mindfully walking on his way to USER-S that morning. He continued to explain how he developed the practice of being mindful over time. He would let thoughts in and let them go, allowing himself to freely let go in those moments of deep breathing. He then led the seminar attendees in a few minutes of mindful breathing. These experiences were not my only introduction to mindfulness practices. One of my first-year coteachers, also a longtime participant at USER-S, practiced mindfulness in the classroom and some days would take out her chime bowl and lead the students in quiet meditation.

These foundation years of dabbling in mindful breathing and meditative practices were to become my cornerstone rituals for surviving during my fourth year of teaching. At first, I would try it on my own but felt my thoughts would wander too much. I then tried different meditative YouTube videos until I settled on meditations by The Honest Guys (2014). This became a ritual. "Rituals are constructed from a combination of ingredients that grow to differing levels of intensity" (Collins, 2004, p. 47) that leads to "outcomes of solidarity, symbolism and individual emotional energy" (Collins, 2004, p. 47). My ritual was to begin my day with five minutes of meditation and five minutes of gentle yoga. Gradually, I increased my time to 10 minutes of meditation and 15 to 30 minutes of yoga. I engaged in these two practices not as a fad but for my survival. There were some days at school when I needed those five minutes. Moments when I experienced high-intense emotions, I would gather my necessities: my yoga mat, cell phone, earphones. Crouched down in between cupboards and carton boxes full of science supplies, for those five minutes, I sat, listened and breathed deeply.

In my earlier years of teaching, I had other ways of coping. I would listen to India Arie's, "Strength, Courage and Wisdom" on repeat or a gospel music mix on those more difficult days. For Afro-Caribbeans and African Americans, religion and spirituality are the more likely options for dealing with stressful situations than seeking mental services (Chatters et al., 2008). Older adults in these demographics are especially resistant to choosing these services and are more likely to opt for prayer and speaking with their pastors to cope with stress rather than pursuing mental services. I had been praying, listening to gospel music and sermons. However, I felt like I was only avoiding dealing with the underlying issues. My immunity needed a complete overhaul.

2.5 *Therapy and Acupuncture*

I had reached out to my therapist as early back in 2016 after a friend referred her to me. I had contacted other therapists over the summer but was not too interested. They were not who I was looking for: I wanted to work with a Black woman, preferably Caribbean. She fulfilled both criteria. However, I learnt that she did not take my insurance and I tabled the idea to see a therapist. Fast-forward to the following school year. I knew something had to be done. I was teaching other people's children (an ode to Lisa Delpit's book, *Other People's Children*). I felt like I was losing the handle on my sanity. I searched my email inbox for her number and called her outside the school building during one of the breaks. I was near panic because I thought I was having a psychotic episode. So much so I was willing to pay out of pocket to see her. My first session with her was on October 10, 2017.

> *Hi Theila,*
>
> *Thank you for your interest in my practice. I can meet with you to discuss the possibility of working together; however, my office days are Tuesday, Thursday and Friday. At this time, I have openings at 6 pm and 7 pm on Thursday and 6:45 pm on Friday, and before 4 pm on Tuesday and Thursday. Please let me know if any works for you.*

My therapist engages in psychoanalytic therapy which has major benefits. However, it is a slower process compared to cognitive behavioral therapy. I was functional at work and that is what I needed. My emotions were still raw although I was not as scared as I was before. One of the things therapy does is stir up (*unwanted*) emotions and memories. The kinds that had been neatly and tightly wrapped and tucked away deep in the unconscious. I then decided to seek out another method: acupuncture. To my therapist's annoyance, I decided to go to acupuncture to help ease the sadness and pain I felt from some of the sessions. Apparently, you are supposed to work through them to offer you release. I was adamant that the process of working through was much more than I could handle, and I needed something else to numb the pain. Acupuncture seemed like the safest alternative.

I remember after my first acupuncture session when I stepped outside the building, breathing in the cold air, I realized my sinuses and nasal passage were clear. It had not occurred to me all day that I was congested. I inhaled a deep-lung-filling gulp of air. Standing there in the cold that late winter evening, I breathed in the frigid air that felt like it filled my entire body. I breathed in deep gulps as if I were without air for a long time. Upon reflection, this experience might have been a metaphor. I was hitting the reset button for a more mentally-well chapter in my life. In that same session, during the in-take process, when my prospective acupuncturist asked what I wanted to work on, I replied without hesitation: my anger. In those successive sessions, I was able to let go of all the built-up anxiety and frustration from that day and the week.

I would liken this experience to a slow pressure release as I mindfully let go of all the lingering thoughts and emotions for that hour.

2.6 *Others' Stories*

Among the myriad of emotions, I was experiencing that year, I also felt a deep sense of shame. Frazetto (2013) argues that shame, a deeply-ingrained emotion conjures up feelings of unworthiness, inferiority, and inadequacy. So, why was I feeling this sense of shame?

I do not have a clear answer. However, I do know I felt like I was failing and was worried all the time others could see through my façade. I, the imposter, was always on the brink of becoming exposed. In her dissertation, Pride (2018) writes descriptively about imposter syndrome, giving it a persona of double consciousness,[3] the 'other' who wants you to remain invisible and be left mired in obscurity, fear and doubt. She describes imposter syndrome as a debilitating state of emotional, psychological and physical duress that kept her emotionally imprisoned, enslaved, "bound and restricted to fear and shame" (p. 4). The imagery captures so palpably the tokenized imposter that shackled me: that is, fear. The one that immobilizes and renders us powerless. The emotional state of fear, the most intense and briefest disrupter to social life, what Collins (2004) describes as an emotional response of "one being coerced or excluded" (p. 129). I was suffering in silence and sometimes it was deafening.

In her chapter on mindfully discussing race, privilege and social justice, Pride takes her readers through a breathing technique to help them mindfully process the intense emotions transferred from writer to audience (Pride, 2018). Here, I too invite readers to pause and take a deep breath.

> *Take a deep breath in through your nose and exhale out through your mouth. Inhale in, exhale out.*

Collins (2004) discusses that emotions are necessary in the build-up that led to some form of solidarity and emotional entrainment. "The emotional-laden cognitions that become ingredients for the upcoming encounter, feelings of membership and solidarity" (Collins, p. 105). The crucial emotional ingredient for me was fear that linked my experience to others' stories and created feelings of solidarity. I began reading the blog posts of the *Anxious Brother*, a fellow Brooklynite, who shared quite vividly about his experiences with anxiety and mental illness. I felt his raw emotions as he opened wounds and extreme pain in the cathartic writing process. I read teacher blogs that talked about anxiety or burnout. I read anything that would give me insight as to what I was experiencing and feel a part of a community.

I once came across an inspiring blog post in *Mrs. D's corner*, a teacher blog that offered lesson ideas and other discussion topics. The blogger detailed how she had to take a break from teaching *to recover from teaching*. Reading her blog post on the train ride to work that morning was an inspiration (the emphasis in bold was in the original article):

> Teaching is tough, and it's okay to take a step backwards. Your decision to leave your current teaching position does *not* define you. Your struggles do *not* define you. Your anxiety or depression does *not* define you. Your decisions to take care of yourself first do *not* define you. Teaching does *not* define you, and neither does your classroom. (Delussey, 2018)

I did not return to the classroom in the following school year. However, I did not leave education, all together. Instead, I am pursuing a doctoral degree at the University of Groningen in the Netherlands. And, I am still teaching in some capacity: I have taught a summer course at Brooklyn College for the past two summers and I work with young children as part of my research project, a Saturday STEAM-enriched program called Roots: "Ik Ben Science." My main focus group in Roots is Afro-Dutch Caribbean children. A similar deficit discourse serves as the backdrop to the academic performance and career aspirations for the Dutch Caribbean community in the Netherlands, particularly in the sciences. For me as a student researcher, I want to center their resilience and aspirations. I, also, want to learn about their love for science and share mine; to explore their interactions and positioning not from a reference point of where they are less than, but more so, what they bring to and impart with others in the space. As for me, I am unclear of where I will plant roots next, but similar to the experience I hope to create in the program, it will be a place where my personhood and humanity are valued and respected.

2.7 *Resetting the Path to Wellness*

> Dear Black Teacher,
>
> Reclaim your true essence. You are more than enough. You are born with a purpose on this earth and you matter. You bring all of yourself to your profession and that is more than enough. You matter and belong in the spaces you choose to lay a foundation. You deserve to be your full self in your profession.
>
> Reclaim the fear and let it become what empowers you. Caste away all your fears and embrace a spirit of love, power and a sound mind. Once

you can move beyond fear and harness the power within you, you can move boldly forward.

Reclaim your humanity. You deserve to be healthy. Mindfully engage with your emotional, psychological, physical and mental wellbeing. If it works for you, practice daily affirmations, meditation and deep breathing. Find what works for you. Find a path to your over-all wellbeing because you are worth it.

In Solidarity,

An Afro-Caribbean Science Teacher

Acknowledgements

I want to thank Konstantinos Alexakos and the members of the research squad for their peer revisions and input. Thank you for pushing me to write. This chapter was made possible through partial support from the 2019 ESERA Travel Award (the European Science Education Research Association).

Notes

1 I want to thank Mariatere Tapias-Avery, a member of the research squad, for making a salient point by asking the question: "What does it mean to be a pretty brown girl?" Does this mean if a child falls outside the narrow definition of what is considered beautiful in the American context, then they are socially ousted from this affinity group?

2 The part of the title "The Tipping Point" is taken from Michael Gladwell's book published by Little, Brown and Company in 2000 and 2002 titled *The Tipping Point: How Little Things Can Make a Big Difference.*

3 W.E.B. Du Bois introduced the term "double consciousness" in his famous book titled *The souls of Black folk* re-published by Dover publications, New York.

References

Alexakos, K., Jones, J. K., & Rodriguez, V. H. (2011). Fictive kinship as it mediates learning, resiliency, perseverance, and social learning of inner-city high school students of color in a college physics class. *Cultural Studies of Science Education,* 6, 847–870. https://doi.org/10.1007/s11422-011-9317-7

Alexakos, K. (2015). *Being a teacher | researcher: A primer on doing authentic inquiry research on teaching and learning.* Sense. https://doi.org/10/1007/978-94-6300-295-0

Avraamidou, L. (2014). Tracing a beginning elementary teacher's development of identity for science teaching. *Journal of Teacher Education, 65*(3), 223–240. https://doi-org.proxy-ub.rug.nl/10.1177/0022487113519476

Avraamidou, L. (2019). Science identity as a landscape of becoming: Rethinking recognition and emotions through an intersectionality lens. *Cultural Studies of Science Education, 15*(2), 323–345. https://doi.org/10.1007/s11422-019-09954-7

Bakhtin, M. M., Voloshinov, V. N., Medvedev, P. N., & Morris, P. (1994). *The Bakhtin reader: Selected writings of Bakhtin, Medvedev, and Voloshinov.* Edward Arnold.

Bellocchi, A., Ritchie, S. M., Tobin, K., King, D., Sandhu, M., & Henderson, S. (2014). Emotional climate and high-quality learning experiences in science teacher education. *Journal of Research in Science Teaching, 51*(10), 1301–1325.

Carter, J. H., & Lochte, H. A. (2017). Teacher blame and corporate gain: edTPA and the takeover of teacher education. In J. H. Carter & H. A. Lochte (Eds.), *Teacher performance assessment and accountability reforms: The impacts of edTPA on teaching and schools* (pp. 7–24). Palgrave Macmillan. https://doi.org/10.1057/978-1-137-56000-1

Chatters, L. M., Taylor, R. J., Jackson, J. S., & Lincoln, K. D. (2008). Religious coping among African Americans, Caribbean Blacks and non-Hispanic Whites. *Journal of Community Psychology, 36*(3), 371–386.

Clandinin, J. D., & Connelly, M. F. (1996). Teachers' professional knowledge landscape: Teacher stories. Stories of teachers. School stories. Stories of schools. *Educational Researcher, 25*(3), 24–30.

Collins, R. (2004). *Interaction ritual chains.* Princeton University Press.

Delussey, S. (2018, May 11). How taking a year off made me a better teacher. *Mrs. D's Corner.* https://www.mrsdscorner.com/takingayearoff/

Ellis, C., Adams, T. E., & Bochner, A. P. (2011). Autoethnography: An overview. *Historical Social Research, 36*(4), 273–290.

Ford, D. Y. (2012). Culturally different students in special education: looking backward to move forward. *Exceptional Children, 78*(4), 391–405.

Fordham, S. (1993). "Those loud black girls": (Black) women, silence, and gender "passing" in the academy. *Anthropology & Education Quarterly, 24*(1), 3–32.

Gladwell, M. (2002). *The tipping point: How little things can make a big difference.* Little, Brown and Company. (Original work published 2000)

Hall, S. (2019). *Essential essays* (D. Morley, Ed.) (Vol. 2, Identity and Diaspora/ Ser. Stuart Hall, selected writings). Duke University Press.

Powietrzynska, M., Tobin, K., & Alexakos, K. (2015). Facing the grand challenges through heuristics and mindfulness. *Cultural Studies of Science Education, 10*(1), 65–81. https://doi.org/10.1007/s11422-014-9588-x

Pride, L. D. (2018). *Using authentic inquiry to unpack emotions and thorny issues within teaching and learning* [Doctoral dissertation, The Graduate Center, CUNY]. CUNYAcademicWorks. https://academicworks.cuny.edu/gc_etds/2717

Rivera Maulucci, M. S. (2013). Emotions and positional identity in becoming a social justice science teacher: Nicole's story. *Journal of Research in Science Teaching, 50*(4), 453–478. https://doi.org/10.1002/tea.21081

Steele, C. (2010). *Whistling Vivaldi and other clues to how stereotypes affect us.* W.W. Norton.

The Honest Guys. (2014, October 7). *5 Minute calming meditation (with guided voice)* [Video]. YouTube. https://www.youtube.com/watch?v=i50ZAs7v9es

Tobin, K. (2000). Repetition, difference, and rising up with research in education. In K. Ercikan & W.-M. Roth (Eds.), *Generalizing from educational research: Beyond qualitative and quantitative polarization* (pp. 151–172). Routledge.

Tobin, K. (2013). A sociocultural approach to science education. MAGIS. *Revista Internacional de Investigacion en Educacion, 6*(11), 19–25.

Tobin, K. (2015). Connecting science education to a world in crisis. *Asia-Pacific Science Education, 1*(2), 1–21. https://doi.org/10.1186/s41029-015-0003-z

Tobin, K., Alexakos, K., Malyukova, A., & Gangji, A. K. H. (2017). Jin Shin Jyutsu and ameliorating emotion, enhancing mindfulness, and sustaining productive learning environments. In A. Bellochi, C. Quigley, & K. Otrel-Cass (Eds.), *Exploring emotions, aesthetics and wellbeing in science education research* (pp. 221–247). Springer.

Tobin, K., & Llena, R. (2012). Colliding identities, emotional roller coasters, and contradictions of urban science education. In M. Varelas (Ed.), *Identity construction and science education research: Learning, Teaching, and being in multiple contexts* (pp. 141–156). Sense Publishers.

Tobin, K., Powietrzynska, M., & Alexakos, K. (2015). Mindfulness and wellness: Central components of a science of learning. *Innovación Educativa, 15*(67), 61–87.

Whiting, D. (2011). The feeling theory of emotion and the object-directed emotions. *European Journal of Philosophy, 19*(2), 281–303.

Yancy, G. (2014). White crisis and the value of losing one's way. In G. Yancy & M. del Guadalupe Davidson (Eds.), *Exploring race in predominantly white classrooms: Scholars of color reflect* (pp. 1–16). Taylor & Francis.

Zembylas, M. (2002). Constructing genealogies of teachers' emotions in science teaching. *Journal of Research in Science Teaching, 39*(1), 79–103.

CHAPTER 9

Transforming African American Cultural Identity through Dance as a Wellness Practice

An Autoethnographic Movement of Self-Recovery

Francie Johnson

Abstract

I am African American. A product of my ancestors brought to the United States, infused with a mixture of bloodlines (African, European, Native American, others?), acclimated in a culture that favors white, upper- and middle-class males, that suppresses my blackness and encourages separation from other African Americans by being classified as exceptional and successful. To function on a daily basis, I assimilated to the dominant value system while negating my African heritage, while at the same time wanting to be proud of who I am. These feelings of anxiety and self-doubt from this internalized racism assault my sense of cultural identity and wellbeing. Realizing that this conflict could lead to self-destructive practices, I sought to change myself. This autoethnography explores my transformative process of using dance and entrainment to reaffirm the value of being African American while combating the negative emotional effects of racism.

Keywords

cultural identity – African American – dance – racism

1 Self-Introduction

Sitting in a circle, I ask my high school dance class: What is culture? Students give numerous answers including food, clothes, customs, traditions, and geographic location. I then ask them, "What is your culture?" Their responses are where they live or what country they are from. A few students say they are from the boroughs of New York City, while others state where their parents came from. I nod, silently acknowledging the importance of national origin in culture.

 | DOI:10.1163/9789004527348_009

> "Where are you from Miss, "asks the 9th grader sitting next to me.
> I reply, "I am from here in the U.S."
> "But from where are your parents?" adds another freshman across the circle with a confused look on his face.
> I calmly answer, "My parents are from here too. I am African-American." They nod in acknowledgment but still seem unsatisfied with my response.
> Another student asks again, "But where are they from?"

During this discussion, I felt as if my students were not only questioning my culture but who I am. It's not the first instance I had to clarify my cultural identity, and each time it's frustrating because being African American is emotionally complicated. I feel proud of my African heritage and the history of creative and strong people, but the negative effects of racism and oppression contradict these sentiments. Theoretically, culture is the set of practices, beliefs, social formations of a group of people that create a sense of belonging and community (William & Sewell, 1999). These shared practices encourage us to live together creating communal language and customs that when practiced help us feel accepted into a group. However, when a group of people or a person like me feel rejected, their sense of culture and cultural identity becomes unstable. Cultural identity is a flexible categorization of culture that helps define who we are as an individual or a group (Hall et al., 2003). Throughout my life, I have formed, remodeled, and reformed my cultural identity. When I was younger, I was unsure of myself and my culture, and even now, I still have insecurities. Smiling mechanically, I tell my students that I am African American feigning confidence and security. Yet my thoughts scream in protest. I am a product of my ancestors brought to the United States, infused with a mixture of bloodlines (African, European, Native American, others?). I was born and raised in the United States, but have no specific country of origin. I am acclimated in a culture that favors white, upper and middle class males, and suppresses my blackness. Encouraged to separate from other African Americans by being classified as exceptional and successful, I strive wanting to help those who fall further behind. These sentiments cause anxiety and self-doubt as I push these overwhelming feelings aside. When I want to clear my chaotic mind of these jumbled thoughts, I do what I always do: dance.

I step back into the dance studio with the light brown, hardwood floors, 6 feet mirrors covering three of the four walls with attached ballet barres, and 30 foot high ceilings. I smile a little picking up the broom to sweep the floors singing with familiar words to the song playing. The short black bristles clear away the prickly thoughts along with the dust and the dirt with each step of my firmly planted feet. The song switches as I store the broom in the closet and percussive drums start to play slowly with a steady, ritualistic pace, stirring my feet to echo the beat. My bare feet shuffle side to side in time to the rhythm, my hips, torso, and arms follow, inciting a sigh as I surrender to the sensations, allowing the music to dictate my movement. Without thinking, I continue dancing to the music. Sometimes my feet imitate the melody of the drums and sometimes go against them. My arms swing from side to side while my torso pushes forwards and backward in counterbalance. My hips circle, my hands reach up and down, and my legs kick high. As the music goes faster, I jump feeling the air under my feet as if suspended just for a moment. I turn and spiral, heart pumping, breathing harder. I find myself doing steps I learned from before and sometimes creating new ways of moving. For a moment I forget about my bad mood, my problems and myself. I just hear the African drums and feel the power of my body and the ancient rhythms that were passed down for generations. I absorb the energy from the African souls that danced these same steps and feel more at ease. As the song ends, I wipe the bit of perspiration from my face and slow down my breath. I feel better, calmer, rejuvenated to think through my problem realizing that dance brought me through another difficult moment.

> Why do I dance? Dance is my medicine. It's the scream which eases for a while the terrible frustration common to all human beings who because of race, creed, or color, are 'invisible.' Dance is the fist with which I fight the sickening ignorance of prejudice. (Welsh-Asante, 1996, p. 24)

The words of choreographer, dancer, and anthropologist Pearl Primus echo my frustrated feelings as I struggle to reaffirm my cultural identity as an African American. Using dance, I navigate the harmful effects of racism and personal insecurities in my efforts to rediscover who I am. This autoethnography explores my transformative process of using dance and races the inherent problems of growing up African American in the United States, and how one individual used the arts to overcome them.

2 Methods of Sharing

To share my story of self-recovery as an autoethnography, I use a combination of authentic inquiry (Tobin, 2018), reflexivity (Bourdieu & Wacquant, 1992), mindful practice (Alexakos, 2015), and kinesthetic knowledge awareness (Conquergood, 2002). These theoretical methods provide the structure and accessibility to highlight the complexity of my journey. An autoethnography interprets a personal experience through a social lens (Puddephatt et al., 2009). It uses observations and direct interactions to explore the human culture centered in these actions (Van Maanen, 1988). Within this scope, my work uses a racial context to trace how my choices are affected by my environment and in return influence my actions. Autoethnography provides an opportunity to explore sensitive topics by understanding the thoughts and feelings of someone involved. For example, within her work, anthropologist Edith Turner (2011) recounts her personal experiences of studying a spiritual, West African tribal ceremony. She and her team eventually became members of the tribal community and video recorded and took field notes of the sacred ceremony. Turner, who is not from that African tribe, may judge the ceremony differently from a tribal member because of their distinctive perspectives. Van Maanen (1998) argues that a researcher's culture, theoretical and methodological framework and experiences influence how and what the fieldworker views, expresses, and understands about the subject matter. Thus, we can expect Turner's account of the event to differ from a tribal member or even someone from her research team as each has their own viewpoint. In this chapter, I intend to discuss and analyze my own stories through self-reflection and authentic inquiry from my own unique standpoint.

Pierre Bourdieu's (1992) defines reflexivity as the means of thinking about how the individual narrative is influenced and influences the larger social context. It also places short term experiences within a larger context to see how they are connected. I reflect on my past to understand how I react to racism and how such influences have affected my more recent life choices. For me, mindfulness is being consciously aware of ourselves in the moment (Alexakos, 2015). Through mindful practice, I have become more cognizant of how my perception of racism and self-identity has changed throughout my life. I am more aware of how dance affects my emotions and enables me to influence them to make myself feel better or strengthen my sense of culture. Mindfulness has been instrumental in helping to document and express my feelings, emotions and experiences of my journey.

Within my process are the ontological component of authentic inquiry and the use of kinesthetic memory. According to Ken Tobin and Konstantinos Alexakos authentic inquiry is a research method that allows participants to transform themselves by investigating meaningful topics (Tobin & Alexakos, 2022). It focuses on finding answers as they arise in the research instead of preconceiving them at the start. Thus, the research began with an open-ended exploration of my racialized identity through self-reflections and dance to reveal the source of my problems to be a mixture of physiological and societal factors. The investigation incorporated Dwight Conquergood's (2002) work on kinesthetic memory as another method of understanding my actions. Conquergood argues that when we experience an event, our body holds onto knowledge as we attach meaning to involved movements whether it is actual dancing or an everyday activity. Thus, we use our bodies to receive, remember, and understand life experiences. After writing down my initial memories, I videoed myself retelling the same verbal responses to reprocess my answers and read my body language in order to gather more insight. This process of researcher-examining my initial responses (Timmermans & Tavory, 2012), allowed me to add forgotten details or clarify misunderstandings within myself. Video recording my responses and analyzing them kinesthetically, brought up hidden emotions and forgotten details. Throughout my story, I specifically focus on these emotional memories as they stand out as important choices. Using these methods I observed how and why I choose to think, act and believe in what I do in learning to live as an African American.

3 Growing up African American

> I say remember the pain because I believe that true resistance begins with people confronting pain, whether it's theirs or somebody else's, and wanting to do something to change it … That is what connects us – our awareness that we know it, have known it, or will know it. (hooks, 1994, p. 61)

The first time I remember the pain from internalized racism was when my first grade teacher questioned who I was. My parents believed getting an education in an affluent, white, middle class school would provide more opportunities and so they worked hard for our family to move to the suburbs of New Jersey. I attended a private school from kindergarten through twelfth grade, where 70% were white middle/upper class students, 20% were Asian and the remaining 10% included Latinos, African Americans, and Caribbeans. My first-grade teacher was an older white woman with short, grey hair and glasses that were held on with an eyeglass chain. On the first day of school, we introduced ourselves, and I told her that my name is Francie, expecting her to continue going down the line, but she didn't. I remember her voice cutting through the silence in the room as she asked, "Are you sure that is your name? You should go home to ask your parents." Not knowing what to say, I quietly sat down, as I felt my heart retreat sadly into darkness. I don't know if I ever told my parents what happened because I felt embarrassed. My name is a combination of different maternal family members that had been given to me to honor our elders and was a source of pride. It's as if she told me that my self-image was wrong and I should become who she wanted me to be instead of who I was. I respected my teacher first because she was white and second because my parents told me to. I dared not dispute her and obediently thought how to remodel myself in her desired image. As the class continued, I noticed that my teacher didn't question the white students and I figured I should be like them. From then on I unconsciously and often consciously did my best to assimilate into white culture and become like my white classmates. I was beginning to understand the complexities of being an African American.

Ron Eyerman (2001) notes the term African American was adopted after the Civil War to acknowledge those who were brought to the United States as enslaved Africans but not fully integrated as Americans. The institution of slavery helped create an inherent identity conflict as African Americans sought acceptance by the same group of people who dominated them. Slavery becomes a collective traumatic experience for African Americans and a foundation for their cultural identity (Eyerman, 2001). Collective trauma occurs when an extreme shock or disruption in routine happens in a group of people which can deeply affect that group's cultural identity (Onwuachi-Willig, 2016). Such trauma creates collective memory as the affected group reaffirms the traumatic event through literature, traditions, celebrations, and cultural artifacts (Eyerman, 2001). I recall my uneasiness during Black History month in school as we read the short section on slavery in our history textbook or feeling sad when looking at movies recounting the cruel treatment inflicted on plantations. These violent images are reinforced when looking at clips of civil rights protesters getting hosed or attacked by dogs in the 60s and 70s and now with videos of police brutality. Onwauchi-Willig (2016) extends the theory of collective trauma to include current, long term occurrences that are a government-approved expected and prolonged interruption of routine; and is known by a wide audience and publicly discussed. Police brutality has become another means of collective trauma because it routinely happens to African Americans in significant amounts, is sanctioned by the government through police practices, and is discussed openly through protests, news in public and private (Chaney & Robertson, 2013). While talking with a friend about the police killings of African Americans, he said, "I can't believe that George Floyd was killed by the police!" My mind replied, "Yes I can," while my head smiled and nodded in agreement. I realize this indifference is a part of the collective trauma that I emotionally endure and a part of the effects of racism. It reminds me that African Americans are not fully accepted as Americans and bores a hole in our cultural identity.

At home, my parents tried to buffer the effects of racism by cultivating a positive image of African Americans. My father was a lawyer and my mother was a college professor, and both were loving and supportive. My parents were civil rights activists who encouraged African American cultural pride through events, such as celebrating Kwanzaa and learning Black History that wasn't taught in the books. We watched black TV shows and movies, read black magazines and books, and attended Afro-centric arts programs, especially in dance. My mother enrolled all three of her daughters in dance at an early age and made sure we took black dance styles, including West African dance. At home, I saw myself as a proud African American but in school I wanted to assimilate to white culture. I created two self-identities that developed into a colonial mindset and purposely began to change my behavior. Frantz Fanon (2008) defines colonial mindset as aspiring to white, middle class culture and believing that the dominant white culture is better than other cultures, including your own which creates an inferiority complex in the oppressed. Double consciousness is another self-inflicted form of racism where the oppressed culture assumes the viewpoint of the dominant culture, which states that they are inferior to whites (Du Bois, 1903). Both colonial mindset and double consciousness are forms of internalized racism that enforce the superiority of the white, dominant culture while subjugating other groups. This inner conflict made it difficult to make friends where I felt that I belonged.

During my childhood, I spent most of my out of school time with my immediate family or my cousins, but a part of me wanted to hang out with friends. I was shy at that age and didn't know how to develop friendships, but I assumed that we must be or act similar to our friends to be liked. I wanted black friends because I thought I should have them since I am African American, but I also needed white friends to fit into school. I decided that I should "act" black to make black friends and "act" white to make white friends. In my mind, acting white is normal because I do it every day at school, but acting black must be different from my normal behavior. Even though I did the same things at home that I did at school, yet mentally it was different and I separated black and white behavior. I compartmentalized my actions into code-switching, noticing and creating two conduct categories. Code-switching (hooks, 1994) is where one adapts behavior or language to function in one culture or another, and helps keep the two versions separate. I tried shifting depending on which race of friends I am with, but wasn't always successful. My black friends often accused me of speaking "white" which is the same as saying that I don't act "black." I developed an inferiority complex because it appeared that I was better acting white than African American. These anxieties manifested in feelings of self-doubt leading to mistakes and eventually failed projects that cycled again into self-blame.

It wasn't until my late 20's that I finally understood that the double consciousness and code-switching were coping mechanisms of living with internalized racism. Because I have only occasionally experienced indirect or verbal racism, I didn't consider myself to be a victim of oppression. After reading theories by African American scholars, I learned how oppression is enforced, how I was entrenched in the system, and understood that I am not suffering alone. I immersed myself in the African American community to buffer the effects of racism and diminish the chances of being racially victimized. I surrounded myself with African Americans who connected to their African heritage by going to African and African American festivals and events. I was inspired by their Afro-centric hair, fashion, and positive attitude. Once I knew what I was feeling, the cause of it, and possible solutions, I could transform. I may not be able to change social conditions in the US, but I can change myself. Initially, I did not dare confront these challenges directly, so I chose an indirect method through dance. When I am moving in dance class I don't have to worry about race or code-switching. My body did what I wanted it to do and I was in control. I could enjoy myself, learn new skills, and overcome challenges. I was happy, especially in doing African dance.

African dance is a way to reconnect to the African Diaspora. Research acknowledges that dance and music are ways to connect with our cultural ancestry (Falola, 2013). Dance is an important aspect of African culture because it conveys social knowledge of all major life events and is a representation of African people (Montiero & Wall, 2011). In Africa, history is passed down through music and dance to convey the rhythms, stories, and belief systems that are shared by the individuals within the community (Green, 2011). These dance steps are taught for generations and still hold onto their original meaning and social customs and practices (Welsh-Asante, 1996). With the 1964 Civil Rights Bill integrated Black studies in the national educational curriculum, African dance became accessible to the United States (Green, 2011). African countries wanting to make their presence known sent national dance groups of their best dancers as cultural ambassadors (Welsh-Asante, 1996). These performances provided African American opportunities to see African dances on stage and even learn them, as dancers from these companies stayed in the US as teachers and dancers from the US went to Africa to study. Asadata Dafora, the National Ballet of Guinea, and the National Ballet of Senegal were some of the first teachers of African dance in New York (Welsh-Asante, 1996). Dance ethnographers, choreographers, and teachers, such as Pearl Primus also lent their artistic and academic voices to share the dances learned from research and voice their sentiments of connecting back to this culture (Primus, 1974). These pioneering dance companies, teachers, and researchers created opportunities for those wanting to learn about African culture and connect to their African roots. Individuals, like my parents, used cultural activities such as African dance to teach themselves and their children about who they are and where they come from. I loved West African dance class the most in hearing the drums, singing African songs, moving my whole body in poly-rhythmic and polycentric ways, and learning about my culture. Studying dances of the African diaspora allows me to learn about African culture and is a source of pride while connecting to African culture that became a basis to reaffirming my cultural identity.

4 Dance as a Tool for Emotional Change

In order to alter my thoughts about being African American, I had to change my feelings about it. Dance becomes an ideal tool to accomplish this because it can bypass physiological and emotional barriers. Stephen Porges' (2007) polyvagal theory asserts that the vagus nerve that runs through the peripheral nervous organs and the base of the brain triggers a physical and emotional reaction. For instance, fear may cause the heart rate to increase or make the palms sweaty. He also argues though that these responses can be changed through retraining. I recall times when I had stage fright and my stomach felt agitated, my heart sped up, and my breath came quicker. Yet after dancing numerous concerts, my fear was replaced with confidence and my body now reacts differently. Before stepping onto a stage, I focus on the applause from the audience instead of the fear of failure and quiet my body. Physical and emotional reactions may be involuntary but can be controlled, changed, or even avoided. I have learned to control and change some of my reactions through breathing slowly, meditating on calming and positive images, and simply acknowledging what's happening to my body and willing it to change. When I begin to question my identity I apply the same process. Rather than dwell on the self-doubt, I focus on my accomplishments, the love from those who support me, and the energy and power from dancing. These positive emotions can temporarily quell my fears and soothe pain even though I know the negative thoughts may resurface.

Using dance to uncover and work through emotions is the basis of dance therapy. Dance therapy emerged in the United States in the 1950s as a clinical practice that focused on bodily expression rather than primarily verbal means (Dosmantes-Beaudry, 1999). Irma Dosamantes-Beaudry published results of her case studies detailing how her clients used trauma inspired movement to work through their emotions until they could verbally discuss them. She found that over the two years of treatment her clients developed self-confidence, the ability to set personal boundaries, and the capacity to interact with others positively. In addition, research shows that dancing can improve mood (Lewis et al., 2016). I use dance as a personalized form of dance therapy to work through my emotions and process problems. As Conquergood (2002) points out, we have kinesthetic knowledge that we can access and which I use to process difficult or sensitive information. When I don't have answers for a dilemma, I can release my emotions or even make a dance about the topic to gain a new perspective. Dance became a metaphor for change. As I improved my dance skills I imagined that my life improved. The self-imposed dance therapy coupled with the physiological effects of dance helped my imagined success become real. The ability to learn, create, and perform reaffirmed my self-confidence and combats feelings of self-doubt and inferiority. While dance in general has these positive attributes, African dance is especially important because it connects me to my African heritage. To reaffirm a positive sense of cultural identity, I altered my individual perception of African American culture through entrainment (Collins, 2004). In entrainment, we associate specific feelings and emotions with different social interactions based on how one feels and how others react to what we do (Collins, 2004). These feelings reinforce or change depending on what happens when we repeat these actions. Using this principle to transform my cultural identity, I changed my habitual patterns of thought from negative to the positive images by reinforcing my connection to traditional African culture. I chose, at first unconsciously and later consciously, to recall more happy thoughts about learning and performing African dance than unhappy moments when I feel stressed or depressed when thinking about my culture. A vital part of my development was surrounding myself with positive African Americans and people and enriching activities. I work, dance, and live in places that value African American culture and have uplifting attitudes. They provide spiritual support, emotional outlets, and reminders that being African American is a good thing. Whenever I feel overwhelmed from the effects of racism, I reinforce my spirit and self-value through African dance and positive members of the black community. This process takes time, but eventually, African dance and culture became a source of happiness and pride.

There is no succinct ending to this story. Transforming internalized racism into self-love is a continuous process. I may not be able to eradicate my anxiety and doubt as an African American, but being connected to supportive communities and friends, gives me the courage to struggle. Surrounding myself with people, who positively embrace African American culture, strengthens my resistance while reaffirming a loving self-image. I will keep telling and retelling my story so others may learn from my experience and understand that they are not alone. Dance will remain a part of my life because it allows me to express who I am and stay grounded amidst the chaos. My heart beats steadily with the rhythms of my African ancestors passed down for generations. My feet touch the ground with the memories of the sacrifices of African Americans that infuse with my body. Together these experiences inspire a creation of movements that represent something new, that represent me.

References

Alexakos, K. (2015). *Being a teacher | researcher: A primer on doing authentic inquiry research on teaching and learning.* Sense Publishers.

Bang, M., & Vossoughi, S. (2016). Participatory design research and educational justice: Studying learning and relations within social change making, *Cognition and Instruction, 34*(3), 173–193.

Bourdieu, P., & Wacquant, L. J. (1992). *An invitation to reflexive sociology.* University of Chicago Press.

Chaney, C., & Robertson, R. V. (2013). Racism and police brutality in America. *Journal of African American Studies, 17*(4), 480–505.

Collins, R. (2004). *Interaction ritual chains.* Princeton University Press. doi:10.2307/j.ctt13x0rs3

Conquergood, D. (2002). Performance studies: interventions and radical research. *The Drama Review, 46*(2), 145–156. https://doi.org/10.1162/105420402320980550

Dosmantes-Beaudry, I. (1999). Divergent cultural self construals: implications for the practice of dance/movement therapy. *The Arts in Psychotherapy, 26.* https:doi.org/10.1016/S0197-4556(99)00011-8

Du Bois, W. E. B. (1903). *Souls of Black folk.* A.C. McClurg & Co.

Eyerman, R. (2001). *Cultural trauma: Slavery and the formation of African American identity.* Cambridge University Press.

Falola, T. (2013). *The African diaspora: slavery, modernity, and globalization.* University Rochester Press.

Fanon, F. (2008). *Black skin, White masks* (1st ed.). Grove Press.

Green, D. (2011). The saga of African dance and Black Studies departments. *Journal of Pan African Studies, 4*(6), 210–222.

Hall, S., Hobson, D., Lowe, A., & Willis, P. (Eds.). (2003). *Culture, media, language working papers in cultural studies, 1972–79.* Routledge.

hooks, b. (1994). *Outlaw culture: Resisting representations.* Routledge.

Lewis, C., Annett, L. E., Davenport, S., Hall, A. A., & Lovatt, P. (2016). Mood changes following social dance sessions in people with Parkinson's disease. *Journal of Health Psychology, 21*(4), 483–492. https://doi.org/10.1177/1359105314529681

Monteiro, N. M., & Wall, D. J. (2011). African dance as healing modality throughout the diaspora: The use of ritual and movement to work through trauma. *Journal of Pan African Studies, 4*(6), 234–252.

Onwuachi-Willig, A. (2016). The trauma of the routine: Lessons on cultural trauma from the Emmett Till verdict. *Sociological Theory, 34*(4), 335–357. https://doi.org/10.1177/0735275116679864

Porges, S. W. (2007). The polyvagal perspective. *Biological Psychology, 74*(2), 116–143. https:doi.org/10.1016/j.biopsycho.2006.06.009

Primus, P. (1974). *The wedding*. Alvin Ailey Dance Theater, State Theater.

Puddephatt, A. J., William, S., & Klienknecht, S. W. (Eds.). (2009). *Ethnographies revisited: Constructing theory in the field*. Routledge.

Sewell, W. H. (1999). The concept(s) of culture. In V. E. Bonnell & L. A. Hunt (Eds.), *Beyond the cultural turn: New directions in the study of society and culture* (pp. 35–61). University of California Press.

Timmermans, S., & Tavory, I. (2012). Theory construction in qualitative research: From grounded theory to abductive analysis. *Sociological Theory, 30*(3), 167–186. https://doi.org/10.1177/0735275112457914

Tobin, K., & Alexakos, K. (2022). Using heuristics to enhance the quality of cultural production. In K. Tobin & K. Alexakos (Eds.), *Transforming learning and teaching: Heuristics for educative and responsible practices* (pp. 1–17). Brill. https://doi.org/ https://doi.org/10.1163/9789004507609_001

Turner, E. (2011). *Experiencing ritual: A new interpretation of African healing*. University of Pennsylvania Press.

Van Maanen, J. (1988). *Tales of the field: On writing ethnography*. University of Chicago Press.

Welsh-Asante, K. (Ed.). (1996). *African dance: An artistic, historical, and philosophical inquiry*. African World Press.

CHAPTER 10

Personal and Environmental Wellness

Eleanor A. Miele

Abstract

This is both a personal and societal story of resignation and rebellion and resilience. Taking care of both ourselves and our environment are emerging as major concerns in our culture, but taking positive action is confounded by societal expectations to put our families and our work ahead of our own health, and to place commerce and convenience ahead of the health of our environment. We are challenged by conflicting messages. How can we find our way back to a healthy path for ourselves and our environment?

Keywords

wellness – resilience – complementary medicine – stress – environmental health

•••

> And we've got to get ourselves
> Back to the garden …
>
> JONIE MITCHELL (lyrics from the album *Ladies of the Canyon*, 1970)

1 Finding Balance in a Stressful World

This is a story of wellness and fear of wellness. A story of resignation and rebellion and resilience. It's a personal story and it's a universal one as well. We all walk through time in one direction, in a constant dialogue with our bodies and our environment, informed by our prior experiences our surroundings and our culture. Whether we consciously listen to that dialogue or not, this

 | DOI:10.1163/9789004527348_010

conversation guides our actions. It is hard to listen. It is harder still to acknowledge when things are going the wrong way. We try to balance our outward and our inward focus, but we often fail. We take care of our jobs, our family and ourselves, usually in that order. Today, taking care of ourselves and our environment are emerging as major issues in our culture, but we are confused. Is self-care just selfish? For both our bodies and our planet it is hard to take the time to even understand what it means to be well.

We are often resigned to following a daily schedule that leaves no room for wellness. We are resigned that we can't make the time to create and eat healthful, nourishing food. We are resigned that we can't make time to exercise, or even sit up straight, get up and walk around, or stretch. We see and read that the planet is in crisis. We are resigned that we are powerless to prevent climate change, accelerating extinction and environmental degradation. We get conflicting messages from myriad sources. We resign ourselves to trust no one – to march ahead doing what must be done, but not doing what we need to do.

2 A Parable

There is an adage about two woodsmen. One is young and the other old. The younger woodsman comes upon the older one sitting on a stump. The younger woodsman laughs at the old man resting, and the older man challenges the younger one to a tree felling contest. Sure enough, throughout the day the older man sat down every hour or so while the younger one felled away. At the end of the day the young man was shocked to see that the older woodsman had felled more trees. "How can it be that I worked all day, and you kept resting, but yet you felled more trees," the younger one asked? "While I was resting, I was also sharpening my axe," the older one replied.

Emerging evidence about the importance of getting adequate sleep for individual productivity support the message of this adage (Magnavita & Garbarino, 2017). An epidemic of stress related diseases such as diabetes, high blood pressure, obesity, digestive disorders, depression, and anxiety is taking an increasing toll on workforce productivity, longevity and quality of life (National Center for Health Statistics, 2010). We need to take care of ourselves. Each of us must find time to sit and sharpen our axes, for our own health as well as our productivity. Increasingly this is being realized in the workplace and large corporations are making time in the workday to support employee health in support of the corporate bottom line (Baicker et al., 2010). But each of us has only one life, and the quality of that time is the true bottom line for each individual.

3 New Threats to Health

The Centers for Disease Control (2020a, 2020b) predicts that climate change will intensify existing health threats and allow new ones to emerge. Increased rates of respiratory and cardiovascular diseases are likely to result due to increased air pollution and an increase in airborne allergens. An increase in food and water-borne diarrheal pathogens and vector-borne infectious illnesses is also expected. These threats to well-being are in addition to an increase in injuries and deaths due to extreme weather events, such as floods, temperature extremes and wildfires. Disasters can have negative impacts on mental health among those with and without a history of mental illness. Anxiety and post-traumatic stress were widespread following hurricane Katrina (Rhodes, 2010) and similar effects follow floods, heatwaves and wildfires. We need to take care of our planet as part of our self-care. But the reality is that we have limited control over adoption of the policies that can reverse our current course, and the status quo merely contributes to the daily stress load of those who acknowledge the gravity of the climate crisis.

4 Embracing the Challenge

I told you this would be a story of resignation, rebellion, and resilience. We need to put an end to resignation. We need to rebel against the personal and societal forces that push us to chronic ill health. We need to nurture the resources that empower us to be resilient in the face of ongoing assaults on our personal, community and global health.

My own story mirrors the awakening of our culture to the common crises of personal and environmental health. Back before Rachel Carson (1962) warned us of the collateral effects of the ubiquitous insecticide DDT on wildlife as it moved up the food chain, I remember welcoming the spray truck attacking the mosquitos. I still recall the strange taste in the air. The publication of Silent Spring in 1962 heralded the beginning of the environmental movement and an awareness of the widespread and unexpected impacts of modern human life. Back then, there were half as many humans on the planet. It is hard to imagine, but only a few generations back, human life was not dependent on gasoline and oil. We are living in a new geological age, the Anthropocene, when human activity has become the dominant influence on climate and the environment (Waters et al., 2016).

Scientists now agree that the planet is experiencing global climate change as a result of human actions. Our industry, homes and businesses generate an unsustainable level of greenhouse gases, inexorably raising the global temperature above natural levels (IPCC, 2014). The effects are difficult to predict locally, but easy to predict globally. There will be stronger storms, more and larger wildfires, coastal and inland flooding, sea level rise, more frequent and hotter heatwaves. Consensus predictions of the effects of climate change have severely underestimated the impacts. How can we even begin to restore homeostasis to the planet, when we don't even agree that there is a problem? It is too easy to ignore the signs of trouble, both globally and personally. I have seen this in myself.

5 Pain Is the Human Condition

When I was a teenager, I remember my sister telling me that her doctor said, pain is the common condition of mankind. I think perhaps I let this become not a comfort, but an excuse to accept, even expect, a life of malaise. When I was just a young girl, I remember waking up every morning cuddled with my cat and nursing a sore throat. I don't think I put the two together until I was in my fifties. I'm allergic to cats! The lasting effect was a general sense that being unwell was the norm.

I started high school in Manhattan in 1969, before the Clean Air Act of 1970 went into effect (Ross et al., 2012). When I crossed Broadway on my way to school, I consciously held my breath crossing the street, so I wouldn't cough from the diesel exhaust of the buses and trucks. How many seconds did I need to hold out before that next breath would be safe?

Soon I went off to college in upstate New York and the clean mountain air cleared my lungs and my breathing was easy. The first time I came back to the city for the weekend, I thought I was breathing little knives. It was a warning I should have heeded. Perhaps a country life would have spared me what was to come. A few more years in the country and I was in pretty good shape, but once I returned to the city for graduate school my coughing started again. I called it my Autumn cough. Whenever the leaves fell, the cough would come back. Of course, never in a doctor's office. My chronic asthma was off the medical radar.

Fast forward several decades. September 11 had come and gone. The metallic tinge in the air was hard to miss, but any respiratory symptoms could be attributed to hay fever. But those symptoms just never went away. One day I found myself with my mother-in-law in the hospital, and my sister in the same hospital on another floor. I was sick, just another cold. I had them constantly since I had started working with elementary school teachers. But now I was carrying a purse bulging with cough medicine, decongestant, antihistamine. I was taking the next dose as soon as the label allowed, but still getting looks from the doctors and nurses ... Coughing constantly, producing constant phlegm. Each time I entered the hospital I eyed the Emergency Room and thought, perhaps I should take a seat ... but I could not allow myself to take care of me.

Every breath was an effort. The coughing never stopped. The constant coughing left my neck and abdomen in constant pain. I couldn't sleep at night for the pain. I was growing weaker all the time. The little cough from my high school years was now constant. I could not get through a single waking moment without coughing. A neighbor who was a physician broke with tradition and took me aside to say I really needed to get my cough looked at.

6 Facing Facts

When my mother-in-law and my sister got out of the hospital, I finally said to myself, now I need to take care of me ... so, I made an appointment with the critical care physician who had saved my sister's life. He was also a pulmonologist with an open practice. I needed to breathe.

Finally, in the doctor's office, I told my story. He listened to me breathe, took my pulse oxygen, and said he didn't see a problem. Just like my family practice doctor, he underestimated my condition. But this time I pushed. I was desperate.

I told him I was a singer, and I could move air, but I felt like I was always working at breathing, and when I relaxed in sleep at night, or walked at a normal pace, I felt like I couldn't get enough air. I told him I had had a constant cough for years and that I often encountered air that triggered terrible fits of coughing that made my head feel like it was going to explode. He said, OK, let's do an X-ray and a pulmonary function test and see what's going on.

The doctor came back with the results of my pulmonary function test and apologized. He looked a little shocked. The test showed that I had both reversible and non-reversible airway constriction. I had asthma and chronic obstructive pulmonary disease (COPD). I had only 70% of the capacity I should have to move air. I couldn't exhale in a single sweep, but stepped down, with two or three distinct plateaus. Those are signs of the constriction in your airway, from remodeling of your bronchial tubes, my doctor explained. Constant inflammation makes the airways hypertrophy, narrowing the airway (Keglowich & Borger, 2015). The asthma could be treated, but the COPD was irreversible and progressive. We needed to stop the constant assault to my body of the constant coughing.

I came home from that appointment with a prescription for the asthma medicine *Advair*. Of course, I looked it up and discovered a long list of side effects that made me hesitate. Fear of having a bronchospasm as a reaction made me anxious. Ultimately, I agreed to try the Advair if my doctor first gave me a prescription for Albuterol, a rapid relief drug for bronchospasm. Once I reluctantly tried the *Advair,* I was shocked to discover that my breathing could actually be better. I looked forward to the next dose, because after ten hours or so I could feel my breath getting tighter and the phlegm begin to form again. I hadn't realized how sick I was. I also hadn't believed that medicine could help.

7 A Step by Step Trip Downhill

How had I let this happen? As a biologist by training, I had always prided myself on using basic biology to inform my health habits. I ate right. I tried to sleep right. I took the stairs, not the elevator. But I had taken on a lot of responsibility. My kids were getting ready for college, so we needed the income to pay for tuition. My father-in-law had passed away and my mother-in-law needed looking after. My sister had chronic health problems, and no support network except me and my husband. My neighbor became ill and a source of constant concern. I loved my job, but the responsibilities kept growing. I realized I was waking up in the middle of the night in panic almost every night. There were things to do, and people were counting on me to get them done.

I realized that I needed to take time to really take stock of my health, to start to listen to my body again. Too much focus on caring for my family and doing my job had left no room for me. I realized that I had forgotten what it was like to be even remotely well. The gradual nature of the changes and my general strength had been masking a progressive illness. I needed to focus on my own wellness, and I wasn't satisfied to allow the medicine to do all of the work.

I thought about how I had been able to effectively cope with such a debilitating illness without it showing … The cough was obvious, but the loss of respiratory function was hidden. Even the pulmonologist didn't think there was a problem on first examination. I realized that I had learned to compensate for my increasing breathlessness in part by drawing on breathing skills I had learned in yoga, choir, and Lamaze class.

8 Old Lessons Relearned

I cast my memory back on a book by Norman Cousins that had influenced my approach to health, back when my sister had had an earlier health crisis. *Anatomy of an Illness as Perceived by the Patient: Reflections on Healing and Regeneration* was first published in 1979. This was the first book by a patient that explored a doctor-patient relationship as a partnership for healing. In it,

Cousins describes taking an active role in his own recovery using humor to distract, entertain and exercise through laughter. He maintained that laughing was his most effective pain killer and credited vitamin C megadoses with helping him overcome a connective tissue disorder. Back then, it was a big production to get access to video in a hospital room, and Cousin's doctor agreed to support his request to have comic movies projected in his hospital room. This book ushered in an age where medicine increasingly recognized and valued alternative and complementary approaches to healing. Cousins, originally a journalist, joined the faculty of UCLA Department of Psychiatry and Behavioral Sciences where he researched the connection between attitude and health and founded the Cousins Center for Psychoimmunology.

9 Becoming a Medical Rebel

My sister had been suffering with an autoimmune disease and I was a biology major spending my spare time reading the medical literature on her condition and the emerging literature on alternative medicine. Back then Rodale Press was bringing ideas about nutrition and exercise to the public with their Prevention Magazine. Prevention was a marginal magazine at the time and its readers were viewed as "health nuts." But I had discovered a lot of surprising information about the power of vitamin C to help with allergic and inflammatory conditions in the stacks of the Cornell library while doing research for a senior seminar on immunology. Rodale articles were based on emerging science and cited the literature. I found their articles to be well-researched.

Later I learned in graduate school that research on benefits of vitamins were buried by pharmaceutical companies because vitamins could not be patented and would not generate revenue that could be controlled. My mind was opened to the concept of alternative approaches to healing using exercise and nutrition and attention to keeping a positive attitude.

As a graduate student I had developed a mysterious illness that resulted in my losing over 15 pounds from my top weight of 106. My physician could find no cause and assumed it was "stress" although my allergist suggested that my bloodwork indicated a possible parasitic infection. I was referred to the student health psychiatrist. Lucky for me, that psychiatrist was an early adopter of complementary medicine and helped me use vitamins to stabilize my condition and improve my appetite. Once I returned to relatively good health, the lesson of the value of good nutrition to maximize health was one I never forgot. Over the years I successfully resolved bouts of neck, back and hip pain with exercise and improved nutrition. Home-made bone broth and vitamin C was my go-to elixir for supporting connective tissue injuries, and it always did the trick. For many years I had been able to control or reverse my health problems with this approach. I developed a confidence in my ability to manage my own health and a deep suspicion of standard medicine.

10 Resignation

Although with my asthma and chronic bronchial constriction I had finally found myself with a chronic condition that I couldn't cure with exercise and nutrition, I knew that complementary medicine could help me reach my best self. My first step after accepting that my condition required standard medicine was to take stock of how I could support my health. One part was minimizing my chances of getting the flu, because getting the flu when your breathing baseline is compromised is a serious problem (Busse et al., 2010). It was, ironically, by doing this that I discovered another hidden health problem that I couldn't deal with without medicine. As I coughed less, I was able to notice that my neck and abdomen had become weak. My family doctor dismissed my concerns after asking me to push back on her hand, but I knew the problem was real. I had chronic neck pain that interfered with my sleeping and my abdominal muscles had become so weak that I had to use my hands to help get into and out of chairs. I struggled to lift a pot of water to make pasta. I even had trouble swallowing. That's old lady muscles, not mine. I had become frail before my time. I mentioned to the nurse practitioner who was administering my flu shot that I had abdominal muscle weakness and trouble swallowing and she said, "have you had your thyroid checked?" Muscle weakness is a common symptom of low thyroid hormone levels (McKeran et al., 1975) but none of my doctors had ever mentioned this, even though I complained of muscle weakness. I had known that my thyroid levels were a little low, but they were still in the normal range. My family doctor didn't think I needed supplemental thyroid hormone "yet", but my holistic psychiatrist agreed that I should start treatment immediately, and what a difference! My ability to swallow started to improve soon after I started to take thyroid supplements and my ability to tolerate exercise improved.

11 A Slow Road to Recovery

I enrolled in a yoga class composed almost entirely of older women with serious skeletal problems and an instructor who taught classes at the Hospital for

Special Surgery in New York. Although I was the youngest in the class, I was also the least capable. I was shocked to realize that I could not command my body to do the simplest things. I could not lie flat on my back. I could not lie flat on my stomach. I could not lift my head from a prone position. The commands went through, but the body didn't respond. My body had contracted, and my neck could no longer align properly above my spine. Little by little, poor posture and increasing weakness had written itself into my muscles and tendons. Some were too long. Some were too short. There was no fast, easy fix for this. No medicine could rebalance my body. It would take a long-term commitment to make incremental progress. Slowly and steadily, I needed to strengthen and realign my muscles. Progress would be millimeter by millimeter. Simply engaging my back and neck muscles to move a little closer to a normal alignment was exhausting and painful. Sometimes I was tempted to give up.

But I realized that every day was an opportunity to move a little closer to healthy alignment and not further away. It had taken years of neglect of my body to get where I was. Each day that I strived to move toward health was one more day that I was not moving further toward frailty and irreversible damage to my bones. Only recently have I learned that I was in excellent company. B. K. S. Iyengar, who helped introduce yoga to the West, credited yoga with saving his life. Iyengar yoga focuses on alignment and utilizes props to help students go into poses safely that they cannot assume without the props. He himself had been weakened by bouts of malaria, influenza, tuberculosis, and typhoid fever and as a beginning yogi at the age of 16 could not assume the poses himself without props. In his obituary, the New York Times (Barry, 2014) quoted Iyengar as saying "My head used to hang down, and I had to lift it with great effort." This quote resonated with me – because I have been there. Iyengar died in 2014 at the age of 95. He was still standing on his head at 83.

12 Building Resilience

Building strength would require building muscle. After every yoga session I would drink a kefir-based potion with vitamin C, cod liver oil, turmeric and ginger followed by a high protein lunch to get extra protein and control the inflammation that comes after exercise. For the first few years I practiced yoga, I was plagued with delayed onset muscle pains that would haunt me for days after a workout. It was hard to keep up with daily realignment exercises through the muscle aches. It was harder still to keep going to class, knowing that 24 to 48 hours later the pain would set in. But I knew I had to keep at it until I could stand up straight again. And today, I have regained normal posture and a healthy alignment of my spine and hips. One day that extreme delayed muscle pain just stopped coming. I go to yoga at least once a week without fail and continue to work on fine points of alignment. I joke that by the time I'm 85, I'll be able to do all of the poses without props. But the point I want to share here is that wellness really does require a continual commitment. No one is ever too sick to benefit from attention to posture, breathing and healthy eating. It's never too late to start improving your health.

Making time to be in nature also helped me on the road to recovery. Once my cough was under control, I could take walks in the park again. A brisk walk and talk helped me feel better both mentally and physically. There was the proof that I could get out there and walk up that hill. Sure, at first I needed to draw on those Lamaze skills, but each time it got easier. I tried to get out to walk in nature at least 3 times a week. Walks in the pine woods and on the beach expanded my personal medicine. Breathing salt air was valued as a cure-all throughout the 18th and 19 centuries. Recent studies show that breathing salt air improves subjective feelings of health, although there is as yet no conclusive research to support this (Hedman et al., 2006). But in terms of my uncontrolled experiment of one, now I can hike for three miles and not get winded. The overall benefits of time spent in nature has been emerging in recent research. Contact with natural environments such as parks woodlands and beaches is associated with better general health (White et al., 2019). Living in greener urban areas has been shown to lower risks of most of the stress-associated illnesses and to correlate with better subjective wellbeing (Maas et al., 2006).

13 Setbacks on the Road

The road to maintaining or recovering health is clear. But it seems that the healthy path is easy to stray from. So many times, over the course of my life, I have taken that step back and realized I needed to take better care of myself. So many times, I have said, ok, great, now I'm fine and I don't need to fuss with all this wellness stuff, only to realize a few years down the road that I am unwell again.

Non-compliance with medication is quite common, especially among those with chronic conditions (Kleinsinger, 2018). There are numerous reasons for non-compliance and many of these also apply to complementary medicines. The cost of complementary medicines can be quite high, and most insurance does not cover these costs. If there are no obvious symptoms many people stop taking their medicines. Taking many different medicines and taking them more than once a day is a constant reminder that you are not well. This all sounds so familiar. Do I really need to keep taking a handful of pills every morning to stay healthy? Then I read the latest article in the news about how supplements are a waste (O'Connor, 2019). I wonder. And I stop taking the supplements that have helped me recover my health.

There is no end date for self-care. It needs to be continuous. Sometimes I wonder whether I have been so unused to feeling well that it actually made me uncomfortable and caused me to sabotage my health subconsciously. Do I suffer from fear of wellness?

14 A Drive from Health to Illness?

If as my sister's old doctor said, pain is the human condition, then are we human if we are not in pain? If misery loves company, will I be alone if I am not miserable? Sometimes when I am feeling my strongest and best, I catch myself wondering if I deserve to feel so well. I see others suffering around me and I feel strangely isolated in my good health. Can one become addicted to illness? Munchausen syndrome is the extreme of this feeling; when a person repeatedly and deliberately acts as if they have an illness when they are not really sick. It has been estimated that 3 to 5 percent of physician encounters involve this syndrome (Savino & Fordtran, 2006). This condition may develop after trauma or illness in childhood. Sufferers have an inner need to be seen as ill or injured. Perhaps there is a continuum of this behavior that is subtly influencing otherwise well people to sabotage their health? If I have been ill most of my life, am I still me without that illness?

In 1970 the neurologist Oliver Sacks (1992), a migraine sufferer, first published his treatise on the subject of migraines, and explored the neuropsychological aspects of the disorder. Sacks observed that many patients develop another compensating neurological condition when their migraines are successfully treated and suggested that migraines may fulfill a physiological or psychological need. For at least some of us, there does seem to be a drive that leads us from health to illness. We must rebel against this drive. Perhaps the inner voice that may question our right to the best health we can achieve must be acknowledged, but we must not let it undermine our resolve to return to the path. Resilience is the quality that lets us keep going despite setbacks. Among the factors that make a person resilient is the ability to see failure as a form of helpful feedback. In my case, I have finally resigned myself to the truth that my health will require constant attention. I have learned from my setbacks and accepted my needs. I have swallowed my pride. I have rebelled against the culture that snickers at those of us who admit to requiring dietary or physical accommodations.

15 Misery Loves Privacy

Another pressure that keeps us from staying on a healthy road is the desire for privacy. We want to keep our health problems to ourselves. Illness is generally seen as a sign of weakness, and we want to project a strong image. Despite the protections afforded by the Americans with Disabilities Act, we tend to keep our health problems to ourselves if they are not visible. And so many disabilities are not. Asthma, for example, is invisible except during an acute attack. Mental illnesses are also invisible, but extremely common. The National Institute of Mental Health (2020) estimates that 17.3 million adults suffered a major depressive episode in 2017 (the latest year for which data is available.) This represents 7.1% of the adult population. It is estimated that 15% of the population will experience depression at some point in their lifetime. Anxiety disorders are even more prevalent. The NIMH estimates that 19% of adults had an anxiety disorder in that same year. But our desire for privacy can be toxic. We can't get the support we need if we can't admit to our health challenges. In the past, I have fallen into this trap. Pride has kept me from being honest about my limitations.

Now I have the luxury of a tenured position and as a full professor I am secure in my employment. I don't worry that my health will be an issue for promotion or retention. From this position of relative comfort and safety, I find that I am free to be honest about my own health issues, and I've discovered that I am not alone. Others struggle, too. But usually in secret. I hope that by being more up front and matter of fact about my struggles, I can encourage others to feel safer to ask for what they need to be productive. I have resigned myself to the need to protect myself from infection, and do so without apology. I will continue to strive for personal resilience. I will forgive myself the attention to my needs. I will take the time I need to recover if I become ill.

16 Wither Now?

I began this essay when COVID-19 had not yet been named, but was merely a vague concern in the West. I am grateful that I have already accepted the need to bow to my physical limitations. COVID-19 has laid bare the truth of how frail we all are. Talk of underlying conditions is in the evening news. Now we have all gained a new awareness of how precarious our health is. We have also seen how quickly our skies have cleared during the "pause" in travel and commerce. We have noticed the birds singing in the quiet of mornings without the rush to work. As a society we have strayed from the healthy path. Modern conveniences and comforts have trumped caring for our environment and ourselves. We have forgotten what environmental wellness feels like, and how tied it is to our own health. I hope that we will all find the path together past the signposts of resignation and rebellion to resilience.

References

Baicker, K., Cutler, D., & Song, Z. (2010). Workplace wellness programs can generate savings. *Health Affairs, 29*(2), 304–311.

Barry, E. (2014, August 21). B. K. S. Iyengar, who helped bring yoga to the West, dies at 95. *The New York Times*, p. B17.

Busse, W. W., Lemanske, R. F. Jr., & Gern, J. E. (2010). Role of viral respiratory infections in asthma and asthma exacerbations. *Lancet, 376*(9743), 826–834. https://doi.org/10.1016/S0140-6736(10)61380-3

Carson, R. (2002). *Silent spring*. Houghton Mifflin.

Cousins, N. (1979). *Anatomy of an illness as perceived by the patient: Reflections on healing and regeneration*. Norton.

Hedman, J., Hugg, T., & Sandell, J. (2006). The effect of salt chamber treatment on bronchial hyperresponsiveness in asthmatics. *European Journal of Allergy and Clinical Immunology*. https://doi.org/10.1111/j.1398-9995.2006.01073.x

Intergovernmental Panel on Climate Change. (2014). *AR5 synthesis report: Climate change 2014*. https://www.ipcc.ch/report/ar5/syr/

Keglowich, L. F., & Borger, P. (2015). The three A's in asthma – airway smooth muscle, airway remodeling & angiogenesis. *The Open Respiratory Medicine Journal, 9*, 70–80.

Kleinsinger, F. (2018). The unmet challenge of medication nonadherence. *The Permanente Journal, 22*, 18–033. https://doi.org/10.7812/TPP/18-033

Maas, J., Verheij, R. A., Groenewegen, P. P., de Vries, S., & Spreeuwenberg, P. (2006). Green space, urbanity, and health: How strong is the relation? *Journal of Epidemiology and Community Health, 60*(7), 587. https://doi.org/10.1136/jech.2005.043125

Magnavita, N., & Garbarino, S. (2017). Sleep, health and wellness at work: A scoping review. *International Journal of Environmental Research and Public Health, 14*(11), 1347. https://doi.org/10.3390/ijerph14111347

McKeran, R. O., Slavin, G., Andrews, T. M., Ward, P., & Mair, W. G. (1975). Muscle fibre type changes in hypothyroid myopathy. *Journal of Clinical Pathology, 28*(8), 659–663. https://doi.org/10.1136/jcp.28.8.659

National Center for Health Statistics. (2010). *Healthy people 2010*. U.S. Department of Health and Human Services Centers for Disease Control and Prevention. https://www.cdc.gov/nchs/data/hpdata2010/hp2010_final_review.pdf

National Institute of Mental Health. (2020). *Major depression*. https://www.nimh.nih.gov/health/statistics/major-depression.shtml

O'Connor, A. (2019, July 16). Popular, but not very effective. *The New York Times*, p. D4.

Patz, J. A., McGeehin, M. A., Bernard, S. M., Ebi, K. L., Epstein, P. R., Grambsch, A., Gubler, D. J., Reither, P., Romieu, I., Rose, J. B., Samet, J. M., & Trtanj, J. (2000). The potential health impacts of climate variability and change for the United States: Executive summary of the report of the health sector of the U.S. National Assessment. *Environmental Health Perspectives, 108*(4), 367–376. https://doi.org/doi:10.1289/ehp.00108367

Rhodes, J., Chan, C., Paxson, C., Rouse, C. E., Waters, M., & Fussell, E. (2010). The impact of Hurricane Katrina on the mental and physical health of low-income parents in New Orleans. *American Journal of Orthopsychiatry, 80*(2), 237–247. https://doi.org/10.1111/j.1939-0025.2010.01027.x

Ross, K., Chmiel, J. F., & Ferkol, T. (2012). The impact of the Clean Air Act. *The Journal of Pediatrics, 161*(5), 781–786.

Sacks, O. (1992). *Migraine*. University of California Press.

Savino, A. C., & Fordtran, J. S. (2006). Factitious disease: Clinical lessons from case studies at Baylor University Medical Center. *Proceedings (Baylor University. Medical Center), 19*(3), 195–208. https://doi.org/10.1080/08998280.2006.11928162

Waters, C. N., Zalasiewicz, J., Summerhayes, C., Barnosky, A. D., Poirier, C., Gałuszka, A., Cearreta, A., Edgeworth, M., Ellis, E. C., Ellis, M., Jeandel, C., Leinfelder, R., McNeill, J. R., Richter, D. d., Steffen, W., Syvitski, J., Vidas, D., Wagreich, M., Williams, M., ... Wolfe, A. P. (2016). The Anthropocene is functionally and stratigraphically distinct from the Holocene. *Science, 351*(6269), aad2622. https://doi.org/doi:10.1126/science.aad2622

White, M. P., Alcock, I., Grellier, J., Wheeler, B. W., Hartig, T., Warber, S. L., Bone, A., Depledge, M. H., & Fleming, L. E. (2019, June 13). Spending at least 120 minutes a week in nature is associated with good health and wellbeing. *Scientific Reports, 9*(1), 7730. https://doi.org/10.1038/s41598-019-44097-3

CHAPTER 11

Living with Depression

Piyanate Chuychai

Abstract

Living life is very difficult for people who have a long-term major depressive disorder. Suffering takes over life, both body and mind. Thus, depression feels much like dying alive. Often life seems out of control and hard to understand with logical thinking. Therefore, many people who have depression might think that only death can stop their pain and suffering. In this chapter, I share my experience with chronic depression for more than ten years, during which I experienced the illness at various levels of intensity, from mild to severe. In the chapter I illustrate how I transformed myself from depression to a person who enjoys learning and living life. Changing lifestyles in various ways and learning about ourselves are important components of self-care and informed living. I explain how I used mindfulness as a tool to help see the truth of life more clearly. My perception of depression changed when I learned to look differently. Overcoming chronic depression and living with it is not easy, but with regular mindfulness practice I found relief from depression and could lead a successful life.

Keywords

depression – walking – diet – mindfulness – self-care – self-harm – prescription drugs

1 An Overview of What Is to Come

I look at my arms which are full of wounds from hurting myself when I was 20 years old. I might hide these wounds from others, but I could not hide from myself – wounds are on both my body and mind. I remember I almost died because of the depression I experienced at that time. I faced difficulties with depression many times in my life but did not understand what caused the depression. I repeatedly asked myself why I had to live during the darkest experiences. I tried to find a way to live and learn with depression, and from time to time to transform my appearance, as shown in Figure 11.1.

 | DOI:10.1163/9789004527348_011

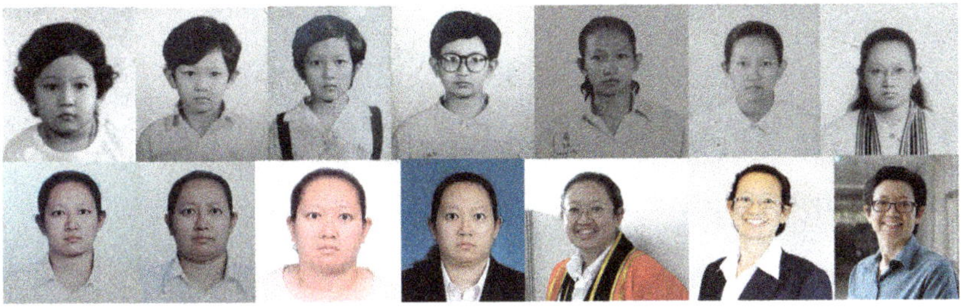

FIGURE 11.1 My transformation during the time

I believe that no one wants to face this illness, and in this chapter, I offer what I have learned for the benefit of readers. There are ways to heal the illness. Even people who are depressed at the moment can be healed and can enjoy living life. I am pleased to still be alive and that I could turn my wounds into the light and learn from my experiences. In the sections that follow I share my experience with readers and hope they learn and benefit from my story.

2 My Early Life

I was born in 1979 in Bangkok, Thailand. As a child, I was a girl who was quiet, shy, and very emotional. I did not have confidence and felt uncomfortable around people. When I met many people at events, I did not know how to interact appropriately. I usually thought I would not fit in with them. Many times, I worried and overthought about the past and future. I rarely felt happy and often felt very lonely. Physically, I was often unhealthy due to allergies and asthma, and I received injections every week or two. My parents worked hard to support a good education for my sister and me, and they treated us well. Their only requirement being that was diligent with our studies.

When I was in high school, I enjoyed being with friends and began to build self-confidence. Normally, there are three levels in Thailand's high school. For me, it was a good time to learn about what I liked or wanted to do. I dreamt of developing myself more in education and social life during this lifetime while spending time with friends during these three years. Sadly, my dreams were broken when I passed the university entrance examination after finishing my second year of high school. I knew I was unprepared for university, and I had to decide whether to stay at school or go to university. My preference was to spend another year with my friends at school. However, my parent and teachers told me that it was a good opportunity to go to the university. I was very sad and confused about what to do. On the one hand, I could follow my preference, and on the other, I could do what the others thought was good for me. Finally,

I did not follow my heart; choosing instead the way that made others happy. Unfortunately, instead of building self-confidence regarding my future, once again I lost confidence. I was depressed and worried for a month before the university started.

My new life began without me planning for it, and I could not imagine how it was going to unfold. I was a physics major – but did not know whether I was good at physics or even liked the subject. I tried to adjust myself to study at the university but sometimes it was hard for me to accept what I had chosen to do. Luckily, I met new friends and they were nice. We helped each other to study and do some activities together. I enjoyed calculation and learning new things. For the most part, I enjoyed the lessons and forgot the disappointments of the past. Sometimes, when I thought about life in high school, I missed it and sadness arose. I still was a worried and less confident person. I never regarded myself as good enough. It was just my character to accept life as it came to me. I did not like my lifestyle but did not know how to change.

During the final year of my undergraduate program, I did a senior project and started to have more stress. I elevated the pressure on myself and worried that my work would not be good enough. The pressure rose a little bit day by day and I did not know how to deal with it. When I presented work in public with stress and anxiety, I could not control my handshaking and trembling voice. I did not like those feelings and suffered. I kept my feelings inside. Actually, the project I did was fine and my advisor appreciated it. From the view of others, I was kind, smart, and excelled in my studies. I graduated with a good grade and my advisor offered me a scholarship to continue studying in the Ph.D. program. Once again, I had to decide.

I hated the feeling of stress, but I wanted to study and to do that a scholarship was necessary. Inside I felt I was not ready and I wanted to slow down my life. There were so many things I thought I could not handle, especially the feelings. My advisor encouraged me to accept the scholarship because he saw my potential to do research. Finally, I applied for the scholarship and enrolled in the Ph.D. program with an uncomfortable feeling.

I tried to tell my friends about my stress, sadness, and anxiety. I told them how much I worried, but they always said that I could do it and should not be worried. I felt that no one listened to me – even my close friends. No one realized that inside I was really painful and suffering. I started to hate myself and everything around me. I did not know what to do since everything seemed out of control. I cried a lot every day and punched or cut my wrist again and again to release the energy or the pain inside. I easily got angry with my parent and friends. From a nice person, I became aggressive. I could shout or scream out so loud if I did not reach my goals. When I calmed down, I really hated myself for being like this. It was also hard to get sleep at night and I did not want to wake up in the morning. I felt depressed and tired all day. My world turned grey and finally dark. It was very difficult for me to live each day. Many times, I thought about plans for suicide. I did not understand what happened to my life.

My parents worried about me, but they did not know what they should do, especially because we had very few conversations since I began at the university. I knew there was something wrong with my body and mind, but I did not want to see a doctor, especially a psychiatrist. It was hard for me to accept, and I still cared about how others would regard a person who had mental health problems. Also, I did not like to take prescribed medicine.

3 First-Time Depression Diagnosis

In 1999, I began my first-year studies in the Ph.D. program. I could not focus on the lessons anymore. My grades were dropping. I often came to class late, missed class, and did not submit assignments on time. Many times, I considered quitting the program. My advisor noticed my unusual behaviors and decided to take me to see someone who could help. He suggested that we would walk to talk to a specialist in the university counseling center who could give me some advice. I went to the center and met the psychiatrist. She asked me to explain my situation and I explained. She told me I was facing an illness called "major depression disorder." This was the first time that I had heard a name for this illness and its symptoms. If the symptoms last longer than two weeks, there was more of a chance that the illness should be discussed with experts, so that they could advise on the best course of action. I completed a checklist about symptoms. I had experienced all the behaviors on the checklist for maybe more than a half year. The doctor informed me that my condition was related to a chemical imbalance in my brain, and I needed to take prescribed medicine. She also gave me a brochure about depression. The brochure contained causes, symptoms, cures to deal with the illness, and suggestions for how people can take care of a patient.[1]

I was sad to hear that I was sick and had to take medicine. The psychiatrist suggested I should come to see her every week. I took medicine and saw her every week. The medicine helped slow down my thought and I felt dizzy sometimes. Every time I spoke with the doctor, I tried to explain my feelings and the situation – but I felt like she never listened and did not tell me how to adjust my lifestyle. Her treatment seemed to be no more than to prescribe a drug and then to see me weekly. I started to resist the treatment. After one month, I gave up and threw away the pills. I stopped seeing the doctor. I thought that I could live on my own and I did not believe that the medicine could help.

After that, the depression got worse during my first year of graduate school. I hurt myself several times. My arms were full of wounds, and I had to cover them by wearing a long sleeve shirt. I destroyed many things such as clothes, telephone, stationery, and books when I got angry. My friends tried to help and talk with me, but it did not help anything. I just cried and said to them that I did not want to live. My parents also tried to help but they were afraid to talk with me. Instead of talking with me, they called the hospital. The doctor sent an ambulance to my house.

I remember that day. Two guys came to my bed while I slept and tied my hands before taking me away in the ambulance. When I saw the doctor, he just talked with me for a few sentences and gave me a prescription. I was so angry with my parents and no longer trusted them. I now had the experience of seeing doctors for depression on several occasions, but the treatments were unsuccessful. The doctors just talked for a few minutes and then prescribed medicine. Every time, it ended up with me discarding the pills because I had no belief that the treatment could benefit me. Also, I could not find a way out. I just tried to live, day by day, without medication. As a distraction, I spent a lot of time and money eating and shopping in an endeavor to relieve my suffering.

After that, my depression was on and off. In 2001, I went to The United States for the first time as a visiting scholar for eight months. I was so excited and liked the weather and environment there – I was located in a small city that was not crowded. I walked from my apartment to the university every day. I learned a lot from the professor there. It was a good time. I enjoyed life and rarely observed the symptoms of depression. I had hope to enjoy life and finish the Ph.D. program. However, when I was back in Thailand, the symptoms returned. Finding a way to live with the depression was always on my mind. I visited the US again in 2003, as a student. There, I found the book entitled *Constructive Living* (Reynolds, 1984). The book talked about what to do about rough times in real life such as shyness, failure, depression, grief, chronic illness, and lack of energy. I learned from the book that we cannot directly control our emotions. Accordingly, we should identify and accept tough feelings and moments. When we learn, those feelings can help us strengthen ourselves. After I read some part of the book, I felt very good and relieved that there might be a way out of suffering even though the book did not directly talk about depression disorder. At least, the way to live life constructively existed and changes in lifestyle can improve the quality of life. Feeling good about reading the book helped me for a while, but I did not do anything that the book suggested in order to live life constructively. When suffering came, I still felt it deep down. My way to relieve suffering still involved eating and shopping. Finally, I graduated from the Ph.D. program, gaining about 20 kg of weight in the process. I totally forgot about severe depression. I did not cry every day, nor did I hurt myself as I had done in the past. However, I still suffered easily and was very emotional. I became a person who did not really know what I wanted to be or what would make me happy in life. I just lived life with fear and kept it inside.

4 Second Episode of Depression

After finishing my Ph.D., I traveled to the US to work as a postdoctoral researcher at the same university I visited when I was a student. I worked with the professor with whom I worked previously. Even though I was familiar with people and places, I started to worry about work because I was not a student anymore. Therefore, I committed to work very hard and produce outputs. It was me who applied the pressure. I continued my Ph.D. work, and there were some new things I had to learn also, mainly about data analysis. My supervisor gave me the freedom to work as usual. He was not strict about the time and did not force me to do anything. Everything seemed fine. I met and discussed research with more people than when I was a student. I was often nervous. I could not easily follow conversations in English, and this slowed down my progress in physics. My stress increased before and during meetings and presentations. The first year of the postdoc flew so quickly. I had a lot of things to do, and I held some stress which I did not recognize.

I asked my supervisor for a two-week vacation to visit Thailand. During the vacation, I experienced familiar feelings of depression. After my return to the US. I watched myself carefully, but it was too late. There were so many things to handle, especially emotions, and situations that I did not anticipate. All behaviors I faced before when I got sick with depression re-emerged. I decided to tell my supervisor. He understood and walked with me to the university counseling center. For me, it was like the replay of a movie. I was in a process of treatment for my illness. I did not know what was going to happen, but I had no choice at that time. My head kept thinking over and over. I could not stop, and it was hard to sleep at night. I started to hurt myself which was not a good sign.

Again, I completed the questionnaire at the counseling center. The test responses indicated that I should meet the psychiatrist immediately. I met the doctor at the clinic the next day. The doctor was kind and asked me to tell her what had happened. I told her my story and cried all the time. I was so depressed. She suggested that I take off work for one week, and then she wrote a prescription. The medicine was anti-depressants and sleeping pills. The doctor made an appointment to see me again in a week. I was back in the loop again – see the doctor and take medicine. I took medicine and felt dizzy.

Because I had taken time off from work, I remained alone in the apartment, with little to do. So, I started to research the depression disorder, seeking information on the prescribed medication, such as what the pill was and how it helped.[2] As I stayed alone, my thoughts kept running on and on. A friend asked me to go out, but I did not feel like doing anything. After one week passed, I was back to the clinic to see the doctor and report my experiences during the past week. I met the doctor and told her about my feelings and activities. As I told the story, I cried all the time. I explained that I did not feel better at all in the past week. The doctor told me that when a patient faced depression many times in life, without receiving the right treatment and medicine, there was a high possibility for the depression to recur. Also, it would take a longer time for treatment than the previous episode. The doctor adjusted the medicine slightly and again asked me to take one week off from work.

Many things happened during the next week off work. I told my family about my illness. My mom sent dhamma books and told me that chanting and praying to Buddha would help. I had a small chanting book from my grandmother, which I had carried since I went abroad. Before I was sick, I sometimes chanted for a short time. For meditation, it was really hard for me. It was no longer than five minutes since my brain kept thinking of so many things and never attained peace. At that time, I could not focus on anything even reading a book. A friend in Thailand tried to tell me about Buddha's teaching, such as emptiness, non-self, and other teachings of Buddha on getting rid of suffering. I did not get it at all. I did not understand how thinking about those teachings could help me relieve suffering. I felt that suffering and myself were the same object, and it was impossible to separate them out. I replied to her, "I might have to find a way out on my own or succumb to suffering forever until my dying day." In that week off, I was getting worse. My thoughts were running, and I could not control my mind. I spent the whole day sitting and thinking on the sofa in the apartment. I had negative thoughts about myself. The situation made me angry, and I hated myself. I was at the bottom of a dark valley again. I did not know what I lived for. I did not want to live anymore. It was difficult to wake up and take a breath, and I lived with these feelings every day. My energy was drained. I did not want to do anything and did not know how to overcome these things. Finally, I reached the appointed time with the doctor. I told her what happened during the week, such as losing focus on daily activities in normal life. She was shocked at how I had progressed so badly. It seemed the medicine did not help and living alone at this time was not good for me. So, she decided to refer me to a nearby psychiatric hospital. She suggested I participate in activities at the hospital. These activities might help adjust my behavior and facilitate a return to normal life. I was so worried about where she was going to send me and what I would encounter next. I asked a friend to take me to the hospital the next day. I also sent an email to my supervisor, who told me to follow what the doctor said and "take it easy."

5 Two-Week Experience in a Psychiatric Hospital

In the morning of the first day at the hospital, I was so nervous as I walked alone inside the hospital and gave the referral documents to the hospital staff. They asked me a few questions, such as whether I hallucinated. I also completed a questionnaire about symptoms of depression. I was so afraid and sad. I cried continuously and could not control my flow of feelings. The staff wrote the word "severe" on the document I had completed. Then I proceeded to another waiting room where several patients were sitting. At 9 am, a staff member gave each of those waiting in the room a piece of paper and provided some oral instructions. There were many questions to be answered, such as completing a check list about how I was feeling today, quantity of sleep, and today's goal. Next, the staff briefly spoke about the activity on that day. I tried to listen but could not catch all that was said. At that moment, I could not imagine what would happen next. I sat quietly and followed the others. I was still afraid and worried about the situation and the people.

I never felt good with my previous psychiatric treatments and did not think they helped. But I had no choice. Accordingly, I completed the questions and set a goal. In the late morning of that day, I participated in my first group therapy session. Every patient, including me, sat on chairs, set in a circle. We could see each other's face. In the room, there was one therapist taking care of us. She introduced herself and also let each patient present themselves and share their feelings – one by one. When someone shared an emotion or story, the others listened quietly. They told their stories, described symptoms, and explained their feelings. Some were sick with a major depression disorder like me, some were sick with bipolar disorder, some had not slept for a week, some were abused since they were young, some were addicted to drugs, some had hurt themselves, and some had made suicide attempts. Finally, it was my turn to share. I introduced myself and, with tears, told my story about depression. I shared the feeling of hurting myself and not wanting to live. Everyone in the room listened intently to what I had to say. The group therapy session was about one hour. The therapist spoke to the group to close the session. After that, she walked close to me and assured, "do not worry, the people here will take care of you."

Lunchtime followed the group therapy session. I followed the other patients to the canteen, grabbed food from the counter, and sat at the round table. One of the patients asked me to join her and the others. I sat with them. As they talked to each other, I was quiet and listened to them. I only spoke out when they asked something about me. After lunch, I attended activities that helped us understand the illness and how they can support our return to normal life. Before 3 pm, the staff called us to together to explore what we learned on the first day. The activities were scheduled from 9 am to 3 pm, and then we all went home. Each day I attended the class. For example, the lesson that I learned for 2–3 days was about studying the nature of the illness, practicing being present, meditating with various techniques, positive thinking, self-esteem, self-accepting, letting go, doing some physical exercises. The group therapy session was held every day for one hour – a session for sharing and listening, feeling and experiencing what you and others have to say.

For 2–3 days in the hospital, everything was improving. I started to talk with others and concentrated on activities better than the first day. I tried to learn what I never knew before, just like a child. I knew that the cause of the illness came from a chemical imbalance in the brain that I had to take medicine. Along with the medication treatment, I also had to improve my habits, such as avoiding negative thoughts, increasing self-esteem, and coping with emotion. The staff taught us almost everything in theory and practice to help us live life. I liked when they taught about negative thinking, and they said that the patients seemed to have a magnifying glass. Some guilt might be so tiny that we could ignore it, but patients could magnify it significantly – the mind increasing its magnitude and potential impact on the body. At that time, I did not understand much because what I felt seemed so real. I just kept what they taught as a piece of information. The group therapy session helped a lot since I felt I was not alone in facing this illness. So many people had experience with depression and tried to find a way out. Once we shared and listened to each other, we could learn something. If we listened carefully with the heart, sharing stories or feelings would resonate inside and become a mirror to know ourselves.

In the late morning of the fourth day, the staff called me to see the hospital's psychiatrist. He introduced himself and asked me my history and symptoms. He inquired about the employment of my father and mother. I told him my father was an accountant before retirement, and my mother was a typist. He smiled and replied that I was smart like my father. The psychiatrist emphasized that I had to take medicine and therapy together. The staff here would help me, but I had to be patient because it took time to heal. In my case, it should not be too long to be back to everyday life. He changed all my prescribed medicines and ended the conservation with the sentence: "*Worry and enjoy are like the uncertainty principle.*"

In comparison to the uncertainty principle in physics, I knew that he meant when we enjoy, we cannot observe worry at that time, but when we worry, enjoyment cannot stand. I found that 15-minute talking with him to be extremely valuable. He was the best medical doctor with whom I ever interacted. I enjoyed talking with him. I had some hope and encouragement for the treatment. During the five days in the hospital, I had very positive experiences with psychiatric therapy. I wanted to share my feelings with my friends in tomorrow's group therapy session. So, I wrote down my thoughts and hoped I would be brave enough to share them in the group therapy session the next day.

In the group therapy session of the sixth day, I already was regarded as the old patient. There was new patient joined us that day. He was so quiet and stressed. He shared that he had a lot of stress at work until he could not carry it anymore and attempted suicide. Everyone shared and listened as usual. I was almost the last one. I shared my feeling and read the message I had prepared with a shaking voice because of the excitement.

Tuesday, September 20th, 2006

Live and Learn

Now I have already spent five days at the psychiatric center. I learn a lot of things from the people there. I am exploring my life. Who am I? What is wrong with my life? I always ask myself why I have to live. I am so scared to live. I am afraid of the people. It is very hard for me to face and talk with other people. I have fear. I want to just disappear from this world. What's the matter if this world doesn't have me? I always question and try to find the answer. I don't know whether I can find the answer or not but at least I learn something. Learning for me is kind of fun. I enjoy learning.

I had negative thoughts about the psychiatric center or doctor in the past but the first five days here make me change my mind. I met many people who have similar feelings to me. We talk, listen, share and support each other. It is helpful. So, we can think clearly and know ourselves better. For me, here is like school. Everyone is my teacher. I feel like I'm going to school again – listening, thinking, and learning. It's also nothing if I won't do it. Practice is important to keep my life away from this illness – depression. If I still live in this world, I have to explore and take care of myself. Be careful and be conscious every moment.

Let me summarize what I have learned in the first five days. I learn that I have to take care of myself before helping others. If I am sick, how I can help others. I also learn that if I am sick and I cannot take care of myself, I

> should need help from others. I learn I couldn't make any major decision while I am sick with this illness. In the past, I made the decision while I was sick. Thus, the problems haven't been solved. They are still problems and I am never satisfied or accept them. That makes me much more confused about the situation right now. In this time, I learn that before I make a decision, I should first fix myself from the illness. Then think clearly about information and possibility that can occur in reality, and make the decision and accept it. That's the way of life – accept what we choose and who we are, otherwise, we never satisfy our lives and we suffer more and more. Furthermore, I learn to have some goals every day. The goal keeps our lives moving. For me, at least I know what I am going to do today.
>
> I have to keep learning day by day and have fun with learning throughout my life. That's my life; otherwise, I cannot survive in this world. Live and learn.

Everyone in the room intentionally listened to me and clapped hands after speaking. I thanked them for listening also. At the end of the class, the therapist said that I was brave and had better progressed a great deal since the first day. She wished I would continue this improvement. At the canteen, the new patient thanked me for sharing the message. After that, other patients, including me, tried to talk with him about not feeling lonely

Already one week had passed. I felt familiar with the people at the hospital. We talked together and learned so many things. I almost forgot that I was a Ph.D. degree researcher, an Asian, weak in English, not clever, and not good enough. I did not have to wear any mask to pretend to be better than I was. We were friends who had similar feelings. I felt that someone on the Earth understood and listened to me. They did not regard me as a weak person, different from the others, or like a monster. From crying a lot and being very depressed on the first day, I could now laugh and easily fit into the group. I increased my conversations with people. The medicine the doctor prescribed, changed from what my earlier doctor prescribed, seemed to fit well with my body because there were no side effects. When one morning, as a test, I stopped taking it my body did not feel good after. Based on this experience I accepted that I needed to take the medicine.

Almost two weeks passed. Everything seemed to go well. I felt better. Intensive activities, taking the entire the day, helped me to escape from my thoughts. At least I did not just sit and repeat negative thoughts. For two weeks I spoke a lot of English, perhaps more than I had spoken in any similar time interval since I had been in the US. I had the courage to speak out to people that I did not know before. My English and human relations improved so much in 14 days.

Finally, I had a chance to see the psychiatrist again. He said that I was getting better and could now go back to live a normal life. However, I must continue the treatment by taking medicine and regularly seeing a therapist and psychiatrist. Most important, I should bring what I learned and practice adapting it into real life. I thanked him and asked whether I could be his patient. He said that he accepted only patients in the hospital. I was a bit disappointed, but I understood. I enjoyed talking to and learning from him.

Although I was glad to be leaving the hospital, I took a short break, sitting in front of the building and watching the tree and grass. The weather was so nice. A gentle wind blew and touched my face. My thoughts stopped. I remember my mind was very calm and peaceful at that moment. I had never felt like that before. For such a long time, this was the peace I was seeking. It was a perfect moment and I stayed like that for a while. Then, suddenly, a thought came to me: "If I leave the hospital, how can I live life? I have to meet people who do not understand my feeling. There is a lot of work to do. How can I cope with it all?" Then fear welled up within me, and the peaceful moment was gone. The light and bright world became grey. I walked back to the building and continued the activity. I met the therapist and told her that the doctor allowed me to leave the hospital, and I was worried about surviving in the real world. I thanked her for all her help here for two weeks. She always took good care of me and all the other patients. She was very kind and always encouraged all of us. In the afternoon of the last day, the therapist approached and said that she was happy to be my therapist. She worked in the clinic outside and could accept new patients. If I agreed, we could work together, and I could be a patient at the clinic, which meant I would see the psychiatrist she worked with there. I was glad to hear that. I decided to be her patient. That afternoon, I said goodbye and thanked my friends at the hospital. In only two weeks I learned so many things and found new hope for living with depression in real life.

6 Life and Treatment after Leaving Hospital

Spending two weeks in the hospital helped me bring myself back to real life. However, living outside was not easy as in the hospital – more complications and many factors to deal with. The main feeling that I remember was fear. I have a fear of living life and meeting people. I didn't trust anyone. Thought and mind were still running and quickly going outside, but it was not hard to control like what happened before. It might be because of the medicine and the training inside the hospital for two weeks. I continued the treatment for depression and met with the therapist and psychiatrist. The following week after I left the hospital, I met the therapist at the clinic and introduced myself to the doctor. She interviewed me the first time we met and increased the dose of the medicine for the anti-depression and sleeping pills. I felt uncomfortable with the new prescriptions, and I reported the effects and symptoms the next time I met her. The frequent meetings enabled her to adjust the strength of the prescribed drugs over a period of 3–4 weeks. I met the therapist once a week, which was more frequently than I met with the doctor.

Every time I met with the therapist she asked me about my symptoms, my development on coping and living in daily life, or any problems I faced. She tried to help me see myself by asking or giving me some homework. She consulted as much as she could. However, she never gave an answer or made any decision for me. She was just like a mirror that I could see myself or my problems clearly or learn to live a better life. For example, she asked me how I looked at myself as positive/negative from several points of view, and my answers were very pessimistic about myself. However, the therapist usually encouraged and told me that I was strong and had more positive sides than I thought. I remembered that, at that time, I had hardly ever worked on positive thinking. Positive thinking seemed to help me. I felt better, released some suffering, and my brain felt light. Somehow, I thought that changing and controlling thoughts were the way to rid myself of depression and bring me happiness. But I was wrong. Negative thinking still keeps coming back and finally taking over again.

Overall, the depression did not disappear, but it got a bit better and was not as bad as in the past. I took medicine every day. Although I learned that nutrition, exercise, and meditation also help with anxiety and depression (Bourne et al., 2004), I still did not change my behaviors. I tried to do some exercises such as walking, but it was very rare. I ate the same food which had lots of fat and sweets, drinking coffee, soda, alcohol, and fewer vegetables. I still worry about many things. I also tried to apply what I learned from the hospital to real life. Unfortunately, it was not fast enough to deal with the problems before me. I also tried to set a goal, observe and take notes about emotion, emergent situations, and how I coped. But eventually, I did these things less often. So, my feelings were up and down depending on the situation. When the symptoms of depression were terrible, the doctor would change the medicine, and we tried to find the reason. In my case, worry and stress have been long-time habits since I was young. Facing disappointments in life and experiencing lots of stress created the illness of depression. It was naive to expect depression to disappear in a short time, since it had been chronic for so long.

In August of 2007, I told my supervisor that it could be last year that I would work here. I thought that full-time research might not be my way. My treatment of depression continued. I saw the therapist and psychiatrist less frequently, but I still had to take pills. Once during a meeting with the doctor, I asked her how long I had to take medicine. She replied, "For your case, you might have to take it forever." I sighed and accepted the condition. She might be right because I did not know how to get out of this long-suffering.

7 Hope for a New Life of Living with Depression

I was back in Thailand in 2008 with feelings of sadness, relief, hope for a new life, and fear. I stayed with my family in Bangkok for two months before starting a new job in Chiang Rai, a province in the Northern part of Thailand. Even for just two months, living in Bangkok was very difficult for me. The city was full of pollution and hot weather. I was allergic to air pollution and uncomfortable with an overweight body, about 90 kg. I still ate a lot of food every day: white rice, meat, sweets, and coffee, but fewer vegetables and fruit. I loved to hang out with friends, listen to live music, and drink alcohol. I was unhealthy in both body and mind. Luckily, I had the medicine left for depression for a while and it helped me with sleep and emotion. Whenever I looked at myself in the mirror, I felt pity. I did not know how to find a way out of the suffering. Mind and body were very painful. For others, they might see me as having a good profile, but I considered myself a failure.

In Chiang Rai, my new job was as a lecturer at the university which was located on a mountain where the air was very nice. I could see mountains and a green environment every day. People were friendly and easy to get along with. I did not tell anyone here that I was sick with depression. When the medicine ran out just before I moved to Chiang Rai, I decided not to continue to use prescribed medication for treating my depression. I knew that it was risky, but I wanted to try living by myself since the situation was different from the past. However, I learned from the past that if I did not continue the treatment, the depression might come back for another episode. With a bit of knowledge, I must do something to replace the antidepressants. What immediately popped into my head was doing exercise and eating nutritious food. Moreover, I should be careful and did not let the depression last for more than two weeks. If it lasted too long, everything would be so difficult to deal with.

I lived in the dormitory of the university. I usually had breakfast, lunch, and dinner from the university cafeteria and drank a cup of coffee after lunch almost every day. I stopped soda first and added a small portion of the vegetable menu into the dish. I kept thinking of exercise and tried to do it someday but, later, I could not do it regularly. I quickly got tired, had asthma, and had leg pain because of my overweight body. For the mental part, if I had an emotional impact, my mind was easily down. Sometimes I heard people argue with loud voices and even though it was not my business, my emotions were perturbed, quickly fluctuated, and it was difficult to return to normal. I often did not know how to stop my emotions, so I just hung out with friends and drank beer. Even though I knew alcohol never helped to make the suffering go, and it could destroy the brain and cause depression,[3] I could not stop drinking because I did not want to remove myself from my social circle that included beer drinking. I assured myself that I should not worry too much since I was not an everyday drinker. I was not addicted.

8 Keep Promising, Keep Walking

In September 2008, one semester had already passed. As a university lecturer there were many tasks to do. I learned how to deal with many new things here. Even though teaching was the activity I liked most, I still had to deal with fluctuating emotions. It was tough when feelings such as depression, anxiety, anger, or stress emerged. It was like I was pulled to hell again. Changing my eating behavior, a little did not help much. The doctor's words in the US echoed in my head: "For your case, you might have to take medicine forever." I felt sad when I thought of her words but I accepted that I would live with depression forever. I told myself I should not be sad. I had to do something to help myself survive the illness. I should do something to replace taking medicine but what was it? I thought, how about exercise? After I considered for a while, I decided to go out for a walk for around 40 minutes every day. This time I was so serious about walking. I promised myself I would walk every day to help live with depression forever until I die. I did not even have some hope for recovery from the illness. I thought just being able to live with it was OK for me. I kept promising and walked around the university every evening. Walking was so boring, so I always carried an mp3 player to listen to music. Someday, if I had to skip walking for some reason, I would walk longer than usual the next day.

After I had walked for several months, it became my habit. When I felt very emotional in some situations, I would go out for a walk to release the bad energy or thought. It helped a little. At least, it was better than doing nothing. People who saw me walk every day appreciated and encouraged me. Surprisingly, many people, including myself, noticed that I was thinner than before. I lost weight at a rate of about 1 kg per month. It was good encouragement for me to continue walking. I expected to lose more weight and get better shape and health. One of my friends taught me how to calculate calories from food[4] and activities[5] related to our weight.[6] I never knew that before, but after I learned from her, I tried to look at the labels of the packages more carefully before I chose something to eat. After one year of walking, I could lose 10 kg. It was so amazing. Losing weight was not my first intention, but it was a byproduct of everyday walking and being a little more careful of food choices. I kept walking and still have some hope of living with depression better. Now losing weight is also my goal since I felt good after losing 10 kg. If I continue walking, losing another 10 kg might be possible.

9 Practicing Mindfulness

About the middle of 2009, a friend Jeff gave me Luangpor Pramote Pamojjo's dhamma CD s.[7] Listening to dhamma talks was not in my thought. It was boring and hard to understand, and I did not know how it helped life out of the suffering. People who could have peace from Buddhism were the only ones who could sit, close their eyes and meditate by following their breath. It was very hard for me. When I sat, closed my eyes, and meditated, my mind quickly wandered away and I thought of something else. I never control it to stay with the object, such as breathing. Thus, it was boring to sit and do nothing for a long time. I had seen my father meditate every day for his whole life—having long chants and sitting for meditation. Jeff kept asking me many times whether I had listened to the CD s or not. Three months later, I chose one of the CD s and listened because I did not want to hear him asking anymore. In the CD, a master named Luangpor Pramote talked about how we could be free from suffering if we truly understood ourselves (both body and mind). We could practice as simple as knowing what the body or mind did at the moment. If the mind wandered off, just know that it wandered and when it is convenient, bring the mind back to the body again. I felt it was very interesting – just knowing ourselves could reduce suffering. I had never heard that before. I knew before that the people who wanted to practice meditation had to learn from the temple for several days to be away from busy life. I asked Jeff whether I could practice while I walked every day or not. Jeff confirmed that I could practice when I walked.

In my second year of walking, I practiced mindfulness as I walked. The method was trying to know what I was doing at the moment, such as legs were moving. When I first practiced, during my 40-minute walk, I could recognize that my body moves only at the start and then again sometime in the middle or near the end. Between that, my mind wandered off and thought about something else and I did not know that I was thinking at all. I was in many stories that I thought and did not know that my body moved. I was surprised. Fortunately, I walked every day, so I could practice knowing body and mind (i.e., mindfulness) every day and have better and better self-knowing during my 40-minute walk, although I did not know how my suffering would go away.

During this time, my emotions are still up and down for my daily life. For example, a tiny mistake could make me so depressed and cry. It was nonsense for the others. Sometimes they wondered what was wrong with me. Depression and I seemed to be close friends. I did not see how it would disappear from my life, but I kept walking anyway, because of my promise to myself. After practicing mindfulness for two months, I decided to stop drinking alcohol because it did not align well with practicing mindfulness. Alcohol made the mind out of the actual feeling at the moment. I promised myself again that I would never drink alcohol again.

In April 2010, I moved to a new house. The environment in that area was nice and so quiet. I still walked and practiced mindfulness along the local road. I was interested in reading some of dhamma books and listening to dhamma talks, but I could not understand them. I still discussed and talked with Jeff about my mindfulness practicing and he said repeatedly that just observing your body and mind as they showed in the moment was all that was necessary. He emphasized that I should not worry about mistakes. If I made a mistake, restart my practice. One day a person gave me a CD of dhamma fiction. I listened to a story just for entertainment. The story was fantastic. There was a scene in the story in which the lady gave food to a monk every day. This resonated with me because each morning I saw a monk walking in our village, and I felt I would like to be like the lady in the story. I could not cook good food at all, but I tried to wake up in the early morning, around 5 am, and prepare some simple things or maybe some fruit or drink for the monk who walked on the same road I walked every day. Since I woke up early, I had more chances to listen to dhamma talks or read some books of various masters.

One day, the monk tried to have a conversation with me after he gave me a blessing. He said to me that "Your mind is already stable. You do not have to close your eyes when you *bhavana* and continuously do it as *a link in a chain.*" At that moment, I replied to him only, "I practice mindfulness while I am walking every day." I was surprised because we had never known each other before and I never told him what I was doing, even about practicing mindfulness. That day, I researched the word "bhavana" on the internet. I had heard this word since I was young but I did not really know what the actual meaning was. What was "we do not have to close our eyes when we "bhavana"? What was "continuous do as a link in a chain?" They were like a dhamma puzzle to me. After some research, the meaning word "bhāvana" itself in Pali was development or cultivate.[8] For example, we can have "citta bhavana" for development of mind or "kaya bhavana" for development of body. In Buddhism, we often heard about two types of bhavana. One is "samatha bhavana" which is the development of tranquility. The other is "vipassana bhavana" which is related to development of insight. Therefore, I found that what I did every morning, mindfulness practicing could be called "bhavana." However, I did not practice continuous like a link in a chain yet because I practiced only 40 minutes a day. But the good news was I have a stable mind – something I did not know. Later, I understood that a stable mind is a mind that was ready to observe the truth at the present moment. Venerable Pamojjo (2012) said that:

> A stable mind sees that the body breathing, or walking, is not us. It is just a body. The mind that is angry, greedy, or anything else, is not us either. The mind is angry, not us. The mind is deluded, not us. The body and mind are doing their work. They are doing what they do, not us. (p. 125)

After that, I also tried to practice mindfulness in daily life and observe life. I noticed that my mind liked to wander off and had a lot of useless thoughts during the day. I rarely focused on what I did. I could see the mind went away on its own without any control. Especially when I listened to dhamma talks, my mind often thought of something else. That was why I did not receive all the information provided by the masters. I repeated those talks, again and again, every morning and related them to my direct experience.

In September 2009, about nine months after I practiced mindfulness, my weight reduced to only 4 kg, instead of 9–10 kg as I expected. Also, the suffering did not seem to reduce yet and I could not see how I could have better lived with depression. One of the lecturers on health science told me that if I wanted to lose more weight, I had to have vigorous exercise to increase my heart rate;[9] walking is not enough. I thought it was hard for me to do heavy exercise because I quickly get tired and hard to breathe due to asthma. I gave up expecting the weight loss but I did not stop walking and practicing mindfulness because of the promise. I continued to observe my mind and body in my daily life. Sometimes I could see emotion when it was raised. I just saw but was not involved. I was so shocked. I had never seen myself like this before. In the past, I was usually involved in the feeling and be someone that received the pain. I could feel the temperature change and the movement of the body, and how the mind fluctuated. I knew this reaction was the result of mindfulness practice. This confirmed the knowledge I learned from dhamma. It was studied not only from others' words in the books or talks but also from our real life. At that moment, I understand how we can be free from suffering if we follow the Threefold Training called morality, concentration, and insight, which I read from the dhamma book when I was young (Bhikkhu, 1996). I am very grateful for Buddha's teaching and believed in the path of suffering-free. I promised myself that I would practice and apply mindfulness in life as much as possible until the last day of my life, no matter how hard it was. Knowing body and mind now turned out to be the goal in my life.

10 When Diet Is Totally Changed

One day I was washing the dishes in the morning. I tried to have awareness while my hands moved. Suddenly, some thoughts popped up in my brain. What did we eat for? The answers came up in my head that we ate for energy to live and for nutrition to maintain and fix our body, no matter for large parts or small parts. I could feel the energy in and out through my body at that time. I think of what I learned from school about nutrition when I was in elementary school and also in the book that I had read. Mood and food are also connected (Bourne et al., 2004). In the past, I just ate what I wanted and never cared about the effect on this body. After that day, my diet was totally changed. I prepared food for myself every day and carefully chose the food. I selected various kinds of food, especially fresh vegetables and fruits. I reduced meat from pork and chicken and selected fish instead. I avoided fried food and sweets. Most of the food I chose was the one that I hated to eat before. That was why my body never received enough nutrition to fix or maintain the parts of the body. For example, I hated brown rice and yogurt since I was young but, at this moment, I could eat them every day. I opened my mind to various kinds of food because I thought the body consists of many organisms with different duties. So, a variety of nutrients were essential for the body. I also stopped drinking coffee because it has side effects on my anxiety (Bourne et al., 2004). I could observe anxiety after drinking coffee without any cause from outside. I always think of what I brought into my mouth and how my body felt. This is like the body tried to communicate something to me. I learned a lot from observation on body and mind.

There was another big change that happened to me. I could not have dinner. I was full in the evening and if I tried to eat something, my body would hurt and feel uncomfortable. It was hard to sleep well if I had too much food. I stopped having dinner and was not hungry at all in the evening. On the contrary, I felt better and relieved. I saw my mind and body better than in the past day by day. For example, how the suffering occurred, what was behind the thought and action, what was beneficial and harmful to my life. To have depression made it easy for me to observe the state of mind and body because of the significant changes of emotion. As a result of diet changes, including cutting out dinner, I lost 2 kg in one month. So, I could reach another 10 kg loss after the end of the second year of walking.

11 New Life Began

Self-observing became my habit. After I awakened in the early morning, I started practicing mindfulness, listening to dhamma talks, and preparing food for the monks. One day, in December 2010, I walked back and forth in my house, then I could feel some chemicals in my brain were injected in large amounts. I had never felt like that before. I did not know what it was, but I could know from my intuition that it made the balance of chemicals in my brain. That means I did not have to experience pain due to chemical imbalance due to depression. This was the first time in my life that I could feel what a normal brain was. I also stopped blaming myself for being weak. I understood that was not about only emotions or feelings, but it was also the condition of the body and chemicals that I could not control, and I should not hold on to such thoughts. It did not mean that all emotions were gone. Depression, anxiety, anger, or sadness were still with me, but it was not difficult to be back to normal. If I encounter a difficult moment that relates to my depression, I try to observe the moment, which may cause suffering. I know and try not to be in the stories (thought) and wait until the event has gone. Sometimes I listen and talk gently and deeply with my child inside to help her heal and grow up. That is the way that I transform and heal my suffering inside, and mindfulness is an important key (Hanh, 2010).

Although I knew that my brain was normal, I did not stop walking and practicing mindfulness. I keep being mindful because the illness can come back again if I do not take care of myself – both body and mind – and there are so many things more to learn. I wrote this message in April 2011 to answer myself in 2006:

> Sunday, April 16th, 2011
>
> At my house in Chiang Rai, Thailand
>
> *Live and Learn Part II*
>
> This was already six months that I have continuously kept practicing the dhamma. I practiced as much as I could while waking up. Actually, it is nothing more than learning myself. I have learned so many things that I

did not know before. I try to have the mindfulness to observe and learn my body and mind. Most importantly, the suffering reduced a lot because I have learned the truth of the nature of my body and mind. This is like I had a nightmare and then woke up to the real world. Now I know who I am. I know what was wrong before and why I really suffered. Now I am ready to face the truth. I do not know how the world would be if I did not exist. But I am already here as a part of nature; I will do my best. Learning is fun and I enjoy learning.

I just realized that I did not understand anything about dhamma in Buddhism classes from school since I was young. But when I started to practice mindfulness continuously, it was like I went to school again and started from the beginning. It was Buddha's school and we had mentors to guide us to the right ways. We are learning by doing in this school. Buddha found the way and taught us 2500 years ago. All students in the school practice and learn via their own experience. The tools are intention, persistence, mindfulness, and wisdom and anyone can learn in this school. We might start from nothing, but we will have more knowledge if we keep doing. We will know the truth of nature, which we call dhamma. True dhamma can be studied from our body and mind. The method is only "knowing the truth of body and mind at the moment–observing them with stable mind and without judgment." I have received a lot of benefits from this practice. The suffering in my mind is lighter. Especially, I do not have to suffer due to depression as an illness anymore since my brain can maintain a chemical balance.

Let me conclude what I have learned in the past six months. I have learned that no one can help me from suffering inside my mind except me. I cannot help anyone if people do not try to help themselves from the suffering. I have learned that everything cannot remain the same and is out of control, so it has to change or transform due to several causes and factors. The suffering comes and goes inside our minds. Nobody brings suffering to us. We create it ourselves because of ignorance since we were born. We only look to the outside but never look back into ourselves. We think that everything, including mind and body, belongs to us. We want to control as we want them to be. We want happiness to last forever and hate the suffering when it comes. It contradicts nature, which no one owns. In the past, we let ignorance play a role in our thought, desire, and action, which brought us to suffering. Today I take my mind to see what the truth is. The proper knowledge grows inside and is ready to be used in time if I have mindfulness at that moment. Whenever the factors are ready to cause the wounds as in the past, I have learned to observe them without judgment and let the wisdom play its own duty. When I have awareness (mindfulness), I heal the wounds accumulated for a long time. I have learned to be at present, try not to attach to anything, and do my best. Mindfulness can help protect me from harm at the moment. I have learned to accept everything that happens – no matter it is good or bad – because I deserved what I have done and there are many conditions involved that I cannot control. There is nothing that I have to regret or consider unsatisfactory. I have learned to keep this body and mind normal, just observe what they think and do, and not hurt myself and others. Next, I will try to live my life with the mindfulness and wisdom I practiced and developed. I will consider carefully before acting. Even though physical suffering cannot be prevented, I will learn to live with it without suffering in mind. Finally, I learned to have a goal in life. My goal is to live every day with mindfulness and try to stay at the moment as much as I can. At least I know what I should do at each moment.

I keep learning this body and mind every day and enjoy learning life as a part of nature. That's the way of my life; although I walk alone, I will keep walking on this way until I die. Live and learn.

12 What Did I Learn from Living with Depression?

The way to live life is very important. From my experience it is important to open your mind, accept and learn from difference, keep doing continuously, and never give up. Eventually, I learned not to refuse prescribed medication. Western medicine helped me pass a difficult time when my depression was severe. But, for me, relying on only medicine can help only to a certain degree. Interestingly, the way to live well with depression is different, depending on each person's condition. Some people might succeed with only medical treatment. Others might need exercise or changes in diet may be required. Some might need holistic change, such as in my case. Of course, I always suggest people see experts if they have a depressive condition that is out of control (or symptoms stay longer than two weeks). Medicine can help quickly bring them back to normal life. But if you keep living life in the same way, the illness can come back and live with you forever also. However, please do not forget that our body can produce natural medicine if we give the body and mind a chance by having the suitable ingredient put into it. If we take care of ourselves by eating carefully and exercising regularly, natural medicine can live with us sustainably. Moreover, learning the cause of our suffering of both body and mind should not be ignored. From my experience, the important ingredient was mindfulness because it made us know and realize what is going on in our lives. So, we can decide how we should live or act in various situations. Nowadays, I still live with several feelings, including depression with mindfulness. I keep learning and adjusting the way of living that is suitable for each lifetime. Suffering and difficult emotions are great teachers to me. Whether they are good or bad, they are precious moments to observe. I learned them through the eyes of mindfulness and wisdom.

Notes

1 Nowadays we can easily find similar information via the internet https://www.healthline.com/health/depression/tests-diagnosis#diagnosis
2 https://www.webmd.com/anxiety-panic/guide/medications-treat-mental-disorders
3 https://www.webmd.com/depression/guide/alcohol-and-depresssion
4 https://www.calories.info/
5 https://healthyeater.com/calories-burned
6 https://www.thebodytransformationacademy.com/blog/how-to-lose-1kg-of-fat
7 https://www.dhamma.com/en/
8 https://en.wikipedia.org/wiki/Bhavana
9 https://www.healthline.com/health/fitness-exercise/fat-burning-heart-rate#fatburning-workouts

References

Bhikkhu, B. (1996). *Handbook for mankind* (First Electronic ed.). Buddha Dharma Education Association Inc.

Bourne, E. J., Brownstein, A., & Garano, L. (2004). *Natural relief for anxiety: Complementary strategies for easing fear, panic, and worry.* New Harbinger Publications, Inc.

Hanh, T. N. (2010). *Reconciliation: Healing the inner child.* Parallax Press.

Reynolds, D. K. (1984). *Constructive living.* University of Hawaii Press.

Venerable Pamojjo, P. (2012). *To see the truth: The teachings of Venerable Pramote Pamojjo.* Suan Santidham.

CHAPTER 12

Reversing Osteoporosis

Lessons in Alignment

Hema Daswani

Abstract

In this chapter I describe how I reversed Osteoporosis using life-affirming foods and practices. I was diagnosed with a severe case of Osteoporosis at a very young age. Through studying and incorporating proper nutrition, yoga, acupuncture, herbs, Jin Shin Jyutsu and Eden Energy Medicine into my life, I learned how to reverse this potentially disabling condition without recourse to prescription drugs. Taking another perspective, I provide insights into how inner energies facilitate the body's ability to heal itself when we return to it with awareness.

Keywords

osteoporosis – osteopenia – complementary medicine – Jin Shin Jyutsu – acupuncture – nutrition – herbal medicine – Eden Energy Medicine

• • •

As energy beings, we have the innate ability to heal ourselves. The key is returning to our still center and reconnecting with this wisdom. When our energies are scrambled, we are akin to an instrument that is out of tune. If we are fortunate, the Universe throws some curve balls at us in an attempt to bring us back into sync.

My visit to an endocrinologist in the fall of 1997 was the event needed to change the course of my life. For a year or so prior, I was experiencing debilitating pain and weakness in my neck and extremities. It's hard to describe the precise feeling. It felt like there was no substance left in my body. Naturally, I was concerned, but nothing prepared me for the prognosis that followed. Looking at me straight in the eye, my physician said "Your case is one in a million – you have the bones of a 90-year-old woman who has smoked all her life. Expect to be in a wheelchair by age 40." I stood there, a deer in headlights – my

 | DOI:10.1163/9789004527348_012

brain furiously trying to process the information. A moment later, an unexpected thought floated up "I love to dance ... I can't let this happen." I was all of 30 years old, my entire life ahead of me. The official diagnosis was Osteoporosis in the hip and spine[1] and Osteomalacia, which is the softening of bone due to a severe vitamin D deficiency. Advanced cases of Osteomalacia can lead to bone pain and muscle weakness. After reviewing my test results, the endocrinologist suspected that the Osteoporosis could be a result of a disconnect in the pituitary/hypothalamic axis in the brain, possibly originating at birth. I was asked to take Fosamax, a bisphosphonate drug prescribed to women 65 and older. Having no knowledge of pharmaceutical drugs, my gut instantly sent out a red flag; the side effects of the medication would probably kill me before the disease itself. I respectfully declined, and instead, started supplementing with vitamin D3 and applying a transdermal patch that provided the tiniest levels of the hormones Estrogen and Progesterone – just enough for me to function.[2]

1 My Early Years

In retrospect, I see an invisible line dividing my life into two distinct chapters: pre and post diagnosis. My early years in Mumbai, India were unremarkable. I came from a family of loving, but authoritarian parents, and two older sisters. I was a highly sensitive child, painfully shy, and lacking in self-assurance, which clearly reflected in my posture. I navigated through life much like a log of wood on water – drifting aimlessly, without a sense of purpose, always taking the path of least resistance. My two joys were Indian classical music and dance, in which I received training since the age of ten.

In college, I chose to study Applied Art, not because of a deep desire to learn design and advertising, but because I was less attracted to the other mainstream choices offered at the time. Five years later in 1989, I traveled to the US to complete my Master's in Visual Communications from Pratt Institute, NYC. Once again, propelled not by a great passion to pursue a career in Graphic Design, but because my middle sister had left for the USA a year prior and I wanted to be closer to her.

Despite my ambivalence, I enjoyed the program at Pratt immensely. Three months after graduating, I was offered a position as in-house Graphic Designer in a medical company. A few years later, I rose to a Managerial position. As my team grew, so did my responsibilities and stress levels. I was having a hard time keeping up, and felt like I was trying too hard. It was then that I started noticing aches and pains in my body, and received the ominous news mentioned above. Since I had refused to take the prescribed drug, and had no knowledge of healing, I didn't have the tools to turn this condition around. All I knew was my current life wasn't working for me, and that something needed to shift. After twelve long years, I finally admitted, that despite my love for graphic design, I needed something else to feed my soul, but couldn't for the life of me figure out what this was! In utter desperation, I turned to prayer. For the next four years, I surrendered completely, asking the Universe for direction.

2 Learning to Trust My Intuition

During this time, I re-started my dance training, despite being on a shoe-string budget. Kathak, an exquisite north Indian dance form comprising of complex and rhythmic footwork, graceful hand gestures, and pirouetted turns, made me feel alive, and provided a means of expressing both the sensual and the divine. One beautiful fall day in September 2001, my friend from dance class announced that her spiritual Guru – an enlightened soul, had arrived in NYC. She spoke about how she had blossomed under her guidance, and urged me to meet her. Without giving me a chance to react, she arranged our meeting. Shri Anandima ji had the kindest, gentlest presence ever! I loved her energy immediately. The very next day, I went through an initiation ceremony called "Shaktipat," wherein the transfer of energy took place – from her to me. My kundalini had been awakened. Kundalini refers to the divine feminine serpentine energy that lies dormant at the base of the spine (Muladhara Chakra). Spiritual liberation is possible when the kundalini is awakened and reaches the Sahasrara (Crown Chakra) through Meditation, Pranayama (breath), and/or yogic/tantric practices. Everything happened so effortlessly, it almost seemed like it had been pre-arranged by my Guru. After my initiation, my daily meditations began. This was a new experience, and extremely challenging at first. My mind was like a monkey – grabbing on to every irrelevant thought. Despite these disruptive moments, I persevered, and 6 months later, in my so-called "meditation cloud," I received a message: "Ask your manager for a 4-day week. Use the extra day to go within. You will find the answers you need." I was apprehensive. I wasn't sure if I should trust this inner voice. Besides, I didn't expect my manager to react kindly to the request. But a force beyond my control drove me to knock on his door the next morning. I explained my health situation and asked if I could step down from the managerial role. His response caught me by surprise! Not only did he express deep concern and granted the day off, but he urged that I stay on as manager. This was music to my ears!

3 Finding Proper Alignment through Yoga

Thus began the story of my unfolding. On my first Friday off, I enrolled in a Hatha yoga class at the Integral Yoga Institute. My instructor turned out to be an evolved and nurturing soul. With each Sun Salutation, Downward Dog, and Shoulder Stand, I felt my resilience growing, my body getting stronger, my mind quieter. After six months, I started my daily practice from home. Over time, I reached a place of greater clarity and focus. As a result, my meditation practices deepened. In 2002, I received another message – "study nutrition."

4 You Are What You Eat

These words, *"You are what you eat,"* spoken by Joshua Rosenthal – founder of the Institute of Integrative Nutrition in NYC – completely changed my perception of food (Rosenthal & Monte, 2002). We can change our thoughts by eating differently! Enrolling in this immersion program in April 2003 provided the perfect segue into the world of health and established the nutritional foundation that I follow to date. Classes were held once a month, allowing me the flexibility to continue working. On the day of enrollment, we were given at least a dozen books to read. My first takeaway was that nutrition is not a cookie-cutter solution. One man's nectar is other another man's poison. Dietary principles from diverse modalities were introduced. These included Ayurveda, Traditional Chinese Medicine (TCM), The Blood Type Diet, and The Power Eating Program. We studied under brilliant individuals such as Paul Pitchford (2003). With each class, we left heavier than we came in – loaded with books, and useful gifts to help us along our healing journey. The array of greens and gluten-free grains we learned about constitute the pillars of my diet even today. We understood why we have cravings and the importance of refraining from refined sugar. Home-cooked meals were provided along with recipes. This allowed me to experience first-hand all that I was learning about food. I felt loved and nourished at every level – mental, emotional, and spiritual. Cooking classes and health-food store tours opened up my world to healthy versions of everyday products, and introduced me to new items such as tempeh and nato. I had never been fond of cooking, but this completely changed my relationship with food. As my knowledge base expanded, so did the desire to share this information. This too, was fulfilled by the Fast Track Program that trained us as Holistic Health Counselors.

5 Discovering the Alchemy of Herbs

Charged with this knowledge – I felt a passion and curiosity like never before! From all that I had learned, TCM held the greatest fascination. In 2004, I enrolled in a 6-week introductory class in Eastern Herbs and Nutrition offered by the Open Center in New York City. At the end of the 6 weeks, I had more questions than answers, so I decided to attend a 13-month extension of the same program. The study of herbs is awe-inspiring! They are categorized by their primary action. For example, regulate Qi or blood, drain dampness, relieve food stagnation, etc. Each herb corresponds with a temperature, taste, and meridians entered and is assigned one of the three properties: aromatic, astringent, or poisonous. I slowly fell in love with this deep and complex science. As much as I wanted to delve into a full-time program in herbal medicine, I made the decision to start with acupuncture.

As part of my exploration of acupuncture programs, I visited California in the summer of 2006. I was also hoping to get some much-needed advice from a seasoned acupuncturist/herbalist – who was the friend I was staying with. After each Open House, I received an acupuncture session at the student clinic. It seemed like a good way to gauge the caliber of the school. After one such session, the Clinic Supervisor handed me a batch of herbs, with instructions on how to brew them. She was convinced that the formula would reverse my condition. Upon reaching home, my friend (the herbalist) emptied out the bag, separated out the herbs, and approximated the weight of each herb group. I heard her gasp! She said that even she couldn't have done better! After writing out the formula, she gifted me a Chinese herb pot, and sent me on my way, with a few words of advice – that I remove all supplements from my diet for 3 months, to give my liver a chance to detox. For years prior, my daily regimen comprised of multiple supplements a day, most of them self-prescribed! After returning to New Jersey, I started receiving weekly acupuncture treatments, and consuming the herbal concoctions twice a day. Six months later, my body aches had completely vanished, and my bone density levels had risen by 5%. The attending physician was speechless and asked which drug I was on! I gave my best smile, but didn't utter a word! I later learned that an average annual increase is 1%. Over time, and with great caution, I added back a few good quality supplements: a fish oil, vitamin D3, vitamin B12 and calcium.[3]

6 Vedanta Taught Me the Art of Living

The years between 2003 and 2007 proved to be intense on every level. Not only was there a burning desire to study everything I possibly could to heal myself but an equally deep-seated spiritual yearning that was not easily satiable. My consistent yoga practice and meditation led me to ask existential questions such as "Who am I?" "Why am I here?" and "What is my life purpose?" On a visit to India in 2004, I attended a talk on "Vedanta," by Swami Parathasarathy. "Vedanta" literally translates to "the culmination of knowledge." This is the ultimate knowledge of the SELF. Derived from the ancient Hindu scriptures (the Vedas), this science defines the Laws of Life and explains that we are all essentially pure consciousness (i.e., awareness). This consciousness is ever-present in all three states: when we are awake, in dream-state and in deep sleep. Most of us identify only with our body, mind and intellect. We think that this is what makes us who we are. The truth is that these are merely faculties given to us while we are on Earth so that we can fulfill our life purpose. They do not exist after we transition. They are in a way, similar to our possessions. Just as we say – "This is my book" or "This is my home" – in the same way, we can say "This is my body," "This is my mind" etc. Once this understanding sinks in, we realize that our body is simply a shell that houses our Atman or Soul. We are so much more than the physical body. When we are sick, it is really the "body" that is sick. Our soul is ever well and free. When we are upset, we can ask the question "Who is upset?" Our immediate answer is "I am upset." The next question that naturally arises is "Who is the "I?" Through a process of self-reflection and questioning, we return back to the answer: The "I" is nothing but consciousness – which is always neutral. It simply IS. One can compare it to a screen on which movies are projected. When it rains in the movie, the screen doesn't get wet. When there's a fire, the screen doesn't get burnt. The screen is the backdrop for whatever is happening. It's almost like viewing life from outside your body – being a witness (or a third party) and responding to events accordingly.

I was blown away by the presentation! This was exactly the knowledge I was seeking! After the talk, I jotted down my name and email in the roster with the hope that I would be contacted if study groups were started in the US. A few months later, this manifested into a reality! From 2005 to 2007, I attended bi-weekly classes. Arthur Schopenhauer's words impacted me deeply. "It is difficult to find happiness within oneself, but it is impossible to find it anywhere else." I began to start paying closer attention to my responses and reactions to external stimuli and looking at life from a bird's eye view. This brought fresh perspective and a certain level of detachment. Books by Sri Ramana Maharshi and Sri Nisargadatta Maharaj (e.g., Maharshi et al., 2010) filled the holes in my understanding. I slowly came to the realization that it is possible to attain a state of equanimity at all times. I was definitely not there yet, but was starting to feel more whole, and complete in myself.

7 Acupuncture Provided Clarity and Deeper Insights

My studies at the Eastern School of Acupuncture in Montclair, New Jersey began in the fall of 2007. I finally quit my job as Manager of Graphic Design, and continued working at the same company two days a week as a Graphic Design Consultant. Before I took this leap, I carefully reviewed my financial situation. No doubt, it meant a significant reduction in my income, but my priorities were clear. I was determined to find the underlying cause to my disharmony and also gain insights into this mysterious science. I decided to attend the program part-time, which gave me additional time to pay the school dues.

Four years flashed by in the blink of an eye! Through the lens of acupuncture, the body is seen as a delicate balance between two opposing and inseparable forces: yin and yang. An imbalance in these two leads to blockages in the flow of qi or vital energy along pathways known as meridians. Acupuncture points that lie along the meridians are portals that regulate the body's vital substances: qi, blood, essence and body fluid, thus correcting many of the body's imbalances. The two types of qi that caught my attention are pre-natal qi and post-natal qi. Pre-natal qi is comprised of Jing or "essence" that we receive from our parents and ancestors at inception. This constitutes our "savings account." Post-natal qi is produced upon the digestion of food, and constitutes our "checking account." If digestion is strong and our emotions and lifestyle are kept in check, our post-natal qi supplies are full. However, in times of stress, or when food is not being properly assimilated, our supplies of post-natal qi dwindle, and we start drawing from our resources of pre-natal qi. This is when signs of aging are noticed – graying hair, flaccid muscles, weak teeth and bones. Interestingly, I was born with a streak of white hair and developed Osteoporosis at age 30, a clear indicator of insufficient pre-natal qi – an extremely rare condition. It became imperative to work, not only with the Primary Meridians but also with what we call the "8 Extraordinary Meridians," as they play a critical role in dealing with chronic, deeper issues and congenital or constitutional issues. The Eight Extraordinary Meridians are reservoirs of qi and blood for the 12 organ meridians.

The five elements found in nature – Fire, Earth, Metal, Water, and Wood, also reside in the body. When in balance, each element engenders or controls another (Figure 12.1). Connected to a yin/yang pair of organs, each element has myriad associations – with emotions, colors, flavors, foods, tissues, etc. The kidneys, belonging to the Water element, are worthy of mention, because of their strong relationship with the formation of bone. The kidneys are the foundation of yin and yang, and govern growth, reproduction and development of the brain. The 8 Extraordinary Meridians have a close relationship with the kidneys. Thus, working with the kidneys and Extraordinary Meridians by nourishing essence, replenishing the body with herbs and foods that build yin (aka fluids/hormones), blood, and essence became essential components of my treatment protocol.

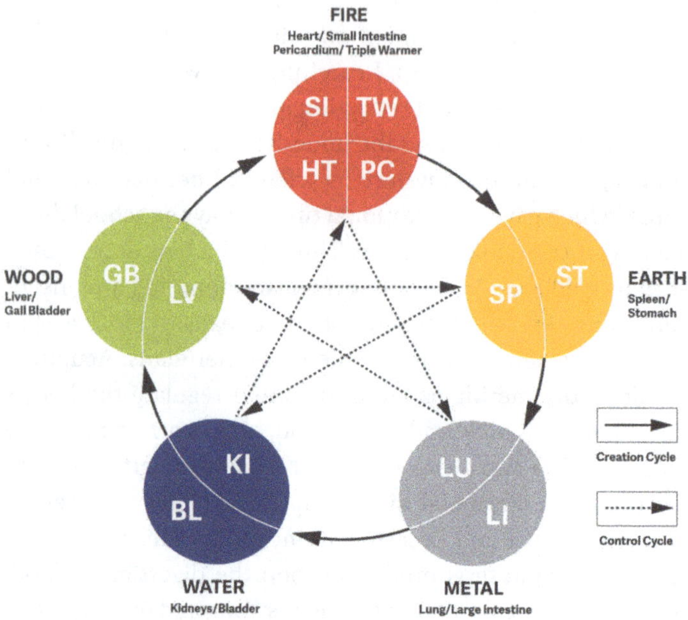

FIGURE 12.1 Five-element cycle

The Eastern School offers a comprehensive program; we were trained in three different styles of Acupuncture: Traditional Chinese Medicine (TCM), Japanese – Kiiko Matsumoto Style of Acupuncture (Matsumoto & Euler, 2017) and Worsley Five Element Acupuncture (Worsley, 2004). When it came time to start treating patients at the School Clinic, I had mentally decided to practice TCM. I did a surprising turnaround however, after noticing a marked improvement in patient outcomes during the Kiiko Style Clinic. Credit for this goes to my teacher and clinic supervisor – Shiaomei Weingarten. Watching this real-time was far more exciting than studying it in a classroom! It was a fun and interactive process yielding exceptional results. Shiaomei shared her pearls of wisdom on treatment protocols, and helped me perfect the application of herbs (aka moxa) on a patient's body; a technique requiring fine hand coordination and patience. It's ironical and amusing to note that all those years when I slaved over my dining table in India, honing my fine motor skills with a paintbrush, were now coming full circle – in the application of moxa! By introducing humor and wit into the clinic setting, Shiaomei lightened the atmosphere, instantly putting me at ease, while instilling confidence. All of the above allowed me to reach a level of comfort in my patient interactions and build trust.

We were also instructed by Kiiko Matsumoto herself! She is one of the greatest, living legends in the world, having studied under Master Nagano and

Master Hukaya in Japan. She eventually developed her own style of acupuncture based on the palpation of the hara (abdomen). She found that different regions on the hara, termed "reflex zones" corresponded with specific organs and meridians in the body. These areas are first palpated. Any discomfort or pressure pain is released by massaging distal points on the same meridian as the reflex zone. If the pain is released, the point is then needled. This style, rooted in interactive feedback from the patient, almost always results in a significant and immediate improvement in their condition. Upon graduating, my practice focusing on Kiiko Style Acupuncture was born on 11/11/11.

8 Reclaiming My Joy with Jin Shin Jyutsu

The official site for Jin Shin Jyutsu (JSJ) is jsjinc.net. Another great JSJ resource is flowsforlife.com. In early 2012, one of my patients inquired if I had studied JSJ. She frowned when she saw the question mark on my forehead, and said in all seriousness: "You are a healer. You should study it – if not to treat others, at least to help yourself." These words got my attention. I attended a 5-day class in Woodstock, NY in the fall of 2012. When I emerged, my mind was swimming with questions. Yet, something inside me knew I didn't need to look any further. I had found my true love!

JSJ is an ancient Japanese healing modality, revived in the early 1900s by Jiro Murai. He passed on his knowledge to Mary Burmeister, who brought this wondrous art to the US in the 1950s. My favorite translation of Jin Shin Jyutsu is "The art of the Creator through the hands of the compassionate." JSJ uses our hands as jumper-cables to harmonize body, mind and spirit. When hands are placed on two locations of the body, they act as magnets, creating what is similar to an electrical circuit between the areas being held, which enables energy to flow through a specific trajectory. Vedanta defines the laws of life; JSJ defines the laws of energy and how it flows through the body. With every exhale, energy descends down the front of the body. With every inhale, energy ascends up the back of the body. Acupuncture follows the same principles as JSJ, although JSJ is much older. Just as acupuncture has more than 300 points on the body, JSJ has 26 such locations called "Safety Energy Locks" (SELs). Each has a specific set of indications and can be seen as portals for moving qi and blood. One can do JSJ on oneself or receive a session from a practitioner. A "hold" consists of placing our hands on two locations of the body. A "flow" is a series of "holds" in a particular sequence to achieve a specific result. I was struck by its simplicity and gentle power. The fact that it could be done anywhere, by anyone, at any time was very appealing. The only things needed are our hands and breath!

It is interesting to note that we are born doing JSJ. All babies suck their thumbs. The thumb represents the stomach and spleen energy which is not fully developed in a newborn. This is why babies can only digest mother's milk. By sucking their thumbs, these two organs are being stimulated.

JSJ explains the connection between the cosmos and the human body as states of energy spiraling down from the formless (Spirit) to form (Matter/Body). These are referred to as "Depths". The deepest depth in our body is 6th Depth. The "Main Central Vertical Flow" addresses this depth, and enables us to access the Cosmic Energy. It is truly a life-giving flow that renews, regulates and detoxifies every cell within. It runs along the midline of the body, activating the chakras (energy centers), organs, and glands. For example, in the first step, the Pineal and Pituitary Glands are activated. This regulates hormonal secretions, sleep and biorhythms in the body, and sharpens memory. I started doing this 9-step flow on myself after my first JSJ workshop. I continued for almost two months, without feeling any different. However, two months later – I remember jumping out of bed with boundless energy. I am not a morning person and despise waking up. Upon doing this flow however, I wake up happy and energized even if I haven't had a full night of sleep. This is all the testimony I needed.

According to JSJ, the body is divided into bustline, waistline and hipline. Each section of the body is further divided in the same way. For example, on the face – the forehead constitutes the bustline; the band across the nose is the waistline; the area across the chin is the hipline. By scanning the body, and making appropriate relationships, a skilled practitioner determines where excess energy is being held, or where the body could use additional energy. Checking the pulse confirms the diagnosis. Corrective flows are then chosen.

Each hand is connected to 72,000 energies in our body; every finger has infinite associations with organs, tissues, tastes, vertebrae, and most importantly – our emotions/attitudes. Figure 12.2 provide some of these associations. The simplest way to create profound changes in our body is to simply encircle each finger, one at a time, for 2–3 minutes each, and stay with our breath. In doing so, one may feel the pulse, a warmth within the body, or movement of energy, such as gurgling sounds, etc. In JSJ, bone formation and development is primarily under the jurisdiction of the heart and small intestine, with the kidneys playing a significant supporting role. The little finger connects to the heart and small intestine. The associated tissue is "bone;" the attitude is "trying too hard." Since the heart is about being authentic, the flip side could be seen as "pretending to be someone that you are not." The index finger relates to the kidneys and urinary bladder. The associated tissue is "muscle;" the primary attitudes are "fear/perfectionism," which are essentially two sides of the

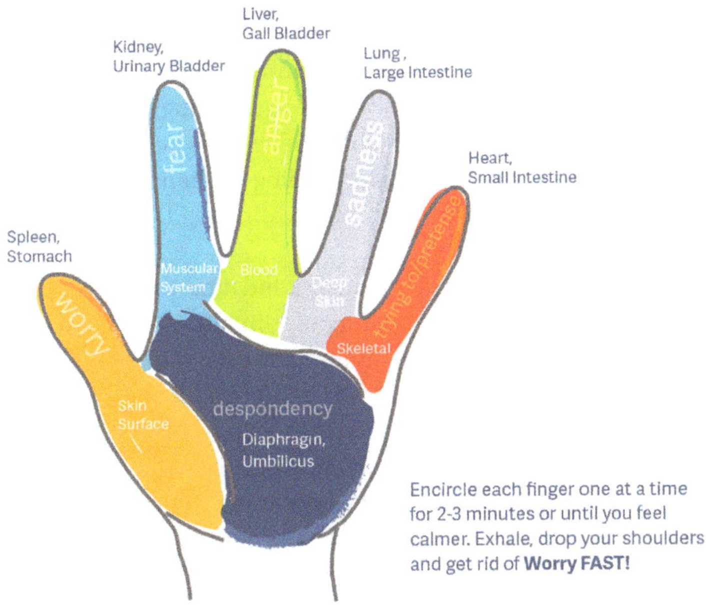

Thumb: worry, vomiting, abdominal pain, indigestion, canker sores, stress, skin projects, insomnia and headaches (base of thumb), when we sit a lot

Index: fear, shoulder/neck/back pain, nausea, menstrual cramps, bladder infections, toothache (hold finger opp to painful jaw), migraines, headache, high BP, sinus infections, muscle tension, self-criticism, shyness, when we stand a lot

Middle: anger, frustration, resentment (stuck anger), impatience, fatigue, flatulence, when we read a lot

Ring: sadness, unable to let go of people or things, breathing difficulties, mucus, earache, tinnitus, cough, skin projects, when we recline a lot

Little: pretense, trying too hard/efforting in life, insecurity, nervousness, bone and heart projects, diarrhea, bloat, when we walk a lot

All fingers: anorexia, auto-immune diseases, lack of focus, learning projects

FIGURE 12.2 Hand emotions

same coin. When one looks deeper, the need to be perfect arises from the fear of not being good enough. All the above resonated with me. I've always been my own worst critic, "efforting" more than necessary, to make sure everything is "just right." Mary Burmeister summed up FEAR as the underlying cause of all other emotions. In reality, however, it is nothing more than "False Evidences Appearing Real."

Today, I consider JSJ to be my most valuable gift. It is pivotal in helping me stay calm, centered and brimming with vitality. The learning is infinite, which keeps me in my joy. When working on a patient, time ceases to exist for that brief hour. By simply being present to my patient, and the pulses, I am a silent witness to the transformation taking place within the body. My hands glide from one location to the next when pulses on both areas being held are harmonized (i.e., when they beat in the same rhythm with equal strength). It's much like doing a dance – the pulse is the music propelling the hands to move from one step to the next. In this way, JSJ allows me to bring to life Kahlil Gibran's words: "Work is love made visible."

Most patients experience perfect peace during and after the session; some experience a sense of lightness – as if floating on thin air, an indication that energy is moving. It can help with almost any ailment, even something as acute as Appendicitis. Here is a story: my patient was in excruciating pain (> 10 on a scale of 1–10). Within 1.5 minutes of doing JSJ, the pain reduced to a 4. A few hours later, her physician confirmed the diagnosis of Appendicitis; but by the time she was taken into the Emergency Room, they found nothing and sent her home. She had continued to do this simple flow the entire time until she was taken into the Emergency Room. Such is the magic of JSJ! The list is endless: Agoraphobia and Post-partum depression were resolved in 3 sessions. Healing after surgery was expedited by 2 months. Chronic projects such as frozen shoulder have been corrected. However, one case that caught me completely by surprise, was when a patient came in with left shoulder pain and right groin pain, but later wrote that the treatment had improved her relationship with her husband. An atmosphere of peace, that was unheard of before the session, had returned to their home. I realized that the chosen flow, namely "small intestine" was just the flow she needed in that moment. The small intestine rules the shoulder and energetically connects with the muscles in the inner thigh. This flow not only resolved her physical projects, but since it is connected to the heart meridian, it also removed heat from the heart and brought back a sense of peace and harmony between the couple. It was after this session, that I finally understood the depth of this magnanimous art.

9 Eden Energy Medicine Brought Balance and Harmony

Eden Energy Medicine (Eden with Feinstein, 2008) came to my rescue during the COVID-19 pandemic. A 3-week visit to see my dad in India in March 2020 ended up being a 6+ month stay! With no courier services available, and therefore no access to my herbs and hormone patches, I wasn't sure how I would manage. I reached out to my friend Kim Gutglueck a week into not having my patches. She introduced me to Eden Energy Medicine at my first JSJ workshop in 2012 and has gently nudged me in this direction ever since. She went through the Eden Energy Medicine Certification Program and is an ardent follower of Donna Eden, a world-renowned Master Healer, who uses acupuncture points and meridians in a unique fashion to help almost any condition. In her early 30s, Eden healed herself of multiple sclerosis, an auto-immune disorder and has a worldwide following today. Her exuberant energy and vitality is contagious! Whenever I spoke to Kim about my condition, she always mentioned an imbalance between triple warmer and spleen.

The triple warmer governs the adrenal gland and maintains the moisture and temperature of the body. It makes us feel safe by regulating hormone and gland secretions within the three sections of the body, hence the term "triple warmer." When the body feels threatened, it goes into "fight or flight mode." In this phenomenon, the adrenal medulla (inner layer of the adrenals), secretes adrenaline and noradrenaline which fires up the sympathetic nervous system causing a cascade of events that allow vital organs necessary for survival to function at their peak, while autonomic functions such as digestion completely shut down. This negatively impacts the spleen, viewed as partner of the triple warmer, responsible for the transformation of food into blood.

Under prolonged periods of stress, the adrenal cortex secretes several hormones, including Dehydroepiandrosterone (DHEA) and cortisol. DHEA is made from cholesterol and is a precursor to estrogen, and protects us against aging. However, since adapting to stress is critical for immediate survival, it is given first priority. Once our body understands that we are not under an environmental threat, it can then focus its energy on reproductive hormones.[4] The higher the stress levels, the greater the amounts of DHEA and cortisol released.

Hyper-secretion of these glands can eventually result in adrenal fatigue, where the body's ability to respond to new stressors is reduced. In order to create hormones, the body requires several building blocks (vitamins, minerals and healthy fats), for which proper digestion and absorption is essential. Thus, finding ways to manage our stress levels is critical, so that the triple warmer can protect our body in times of real danger, instead of being in warrior mode all the time. Later in this chapter I provide a link to a video that explains this concept and contains an exercise for calming the triple warmer (see "Tips for preventing and reversing Osteoporosis" under "Donna Eden").

Another important role performed by the adrenal cortex, especially in this context, is the production of different types of estrogens, when its production stops in the ovaries. One way to help this energy system is to sleep by 10:00 pm. Melatonin, the hormone produced by the pineal gland in the brain is stimulated at night and when it is dark. It controls the biorhythms of the body, such as the regulation of sleep cycles and female hormones. In order to create melatonin, the body needs the same building blocks mentioned earlier. If these are being robbed by the adrenals in response to stress, one is unable fall asleep.

Eastern Medicine sheds light on why we need to sleep at the correct hour. In yin/yang terms, night is a "yin" time, whereas daytime is considered "yang." By sleeping early, we preserve our yin. In eastern medicine, every organ has a two-hour time slot to recharge, enabling it to function at its peak (Figure 12.3). Envision a flock of geese with one goose leading the flock. The goose at the helm is akin to the organ in charge. The time between 9 pm and 11 pm is governed by the triple warmer. Getting to bed on time ensures its optimal functioning. On the opposite end of the biological time clock (i.e., 9 am to 11 am) is the spleen (which is at its weakest time). It's therefore easy for the triple warmer to steal energy from the spleen, which further impairs its functions. Going to sleep late on a regular basis depletes the body's yin and can lead to hot flashes, night sweats, and heat sensations in the feet, hands and heart.

While still on the topic of the biological time clock, it's worth mentioning that the tag team of the pericardium and triple warmer represent the deepest

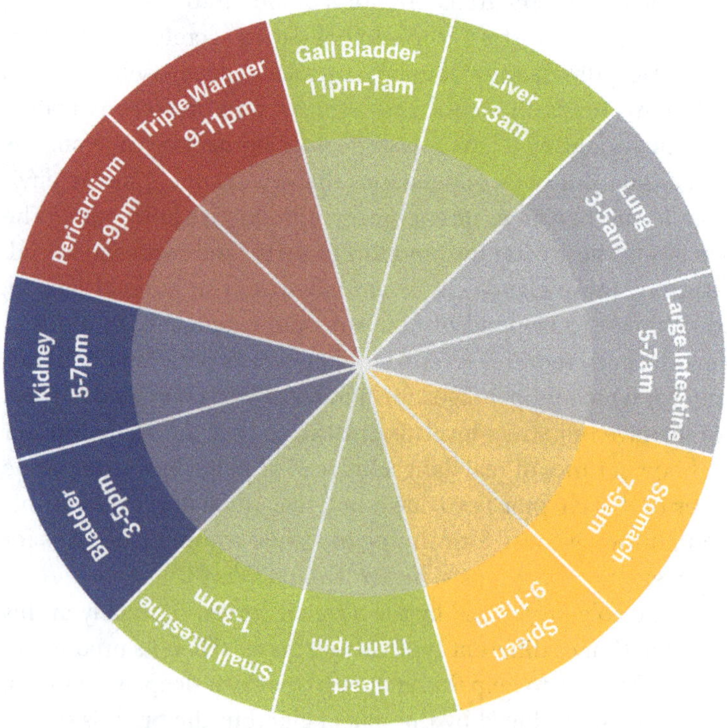

FIGURE 12.3 Time clock

energies in our body (6th Depth) and have a direct connection with the Cosmic energy (7th Depth), which heals, re-charges and revitalizes us on every level. If you look at Figure 12.3 closely, you will see that this duo also acts as a bridge between the urinary bladder/kidneys (3 pm to 7 pm) and the gall bladder/liver (11 pm to 3 am) – the organs that play a critical role in hormone function and detoxification.

Getting back to my story: during the first few days without my hormone patch and herbs, I experienced bouts of depression, night sweats and aches and pains all over my body. As the week progressed, my world slowly began getting darker, while the pain grew steadily worse. Kim then came to my rescue by sending two life-saving Eden Energy Medicine exercises to stimulate the production of estrogen. Massaging the adrenal and cortisol reflex points on the abdomen did the trick! Within two days, I started feeling normal again. It was nothing short of a miracle! Details of these exercises can be found in the "Tips for preventing and reversing Osteoporosis" section under "Donna Eden."[5]

10 A Time for Reflection

It has been 23 years since my diagnosis. I now have Osteopenia, which is "low bone mass" or "low bone density." It is the first stage of Osteoporosis, considered normal for women my age.[6] Yes, my bones are stronger, my spine taller, but more importantly, my entire being has undergone a metamorphosis. I am eternally grateful to my Guru who put me on this path of learning and healing and to all the wise and wonderful individuals encountered along the way who have helped shape me into who I am. I finally feel closer to being a woman of substance.

Today, life offers the variety and stimulation I need to thrive. Weekends allow me the luxury to pursue dance and music. Unbeknownst to me, both have discreetly supported my journey all these years. I recently learnt that soulful music helps regulate hormones. Dance does much more than simply providing a means of expression. The footwork anchors me firmly to the Earth, while the pirouetted turns align my chakras by bringing me back to center each time.

I continue my consulting role as Graphic Designer two days a week. I work with patients the remaining time, using Jin Shin Jyutsu, acupuncture and nutrition. Balance is thus achieved between sitting and standing, thinking and creating and sometimes doing NOTHING. I embrace the study of various alternative healing modalities whenever possible. Other healing modalities I have studied include: Pranic Healing, Mudras, Reflexology, Bach Flower Remedies, and healing with Essential oils.

Understanding how different therapies intersect and discovering new relationships helps me connect the dots better, and is a source of unbounded joy and exhilaration! The human body is, after all, the most intricately designed matrix ever! Viewing the body holistically, has therefore myriad advantages over Western medicine. Mary Burmeister (Pfleuger & Wenninger, 1997), summarizes this beautifully in the following statement:

> Wisdom always recognizes the wholeness, while ignorance sees the importance of parts. (p. 12)

Now it's time to share some of what I've learned along the way, starting with some basic nutrition facts, along with specific recommendations to prevent and reverse Osteoporosis.

10.1 *Basic Nutrition Guidelines*

10.1.1 First Understand Your Internal Climate

Are you hot, cold, too dry or too damp? This can be determined through tongue and pulse diagnosis by an acupuncturist and/or herbalist. For example: If you have a pale tongue, there's a good chance you don't have strong digestive fire and therefore, may not be able to digest raw greens (salads).

10.1.2 Eat According to the Seasons

As energy beings, we are an extension of nature. Consuming locally grown, GMO free, organic produce aligns our bodies with the bio-rhythms of nature.

10.1.3 How You Eat Is as Important as What You Eat

According to Lino Stanchich (1989), you are how you eat, and the stomach doesn't have teeth. Digestion of carbohydrates begins in the mouth by the secretion of the enzyme – amylase. Eating slowly makes us feel satiated sooner than if we gulp our food. Chewing well is key. The more we chew, the better our food is assimilated. On this point, Stanchich cites James Loehr and Jeffrey Migdow (1986):

> The glands in your mouth produce two kinds of saliva. When we are relaxed, the parotid gland produces saliva that contains digestive enzymes and is watery; it easily digests food being chewed. Under stress, however, the sublingual glands exude a thick saliva that is devoid of enzymes. Clearly, relaxing before a meal is the first step towards ease of digestion. (Stanchich, 1989, p. 34)

When eating, just eat: don't talk, walk, read, watch TV, drive a car etc. The brain supplies blood to support digestive function, hence less blood is available for digestion.

Align your posture: While sitting, elongate your spine up as though a cord were attached to the crown of your head.

Bless your food: Say a little prayer before eating, asking the food to become one with you.

10.1.4 Food Needs To Be Cooked on the Stove or in the Stomach

The fire in our body that helps to digest food comes in the form of enzymes and stomach acid. Unfortunately, we have finite supplies of enzymes and acid, which decrease with age. This is why we gain weight around our waistlines more easily after the age of 40. If you have a pale pink tongue, it is preferable to lightly sauté greens and vegetables, rather than eating them raw.

10.1.5 The Question of Water

More than 70% of the Earth's surface is composed of water. Similarly, our bodies are comprised of a significantly large percentage. Although the exact amount differs in each individual, and also varies according age, gender etc., water is the primary component of blood plasma and is fundamental for all biological functions, such as carrying oxygen and nutrients to all our cells, regulating body temperature, flushing waste and toxins from urine and skin, lubricating joints, relaxing muscle tissues to name a few. Staying hydrated by drinking pure water that has a similar pH as our blood is therefore crucial for our overall wellbeing. The pH of our blood ranges from 7.35 to 7.45. Bottled water is usually acidic (with a pH of lower than 7.35). There are just a handful of brands that sell alkaline spring water. As far as water filters, a solid carbon block filter is usually enough. Avoid reverse osmosis filters, as trace minerals are depleted over time.[7]

10.1.6 How to Consume Water

According to Ayurveda, it is best to sit while drinking water,[8] and to drink it slowly, or else it defeats the very purpose – which is to hydrate our cells and tissues. Instead, it passes through our body quickly, and one is left feeling thirsty again. It can also cause arthritis due to fluid accumulating in the joints. There are several other reasons, so grab a seat the next time you wish to drink.

Drinking a few glasses of warm water first thing in the morning, with a drop or two of a pure brand of Lemon Essential Oil (such as Young Living) is a great way to get the bowels moving and purge toxins. Avoid water/drinks with a meal, as you end up diluting your precious digestive enzymes. A glass of warm/hot water 40 minutes after a meal is recommended to aid digestion.

11 Tips for Preventing and Reversing Osteoporosis

11.1 *Avoid Refined Sugar*

Refined sugar is an addictive substance that is present in almost everything. Since it is extremely acidic, it causes calcium (an alkaline mineral) to be leached out of our bones in order to balance the pH level of our blood. Below are ways to reduce the consumption of refined sugar.

Simple ways to reduce sugar (adapted from Rosenthal & Monte) are described in the subsections below.[9]

11.2 *Increase Primary Foods in Your Life*

Primary foods don't come on a plate. Healthy relationships, regular physical activity, a desired career, a spiritual practice that fills our soul and satisfies our hunger for living are some examples. When primary food is balanced and fulfilling, the fun, excitement, love and passion of our daily life feeds us, so that nutrition is secondary. We are more likely to make the right food choices when we are satisfied with life.

11.3 *Cut Down Salt to Lessen Your Cravings for Sugar*

Salty foods cause a contraction or tightening of the body's fluids and tissues, while sweet foods do the exact opposite. If you overindulge in salty foods, your body usually craves sweet foods as a way to maintain balance.

11.4 *Add Sweet Vegetables in Your Diet*

Rather than depend on sugar, our craving for sweet treats is reduced if we add sweet vegetables such as carrots, onions, beets, winter squash, sweet potato and yam. The less popular vegetables that are semi-sweet include turnip, parsnip and rutabaga.

11.5 *Start Your Day with Complex Carbohydrates, and Moderate Amounts of Protein and Fiber*

Complex carbohydrates release their sugars gradually in the system, so you won't spend the day with erratic blood-sugar levels. Adding some protein and fiber will help maintain this balance.

11.6 *Become a Food Detective*

The following suggestions are adapted from Ann Louise Gittleman's (2008) book on reducing dietary sugar. Three-quarters of the sugars Americans ingest are "hidden" in processed foods. Develop the habit of reading labels. The lower the number of sugar grams, the better off you are. One teaspoon of sugar contains 4 grams of sugar. We need two teaspoons of sugar in the bloodstream at any given time. A 12 oz drink of Coke has 39 grams of sugar or close to 10 teaspoons. A quick way to discern sugars on a label is to look for the word "sugar" in any form and for words ending in "ose."

11.7 *Avoid Cows' Milk*

Joshua Rosenthal and Tom Monte (2002) explain that it is a myth that cow's milk makes your bones stronger. I'm a perfect testimony: I drank 2 glasses of milk a day for the first 23 years of my life and yet ended up with the worst case of Osteoporosis by age 30! Cows' milk is meant for calves. Yes, it's true that milk is a great source of calcium, (specifically calcium caseinate). However, since it is bonded to casein, it is not easily absorbable. Cows have four stomachs to break this down. The reason why cow's milk is rich in calcium, is because cows eat greens, so why not simply eat the greens? The majority of the world's population does not depend on dairy foods for their calcium needs. They also ingest less than half of the quantity of calcium than in America, yet they have strong teeth and bones. Additionally, cows' milk is extremely acidic and decreases the pH of the blood. In an attempt to return to homeostasis, the body pulls the alkaline mineral – calcium from our bone!

11.8 *Miracle Greens to the Rescue*

Rosenthal and Monte (2002) argue that most of the food groups we consume are acidic – sugar, milk, grains, legumes and meat, to name a few. What we really need are dark green vegetables to provide the alkalinity that reverses the acidic environment. Among these, are dandelion greens, kale, arugula, broccoli, bok choy, escarole, collard greens and mustard greens. Other alkaline foods include seaweed, sprouts and sprouted beans, miso and salt.

It is noted that certain dark green vegetables, some of which are rich in calcium should be avoided since they contain oxalic acid which reduces the absorption of calcium to a negligible amount. These include spinach, rhubarb, swiss chard and beet greens. If you really wish to consume these greens, cook them with other dark greens such as collards and kale.

11.9 *Eat Foods That Replenish Yin and Nourish the Kidneys*

Drew DiVittorio[10] listed the following foods as examples that replenish yin and nourish the kidneys: apple, asparagus, cheese, honey, kidney beans, lemon, malt, mango, milk, pear, pineapple, pomegranate, string bean, tomato, watermelon and yam.

11.10 *Avoid Nightshades*

Nightshades are a group of vegetables that grow at night. In people allergic to nightshades, calcium is deposited into soft tissue instead of bone, causing arthritis. Eggplants, all peppers, tomatoes, potatoes are some examples of nightshades.[11]

11.11 *Get an Adequate Supply of Vitamins and Minerals*

In order to create hormones and bone, the body needs certain building blocks. It is critical to include healthy fats in your diet, along with foods rich in vitamin B12, B3, B5, B6, vitamin C, folic acid, magnesium, zinc, potassium and calcium. Be sure to use good quality supplements if extra supplementation is required.

11.12 *Get Enough Sunshine*

The Sun has life-giving energy – it nourishes, strengthens and renews every cell in our body and is essential for our physical and mental wellbeing. Vitamin D, crucial for calcium absorption and overall bone health is best absorbed through the skin, so it's important to get 20 to 30 minutes of sunshine daily. Equally important is to include foods rich in vitamin D. People who are homebound are severely deficient in this vitamin and should supplement with at least 1000 IU daily.

11.13 *Gluten and Celiac Disease*

Gluten is a protein found in wheat (includes spelt, kamut, triticale and all varieties of wheat), barley, farina, bulgur and rye. Many of these grains are genetically modified, which causes a host of problems. Eating foods containing gluten can cause celiac disease in those who are susceptible. In such cases, the immune system responds by attacking and damaging the lining of the small intestine, which is responsible for absorbing essential nutrients from food into the bloodstream. This can lead to Osteoporosis. The only treatment for celiac disease is to follow a gluten-free diet, by consuming grains such as quinoa, rice, oats, teff, amaranth, and buckwheat.

11.14 *Consume Bone Broth*

Bone broth is rich in vitamins, minerals, antioxidants, and amino acids. Adding a tablespoon of Bragg's Apple Cider vinegar while cooking, draws calcium out of the bone and into the broth. Drinking a cup or two a day or using the broth[12] to make soups can rebuild the lining of the stomach and small intestine, thereby eliminating "Leaky Gut Syndrome," while providing the nutrients needed to reverse Osteoporosis.[13]

11.15 *Sleep at the Correct Hour*

While it is important to get between 7–8 hours of sleep, it is equally important to sleep at the correct hour. For all the reasons stated earlier, sleeping by 10:00 pm preserves the body's precious yin fluids and hormones, allows the triple warmer a chance to rejuvenate, while enabling the detoxification organs to optimally perform their functions. The use of electronic devices at night should therefore be avoided as the blue light emitted interferes with the production of melatonin.

11.16 *Get the Right Exercise*

Even though bone seems hard and inflexible, it is living tissue that responds well to exercise. The best kinds of activities are weight-bearing and resistance exercises. Weight-bearing exercises such as walking, climbing stairs and dancing force you to work against gravity. Resistance exercises, such as lifting weights, can strengthen bone and muscles that support bone, enhancing balance and flexibility, while preserving joint mobility. All the above reduce the likelihood of falling and breaking a bone, especially among older people.[14]

A consistent yoga practice twice or thrice weekly is an amazing way to center yourself while preventing and reversing Osteoporosis! Being aware of our breath during Pranayama, shifts the body from sympathetic to parasympathetic mode. This is a restorative state where deep healing takes place. Stretching exercises increase flexibility. Twisting exercises are great for digestion. Some poses that help to strengthen bone are Downward Dog, Dolphin and Dolphin Plank Pose, Bridge Pose, Extended Triangle Pose, Extended Side Angle Pose, and Warrior Pose. There are many others. It is best to work with a skilled yoga teacher and work your way up gradually. Tai Qi and Qi Gong are other wonderful ways to enhance the flow of qi and blood through acupuncture meridians, while promoting focus and concentration.

11.17 *Improve Your Posture*

The spine is the central axis of our body that keeps us upright. Lengthening and strengthening our spine is crucial, as our muscles are tethered to it; our nerve endings stem from it. Poor posture, collapse or damage to the cervical vertebrae can cause us to lose height and develop a "Dowager's Hump." When the spine bends, lung function gets compromised and depression could set in. The book that helped me immensely is "8 Steps to a Pain-Free Back" by Esther Gokhale (Gokhale with Adams, 2008). Gokhale illustrates the correct way to sit, stand, sleep, etc. More information can be found at gokhalemethod.com.

11.18 *Establish a Daily Jin Shin Jyutsu and Donna Eden Routine*

Find some quiet time in the day to reduce stress and recharge your energies by doing simple JSJ holds and flows and Donna Eden exercises. The effects are cumulative. Over time, you will notice positive shifts in your body, mind and spirit.

11.18.1 Jin Shin Jyutsu

Holding the little finger and index finger (separately) is a simple and powerful way to dissolve fear and return to your authentic self, while helping your bones. You could hold the other fingers too. Over time, you'll find yourself intuitively encircling the finger that needs the most attention.

Crossing your hands and holding the area just below the clavicle (home to SEL 22) regulates calcium metabolism (Figure 12.4). This helps reduce fears/phobias and enables us to adapt to any situation.

As mentioned earlier, the Main Central Vertical Flow is a life-giving flow, complete in itself.[15]

Other flows that can help are the kidney, spleen, liver, and small intestine.

11.18.2 Donna Eden

All the exercises mentioned below can be easily located on YouTube. They are extremely simple and can be done fairly quickly, once you learn the routine.

A 5-minute daily energy routine is a great way to revitalize yourself.[16] This exercise and the one below, came to my rescue during the COVID-19 pandemic.[17]

In preparation for the exercise:

- Do the triple warmer smoothie
- Sedate the liver meridian
- Triple axis hold
- Find the navel and move an inch above and an inch out on both sides. These are the adrenal reflex points. Massage firmly for 15 seconds. For the cortisol

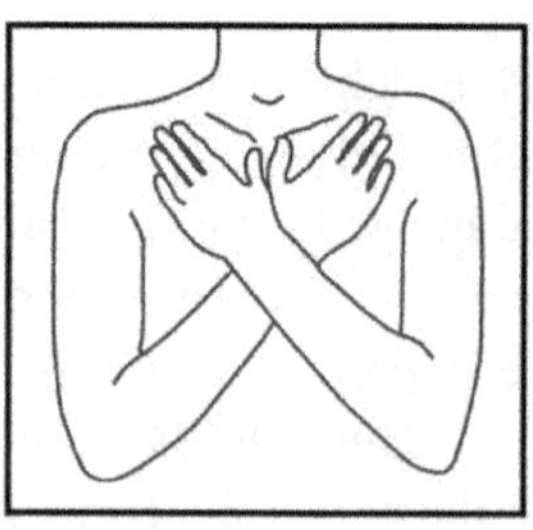

Cross hands and place under opposite collar bone to alleviate fears and phobias, and help you adapt to any situation.

FIGURE 12.4
SEL 22

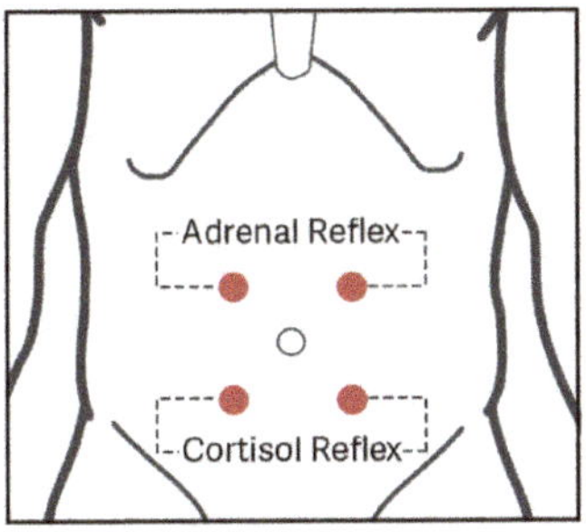

FIGURE 12.5
Adrenal cortisol points

reflex points, move down an inch and out an inch on both sides of the navel. Massage firmly for 15 seconds (Figure 12.5).
- Then, with your left hand flat, lightly place your second, third and fourth fingers on the left temple, just above the eye socket. Place the index and middle fingers of the right hand in the crease behind the right knee. Relax and hold this for about 4 deep breaths. These are the neurovascular points for the triple warmer and gall bladder meridians. This combination stimulates the adrenals to produce estrogen.

YouTube resources are available to regulate hormones[18] (thyroid, cortisol, adrenals) and alleviate stress[19] and to calm the triple warmer and soothe anxiety.

11.19 *Work with a Good Acupuncturist and Herbalist*

Acupuncture and herbs work synergistically to balance the body's yin/yang energies, opening up blocks within meridians, breaking up stagnation, aiding elimination, while detoxifying, and strengthening the immune system. Acupuncture works well in cases of excess, while herbs replenish the body in cases of deficiency. By checking the tongue and pulse, the herbalist prescribes a custom herbal formula based on the constitution, the underlying disharmony and the symptoms presented by the patient.

11.20 *Prevent Tooth Decay and Bone Loss in the Mouth*

The following section is particularly for those of you who, like myself, have experienced extreme loss of bone in the jaw. In consultation with holistic dentists and Jed Schwartz – my JSJ mentor, I have developed the routine below. It keeps even this severe problem at bay. If your dental problems are not as severe, you can select elements that suit your need.

What you will need:
- A tongue cleaner.
- Organic sesame oil.[20]

- Philips Sonicare DiamondClean toothbrush. Recommended by periodontists, it has multiple pressure settings and a 2-minute timer that beeps at 30 second intervals.
- Uncle Harry's Toothpaste is an amazing product containing pure sea salt, essential oils and other ingredients that help re-mineralize teeth, control bacteria and alkalize the mouth. Any toothpaste can be used with minor modifications: if sweet, add the following to the toothpaste in a small dish: a pinch of sea salt, baking soda and a drop of hydrogen peroxide. In the interest of saving time, you can pre-mix equal quantities of baking soda and sea salt and keep this in a container. Omit the salt if the toothpaste already contains salt.
- Hydrogen peroxide solution (5–7% concentration) acts as a mild antiseptic. It releases oxygen which creates an alkaline environment in the mouth.
- Proxy brushes: buy the correct size, depending on the space between your teeth.
- Floss.
- Waterpik/water flosser.

11.20.1 General Guidelines

Massaging gums:
- The act of massaging stimulates gums and teeth and cannot be overemphasized. Before brushing, apply a small quantity of toothpaste/mixture on index finger and massage anterior (front) and posterior (back) sides of gums and teeth, spending more time on affected areas. For teeth in upper quadrant, firmly pull gums downward using index finger and thumb. For teeth in lower quadrant, pull gums upward.
- Brushing: Apply paste on toothbrush and brush for 1–2 minutes, spending a few seconds on each tooth. Use downward motion for teeth in upper quadrant and upward motion for teeth on lower quadrant.

Morning routine:
- First thing in the morning on an empty stomach, swish oil in mouth for 20 minutes. Rinse with warm salt water. Brush off excess oil using a regular toothbrush.
- Massage gums and brush with Philips toothbrush.
- Scrape tongue using tongue cleaner.

Night routine:
- Clean between teeth using Proxy brushes.
- Floss.
- Massage gums and brush with Philips toothbrush.

- Use a Waterpik. Fill the reservoir with warm to hot water (as hot as you can tolerate) and direct the water flow to the areas just under the gums to release any hidden food particles. Be careful not to use a high pressure. This may cause gum pockets which could lead to other complications.

Recommendations:
- Brushing/flossing after eating is recommended. Or swish with a teaspoon of hydrogen peroxide solution in a glass of water. For toothache or loose teeth, massage gums with Uncle Harry's toothpowder once or twice daily. I have found that this strengthens teeth and reduces pain. Sucking on a clove can help with a toothache as well.

12 Coming into Alignment

No matter what healing modality one turns to, each strives for better alignment. We all know that proper alignment is key in yoga. One cannot undermine the role of the spine in this regard, especially in the context of Osteoporosis. While gravity weighs heavily down on us, keeping us rooted to the earth, our spine rises boldly and gracefully and holds us upright; each vertebra a rung on the ladder that rises towards the heavens. By elongating our spine while practicing pranayama, we unite our breath with our body, mind and heart, and come into alignment with our Higher Self. Breath is our ultimate connection to the Cosmic Energy. According to Ramana Maharashi *breath control is a means for mind control.*[21] When the mirror of our mind is polished, and the dust is wiped clean, it is possible to realize our true nature and BE in our joy.

Obstacles are sent to us for a reason. By taking a moment to pause and explore these as opportunities rather than road blocks, we expand our consciousness and come closer to our essence. My diagnosis turned out to be a blessing in disguise as it forced me to look within, turn my life around and find joy in everyday living, all while reversing end-stage Osteoporosis to Osteopenia. Instead of ending up in a wheelchair, I found my wings. I wish the same for you.

Notes

1 1997 Dexa Bone Mineral Density results: Spine age-matched Z score: −3.7; Hip age- matched Z score: −3.1.

2 Details about the transdermal patch, which was used in 1997, are: "Climara Pro .045/.015." Today, I use "Estalis Continuous 50/140," which is manufactured by Novartis.

3 Fish oil: Blue Ice Royal Blend Fermented Cod Liver Oil and Concentrated Butter Oil manufactured by Green Pasture; Vitamin D3 liquid 1000 IU or 2000 IU: Bluebonnet; Vitamin B12, Calcifood Wafers and Biost – non-plant based, supports skeletal health: Standard Process.
4 See https://drjockers.com/10-tips-boost-dhea-levels/
5 For more information about regulating other hormones, please refer to Eden's book (Eden with Feinstein (2008). *Energy Medicine for Women: Aligning Your Body's Energies to Boost Your Health and Vitality*. Penguin.)
6 In 2018 my Dexa Bone Mineral Density results were: Spine Age-matched Z score: –1.9; Hip Age-matched Z score: –1.5.
7 Detailed information on water and water filters, compiled by Lawrence Wilson, can be found at this URL: https://drlwilson.com/ARTICLES/WATER.htm.
8 https://recipes.timesofindia.com/us/articles/health/why-standing-and-drinking-water-is-a-bad-habit/photostory/63299255.cms
9 Adapted from Rosenthal and Monte (2002): pp. 6–8, salt/sugar cravings; pp. 33, 73, sweet vegetables; pp. 101–104, Primary Foods, pp. 64–68, milk; p. 77, dark green leafy vegetables.
10 https://www.opencenter.org/drew-divittorio/
11 https://healthproadvice.com/pain/Is-There-a-Connection-Between-Nightshade-Vegetables-and-Joint-Pain
12 Link to make bone broth: https://wellnessmama.com/5888/bone-broth/
13 Link about benefits of bone broth: https://wellnessmama.com/444231/bone-broth-diet/
14 https://www.bones.nih.gov/health-info/bone/osteoporosis/conditions-behaviors/celiac
15 https://www.youtube.com/watch?v=LKoIxn8eJj4
16 https://www.youtube.com/watch?v=Di5Ua44iuXc&t=3s
17 This YouTube video shows how to stimulate estrogen production: https://www.youtube.com/watch?v=CLLXrA3I1_0
18 https://www.youtube.com/watch?v=39vNM4pPH30
19 https://www.youtube.com/watch?v=EccGn1CNdz8&feature=youtu.be
20 See www.banyanbotanicals.com. Instructions on oil pulling/use of the tongue cleaner can be found in this pdf: https://www.banyanbotanicals.com/info/uploads/Elements_of_Ayurveda_Tongue_and_Oil_Pulling_Guide.pdf
21 https://sriramanamaharishi.com/meditation/breath-regulation-helps-meditation/

References

Eden, D. with Feinstein, D. (2008). *Energy medicine for women: Aligning your body's energies to boost your health and vitality.* Penguin.

Gittleman, A. L. (2008). *Get the sugar out.* Three Rivers Press.

Gokhale, E. with Adams, S. (2008). *8 Steps to a pain-free back: Natural posture solutions for pain in the back, neck, shoulder, hip, knee, and foot.* Pendo Press.

Loehr, J. E., & Migdow, J. A. (1986). *Take a deep breath.* Random House.

Maharshi, R., Maharaj, N., Swami, A., Muruganar, O., & Vasistha, S. (2010). *The seven steps to awakening*. The Freedom Religion Press.

Matsumoto, K., & Euler, D. (2017). *Kiiko Matsumoto's clinical strategies: In the spirit of Master Nagano*. KM & DE Books.

Pfleuger, L., & Wenninger, M. (1997). *"What Mary says, ..."* Jin Shin Jyutsu Inc.

Pitchford, P. (2003). *Healing with whole foods: Asian traditions and modern nutrition* (3rd ed.). North Atlantic Books.

Rosenthal, J., & Monte, T. (2002). *The energy balance diet: Lose weight, control your cravings and even out your energy*. Alpha.

Stanchich, L. (1989). *The power eating program: You are how you eat*. Healthy Products.

CHAPTER 13

Learning from Alternative Methods of Care and Wellbeing of a Loved One

Exploring the Potential of Jin Shin Jyutsu

Andre Poole

Abstract

What we do for ourselves sometimes comes out of what we do for a loved one. What we learn for ourselves sometimes comes from the necessity to help a loved one. In this chapter I reflect on the lived experience of my daughter's occasional struggle with gastrointestinal discomfort in conjunction with my parallel experience as her father with a desire to make her pain go way. I describe how experience led me to search for alternative and complementary methods to bring about relief. The path to finding an alternative led me to consider Jin Shin Jyutsu as a possible solution.

Keywords

parenting – health and wellness – Jin Shin Jyutsu – parent | researcher – complementary systems of wellness

1 Parenting Pain

Family life, as an activity, can be filled with events and experiences that force many different reactions on a family. There are births and deaths, primary through postsecondary schooling, marriages and separations, lean years and fat years, sickness and health, all from people who are central and others who are peripheral. Most often, the relationship that we cherish the most is between parent and child. I loved my mother dearly, and it hurt terribly to watch her receive a cancer diagnosis, given what I have come to accept as only marginal care and succumb to the disease within six months. Conversely, my father receiving a cancer diagnosis has been challenging in a different way. I have witness him receive excellent modern care through access to health insurance while witnessing, daily and firsthand, the effects of intense treatment.

 | DOI:10.1163/9789004527348_013

Thankfully, he is still with us, but I recognize how that could change with one diagnosis or change to his treatment. This is where the fear begins and lives.

Life begins with the love of parents – those who love us first. I fear for my daughter (hereafter JP); not because she is in any danger now, but I fear that I have passed on the potential for something that has been potentially passed on to me. Every unexplained pain does not bring neuroses in me but a recognition of the potential for pain that I wish to spare JP.

Currently six years old, JP has complained of gastrointestinal pain/discomfort for several years. Her situation began as problems with constipation. We monitored her diet and made changes we thought would help. Prune juice became a regular shopping purchase. Old wives' tales and spoken traditions found their way into practice. Rubbing her stomach and drinking water during bowel movements became the normal routine for us. Sleep cycles are broken, and school days become a 'daze in school' as my concentration during my own doctoral studies became increasingly less important.

The first painful experience for us (meaning those that live with her) was when we had to give JP a suppository. Three adults in the bathroom; two in the tub, with the other holding a crying and trembling toddler suffering from the discomfort of this inability to pass her stool. Here we are, having to deliver more pain to bring forth relief. The experience was painful – for everyone in that room. Tears followed pain. The emotions and tensions ran high as the sympathy and empathy seemed to create their own humidity in the space. JP's rank, sticky, black stool became a welcome sight – seemingly the best thing we had ever seen. JP crumbled into her grandmother's arms, crying and tired from the effort. The pain was followed by relief. The relief was followed by fatigue and a strange night's sleep.

I could not help being concerned that constipation was to be an obstacle throughout JP's life – along with routines to prevent, mitigate, and manage discomfort and pain.

JP's symptoms would continue sporadically for some time until we sought help from a specialist. Without any easy answers in front of us, traditional Western medicine led JP to a specialist. Stool softeners and maintaining good hydration were advised and used for the next few months with only minimal effect.

Eventually, JP was tested for Hirschsprung's disease, a condition that affects the colon and may cause problems with bowel movements (Mayo Clinic Staff, 2018). Here, fresh from celebrating her second birthday, outpatient surgery was looming. There was no worry because JP was always so delightful despite her challenges. Watching her giddy from the pre-sedative was just the levity we needed. I was left with my thoughts as my wife left with JP and the operating team into the operating room. During the procedure I do not recall much of

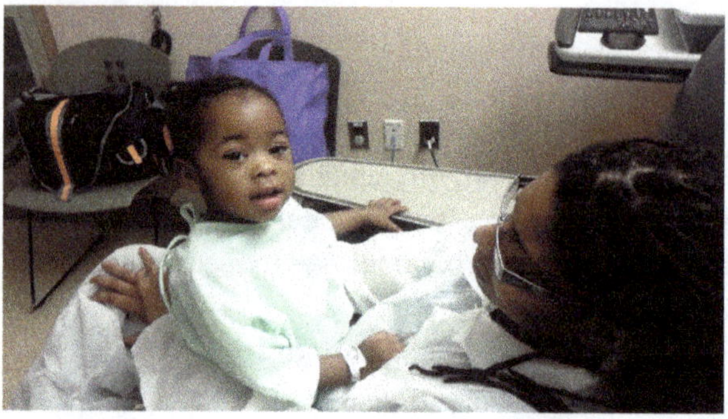

FIGURE 13.1
Sedation prior to Hirschsprung's test

the time I had alone, but it seemed like waiting for a train that was not coming. Looking down the tunnel hoping to glimpse the headlights of the inevitable arrival that would take me from the prison of my own worry.

Thankfully, the results were negative. But this diagnosis brought me little comfort. If Hirschsprung's disease has been ruled out, could the problem be something worse?

2 Denial and Desperation

Over the next two years or so, JP's gastrointestinal discomfort and pain seem to settle down. JP exhibits the typical behavior of a child her age. She is energetic, curious, and thoughtful. She is happy and thriving. Formal schooling begins and her teachers noting her best qualities, including good behavior, politeness, and strong academic performance. JP's reading proficiency has been measured to be two grade levels above normal and math proficiency is also above her current grade level. She enjoys physical activities such as music and movement classes while deriving (much) less pleasure from musical activities (such as piano and violin). Have the moments of worry slipped into the past? Outside of the occasional, but not regular, tummy trouble there wasn't much to report … until there was.

JP started having some pain that was happening too frequently for it to be nothing. Her primary care physician again sent us to a specialist. Simple blood screenings were followed by stool samples. Urine tests were followed by radiological exams. Each time no problems were found. The doctor then expressed that her problems may need a different specialist: a psychologist. The potential of her health issues being psychological or behavioral was a notion we resisted but did not rule out.

This went on for some time, until after JP turned five years old and was given a hydrogen breath test. We had no idea what this was about or what the test would indicate, but this was the next thing to do. The results came back positive.

2.1 *"Positive?"*

What could this mean? The positive test showed evidence of a small intestinal bacterial growth (SIBO) (Ghoshal, 2011), which probably originated after a course of antibiotics for an unrelated condition. The timing of the return of discomfort seemed to match this interpretation.

I had forgotten all about the antibiotics … those damned liquid antibiotics destroyed her gut biome and allowed for an E. coli related growth to take hold. We felt very guilty about the situation but had to use the information as a learning experience. A painful learning experience at JP's expense.

As JP's sixth birthday approached her doctor recommended a more invasive and comprehensive exam based on the ongoing set of symptoms. Soon after that, JP had an endoscopy and colonoscopy, which showed evidence of two small non-bleeding erosions (gastritis). Once again, we felt some relief at a diagnosis of a problem, but now this also left us with questions about possible cause and outlook. These unanswerable questions were, and still are, something that we struggle with mentally. I am glad that she does not struggle with those thoughts, but what awareness she does have of the situation seems to indicate that she has handled herself more maturely than I could have expected. JP has not been, or at least not shown or verbalized, in any serious way, any resentment or anger with the situation. Even as I (rudely) eat some of my favorite foods that she is now unable to eat due to an ever-changing diet, she is pleasant and happy with what she is given.

3 Outside of the Box

JP has, however, become hypersensitive to her stomach troubles. Any pain in her abdomen may become more of an issue than any reaction may have been normally. Simple gas pain becomes a flashing yellow light for the household.

One of my issues outside of all of this is that JP is not a sickly child. She eats healthy foods and has a balanced diet. She was born with an umbilical hernia, which is a hereditary trait via her mother, however this condition is an asymptomatic issue. We have tried eliminating specific foods and adding probiotics and vitamin supplements. We try to keep JP as hydrated as possible through using water bottles with volume measurements in order to keep track of her water intake. I have even tried to bring her in to my own (sporadic) meditation practices. The meditation wasn't foreign to her as she was also exposed to the practice in her time at a college campus-based day care center.

It was at some point in the fall of 2017 that the idea of using another non-Western practice became a serious possibility.

While sitting in on a doctoral-level class held by Professor Ken Tobin, of the CUNY Graduate Center's Urban Education program, the topic of using alternative and complementary methodologies in general health and wellness practices came up into the conversation. While this was not the first time such a conversation had come up in a class that I have been a part of, either with Prof. Tobin or another professor, this time the conversation had become quite personal and pertinent. Now I became interested as both parent and investigator/researcher. I need to help my child.

Ken introduced Jin Shin Jyutsu (JSJ) several times in class over the next few semesters but, admittedly, I was slow to embrace JSJ in the same way I was slow to embrace mindfulness meditation techniques. One day in, or possibly after, class Ken graciously offered to have a JSJ session for JP one weekend. We took him up on his offer, and her JSJ session began. The parent in me wanted to give my child some relief while the teacher | researcher in me wanted to see some change in her.

I do not mean to cast her situation as something dire, while nothing on the order of a "Lorenzo's Oil" situation, I am afraid that her body will not be able to take care of itself over time.

We began very simply; Ken would talk to her while going through the various holds/flows, explaining what he was doing not only to her but to me. Eventually, we started using fingertip pulse oximeters and cameras to examine more closely what was taking place and what effect the JSJ had on JP physically/physiologically.

The social scientist in me was intrigued by the possibility of finding some kind of cause | effect relationship or an intervention that would be effective as a path to wellness. The parent in me just wanted my child to feel better in both the short and long terms.

We began very slowly by originally discussing what JP may experience and what Ken was proposing. She had also had some small JSJ practices through my experiences with it via a set of flash cards and book (Riegger-Krause, 2014) that I had purchased some time ago. I wanted her to know that Ken and (most importantly) I were exploring ways to help her without the need for a

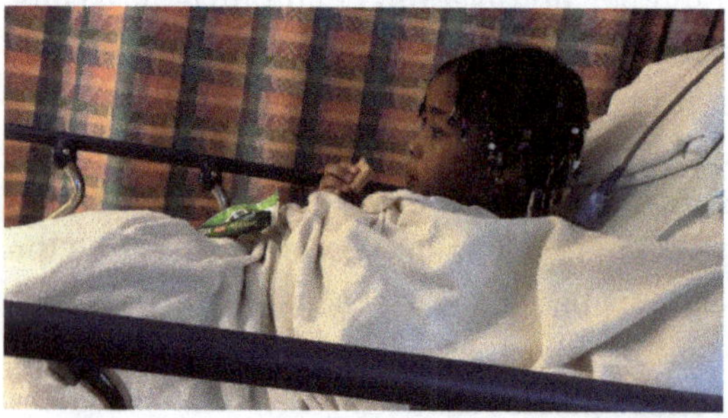

FIGURE 13.2
Recovery after an endoscopy and colonoscopy

pharmaceutical solution. JP had questions but was never worried. In some ways, she was eager to try something new and she enjoyed the first experience as a simple trip to New Jersey.

Ken welcomed JP to the space he established for his personal JSJ practices with open arms. Some weeks prior I had begun some JSJ work with him to try and address some of the issues/projects I was dealing with in my own personal wellness. JP jumped right in and was eager to try it out. She engaged Ken in conversation almost immediately about her martial arts experience to which he commented about his own practices. The conversation continued across various topics throughout JP's first session. Conversation helped to create a social bond, not only with Ken, but with the JSJ itself. Rather than looking at JSJ as a treatment, JP could look at the time spent receiving the treatment as a component of personal wellness; another path to feeling better.

4 Problems versus Projects

An essential aspect of all of this, JP's wellness and researching complementary methods of achieving better wellbeing, is a perspective taken throughout the process and beyond. The point of view many people take when a personal health hardship enters into daily life is to call it a problem. I have certainly been guilty of this all of my life. After all, problems are things or events meant to be overcome. Right? They are bumps in the road to pass over, hopefully, with minimal permanent repercussions. Aren't they? The Oxford English Dictionary (n.d.-a) defines 'problem' as:

> NOUN
> 1. A matter or situation regarded as unwelcome or harmful and needing to be dealt with and overcome.

In my opinion, viewing issues with wellness as problems only serves to deepen the idea within a deficit perspective. In other words, when viewed as a 'problem' the condition or situation that is being encountered, while unwelcomed, is seen as an adversary; an enemy that needs to be vanquished. Conquered. Defeated. This view approaches the condition or situation from a deficient place; the current situation must then be lesser than the desired state. 'Problems' can stay in place unaddressed and unresolved. I conceptualize it as that lingering, but faint, moist smell in a basement: something that can be investigated or ignored. The acceptance or denial of a 'problem' makes no difference within this view, only the problem's prevalence or presence.

Conversely, looking at how one works through 'what ails them' seems to be a point of view that is less about the victory | defeat dichotomy and more about the continuum of just being a living being.

As 'projects,' these experiences with complementary wellness interventions align with the idea that wellbeing, of any sort, is a continuous process. This was the view of Mary Burmeister (Higgins, 1988) as a way to use language that was not dependent on diagnostics.

Wellness becomes less about immediate or short-term events and more about how we will be over long periods of time. Viewing the word 'project' as a verb creates images of moving in an outward, forward moving direction. Preferably, instead of allowing that lingering, but faint, moist smell continue to be there without investigation or intervention, an active decision is made to find a cause, plan a remedy, and put that plan into action that hopefully prevents the smell from coming back.

The difference between the 'problems' and 'projects' could also be seen as the difference between treatment and lifestyle. Injuries receive treatment. Wellness is a conscious decision without regard for cause, severity, status, age, religion, or gender. Wellness is experienced and can often be observed by others. JP is just beginning her life and I want her to have a long one. So, while I can still make decisions for her, I choose to have her broaden her exposure to many forms of pursuing good health.

5 Searching for New Clues

So far, I've looked at this through the lens a father would take: mainly subjective and filled with emotions. However, what does the in-the-moment data show? Admittedly I was, and probably always will be, unsure about what the data may determine. I am not looking at it from a skeptic's point of view but more of a fearful one – a place of hoping for answers but afraid of not getting any.

I decided to look at some of the experiences of others in my research squad, mainly Ferzileta Gjika (2017), based on their own practices in and around JSJ. Ferzileta's experience with her own emerging practices set-along her children's health concerns (2017, pp. 340–341) played a part in how I chose to proceed. Also, in my review of other literature where practitioners have shared experiences with family members (Miniello, 2017, pp. 281–284) I found both comfort and encouragement in the journey of caring for a loved one.

What I decided to do was to see how JP was responding to JSJ using fingertip pulse oximetry. This was a technique that I became exposed to during a study conducted at Brooklyn College with Ken Tobin and Konstantinos Alexakos (Alexakos, 2015).

During the Brooklyn College Study, a few of us were tasked with learning about and reviewing data gathered using the oximeters (Calderón, 2016) amongst various other tools and techniques (Poole, 2016). While oximeter data has the potential to be used as a tool to find very subtle cues physiologically (Calderón, 2016) we were looking to see if there any 'spikes in the curve' during different flows. These spikes would then be used as markers or events for further examination. In addition to the use of the oximeter, we video recorded some of the sessions as a way of capturing any relevant conversational portions where JP was expressing anything she experienced.

6 Ebbs and Flows

The voice inside of my head kept repeating the same "how would any of this make a difference?" While encouraged by what I had read and heard I needed to know more before I went looking for effects. I decided to look to the (aforementioned) prominent resource that kept re-emerging: a set of JSJ hands-on practice flash cards (that accompany a book) from Waltraud Reigger-Krause.

"Health Is in Your Hands: Jin Shin Jyutsu – Practicing the Art of Self-Healing" (2014) became a useful resource in my attempt to conceptualize and materialize my nascent understanding of JSJ and constituent energy flows. All of this brought me, and by extension my daughter, to an intellectual and parental impasse: Would the quantitative effects be noticeable and important and complement the qualitative effects? Learning about the flows, especially the foundational, and their intended effects would become important to this entire endeavour. As Gjika (2017) did before me, I began with what seemed like the beginning.

The main central vertical flow (MCV) is designed to aid with feeling centered and calm as the pathway of energy flows down the middle of the front of the body then up back of the body (Riegger-Krause, 2014). Harmonizing any flow can be described as a series of holds along a series of spots on the body, also known as Safety Energy Locks (SEL s). These locks are spots where energy 'blockages' could occur. Blockages in universal energy are linked to disharmonies which can lead to health issues.

The MCV can be described as a seven-step process where the fingers on the right hand are placed lightly on the top of the head while the left hand is placed and periodically moved through a series positions along the centerline of the body: the middle of the forehead, the tip of the nose, the top of the sternum, the middle of the sternum, the solar plexus, then the pubic bone, The final movement is the right hand from the top of the head to the tailbone while the left hand remains on the pubic bone.

During the session for which we collected data, the treatment began with the MCV, which is designed to harmonize the energy that enters the body along the pathway.

The flow up the back is associated with the inbreath and the flow down the front, with the outbreath. All other organ energy flows are derived from the main central vertical flow, which is regarded as the primary flow of Jin Shin Jyutsu. The duration of the main central vertical flow was 9:10 (m:s). The first two tables show that the main central vertical flow was followed by four organ function energy flows: spleen, stomach, liver, and umbilicus. The time for each of these flows is provided in the tables. The session concluded with what was referred to as a wrap up, which consisted of holding left and right safety energy lock 4 (i.e., at the base of the skull; Riegger-Krause, 2014), until harmony was evident in the pulses (Tobin & Ansari, 2017). In this case the wrap up had a duration of 2:20 m:s.

To obtain a baseline against which the above results could be compared, JP wore an oximeter while she completed her mathematics homework. The results obtained during this interval of a little more than 17 minutes are provided below.

- Time for the homework activity was 17 minutes and 20 seconds.
- Mean pulse rate was 99.0, standard deviation of 6.6.
- Mean blood oxygenation was 97.5, standard deviation of 1.2.

The first observations made were the oximetry results during the JSJ flows, in relation to the baseline (doing homework). The pulse rate declined steadily during the flows, finishing appreciably below the baseline average of 99 bpm. Apart from the stomach flow, in which the average blood oxygenation was 95.8%, the baseline level of 97.5% was similar to the averages obtained during the Jin Shin Jyutsu universal energy flows. So, what is this telling?

In Tables 13.1 and 13.2 the oximeter data are analyzed separately for six different phases of the treatment, during which different organ energy flows were administered.

In a conversation about the data with Ken he noted that any causality cannot be implied since a correlation coefficient shows the strength of a relationship. In this case, as one variable increased, the other decreased. It is difficult to make a determination as to what this could mean without further investigation.

TABLE 13.1 Jin Shin Jyutsu flows: pulse rate analysis

Flow	Mean: pulse rate (bpm)	SD: pulse rate	Duration (m:s)
Main central vertical	91.6	4.7	9:10
Spleen	87.5	3.7	5:05
Stomach	84.2	4.1	9:55
Liver	84.7	4.5	8:20
Umbilicus	83.8	10.0	9:50
Wrap up	83.1	4.3	2:20

TABLE 13.2 Jin Shin Jyutsu flows: blood oxygenation analysis

Flow	Mean: blood oxygenation (%)	SD: blood oxygenation	Duration (m:s)
Main central vertical	97.7	1.6	9:10
Spleen	97.8	0.6	5:05
Stomach	95.8	2.3	9:55
Liver	97.1	0.8	8:20
Umbilicus	97.7	1.6	9:10
Wrap up	97.8	0.6	5:05

7 Moving from What Does It Mean to What We Do?

Our family went into JSJ treatments with a completely open mind and an open heart. I was/am hoping to gain a better understanding of what Jed Schwartz calls the "energetic blueprint to harmonize the flow of energy, and the result is that the physical body will correct or harmonize itself" (Schwartz, 2017, p. 307). That may seem contradictory to what may have been stated earlier about preferred outcomes and objectivity but I truly had no expectations of understanding the process nor the theories at first. However, as I look at what is there statistically, there are some questions that anyone would have based on what is seen in the data and what JP's history has been.

Most obvious is that across all of the flows, the stomach flow easily displayed the lowest blood oxygenation (95.8% vs. a 97.2% average and 2 SD from

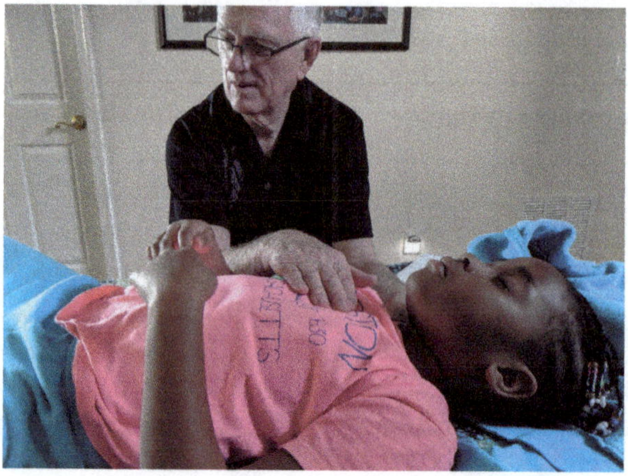

FIGURE 13.3
A JSJ treatment

the mean) percentage and the second highest standard deviation. What could this mean? Does this result have to mean anything? How can I mitigate these effects without the need for pharmaceutical or invasive remedies?

Viewing this situation as a project rather than as a problem, as stated earlier, was the first step to taking ownership of JP's wellness. Additionally, teaching JP that JSJ can be one part of an overall wellness protocol that would last (hopefully) throughout her life.

During a reflective writing session, I came to ask myself a question: For whom do we do things? I wanted to know or operationalize for myself what wellness is. JP's situation had me not only thinking about her health but her wellness. As I was writing I came to realize that, like all parents, the wellness of our children is a selfish endeavor (Poole, 2016, pp. 124–125) because we love them, need them, and need them to be well, not only for them but for our own sense of wellness, wholeness, and emotional wellbeing.

As opportunities arise, I have tried to practice JSJ with JP but due to the rigid sleep schedule we keep her on, extra-curricular activities, and the reserved academic time we try to adhere to it is often difficult.

8 Seeking Meaning

However, in the months since she began JSJ, her stomach problems have not been an issue. I do recognize that I cannot claim that this is a causal, or even coincidental, relationship but I cannot rule out that the JSJ has had an effect in her wellness. The sheer number of variables alone would make it difficult to reach any determination.

Going forward I may seek out others, in addition to Ken, with more proficiency in the interpretation and implementation of JSJ with the hope that my own understanding and practices can be improved to help my daughter maintain and enhance her sense of wellness and wellbeing.

9 Hopes, Fears, and Parallel Paths

> project
>
> NOUN
>
> 1. An individual or collaborative enterprise that is carefully planned to achieve a particular aim. (Oxford Dictionaries, n.d.-b)

During my investigation of both JP's emergent journey alongside my own emerging practice I had to consistently consider whether this is a desperate reach or some-thing that has actual benefit. JP would also go with whatever we, as her parents, ask of her. She has had to change her diet several times at our insistence and at the direction of traditional medical professionals. I do recognize that diet is, of course, a primary means of achieving and maintaining wellness. However, I also do recognize that each of us is built a certain way and that what may be beneficial for one person may have deleterious effects on another.

Also, to be honest, there is a part of me that wonders if there is a level of attention-seeking behavior at play here. While I do not believe that this is a measurable component of what JP reports to us when experiencing discomfort, my experience working with children doesn't allow me to rule it out completely.

Honestly, I am not sure what some of this means. Is there something here, and if so, what is it?

What I dislike about JP's wellness experience so far is the lack of evidence. When we were deep into this investigation, she was not old enough to properly articulate what she is feeling nor has traditional medicine provided a concrete, satisfactory cause.

However, my lack of faith in any one system leaves me open to second-guess everything – except in the ability, innate or not, for harmony to enable natural systems to mend themselves over time.

What I do know is that this is important. Wellness should not be viewed as a luxury item or something that we can 'do later.' This entire undertaking for our family was to move JP into a place where she would be able to maintain her own wellness through her own actions by hopefully forming good habits. As parents, there is nothing more important than seeing our children grow and develop. Introducing JSJ, for us, has been part of that process of building good habits, recognizing the relationships between actions and results, and understanding that feeling good is a personal responsibility. Taking on wellness projects, and approaching them as real, tangible endeavors is part of what we do now.

What I have discovered, or better put – realized, is that this is not JP's journey alone. My journey through (and not to) wellness moves along the same continuum as hers. One experience during a session of the main central vertical flow, my feet suddenly became very hot. I have come to dub it as my 'hot feet' moment (Poole, 2019, pp. 82–84). It was a strange moment that left me confused and unsure about these experiences with JSJ. To this day, I have difficulty describing what happened with any great detail. Even upon reflection and within subsequent JSJ practices, I have not had a moment of similar intensity. I wish that I had the (self)awareness to notice posture, breathing, and other subtle indicators (Schwartz, 2017, p. 308) that may manifest themselves as signals of wellness.

Now nine-years-old, JP's gastrointestinal wellness journey has become more stable in the time since this investigation, projects have shifted into other areas, such as appetite control and moderate weight gain. Our pediatrician has had some recent concerns about the latter issue regarding the relationship to JP's body-mass index (BMI).

However, reading through the experiences of others who have utilized JSJ as a part of their journey (Proscia, 2017) or methods of wellness (Tobin & Ansari, 2017) has given me hope for her and new enthusiasm for my own journey and JP's journey. I have sought out the more experienced practices of others through workshops, seeking out videos for reference, and practicing JSJ on my own. In opposition to the previously mentioned definition of "problem," the overarching point of all of this is to have JP's health project be just that, a project (as per the dictionary definition above), something ongoing and with a worthwhile outcome.

References

Alexakos, K. (2015). *Being a teacher | researcher: A primer on doing authentic inquiry research on teaching and learning.* Sense.

Calderón, O. (2016). Oximetry: A reflective tool for the detection of physiological expression of emotions in a science education classroom. *Cultural Studies of Science Education, 11*(3), 653–667. https://doi.org/10.1007/s11422-016-9731-y

Ghoshal, U. C. (2011). How to interpret hydrogen breath tests. *Journal of Neurogastroenterology and Motility, 17*(3), 312–317. https://doi.org/10.5056/jnm.2011.17.3.312

Gjika, F. (2017). Being and becoming mindful. In M. Powietrzyńska & K. Tobin (Eds.), *Weaving complementary knowledge systems and mindfulness to educate a literate citizenry for sustainable and healthy lives* (pp. 331–344). Sense. https://doi.org/10.1007/978-94-6351-182-7_21

Higgins, M. (1988, March/April). An interview with Mary Burmeister, Master of Jin Shin Jyutsu. *Yoga Journal, 79*, 24–29.

Mayo Clinic Staff. (2018, January 26). *Hirschsprung's disease – Symptoms and causes*. https://www.mayoclinic.org/diseases-conditions/hirschsprung's-disease/symptoms-causes/syc-20351556

Miniello, M. (2017). Jin Shin Jyutsu and our hands. In M. Powietrzyńska & K. Tobin (Eds.), *Weaving complementary knowledge systems and mindfulness to educate a literate citizenry for sustainable and healthy lives* (pp. 265–289). Sense. https://doi.org/10.1007/978-94-6351-182-7_17

Oxford Dictionaries. (n.d.-a). *Problem | Definition of problem in English by Oxford Dictionaries*. https://en.oxforddictionaries.com/definition/problem

Oxford Dictionaries. (n.d.-b). *Project | Definition of project in English by Oxford Dictionaries*. https://en.oxforddictionaries.com/definition/project

Poole, E. A. (2016). Seeing emotions: A review of micro and subtle emotion expression training. *Cultural Studies of Science Education*, 1–13. https://doi.org/10.1007/s11422-015-9698-0

Poole, E. A. (2019). *Know(ing) thyself: examining complementary practices of health and wellness through a teacher's standpoint.* City University of New York (CUNY). https://academicworks.cuny.edu/gc_etds/2982

Proscia, P. A. (2017). Coming Face to face with fears: Journeying to wellness. In M. Powietrzyńska & K. Tobin (Eds.), *Weaving complementary knowledge systems and mindfulness to educate a literate citizenry for sustainable and healthy lives* (pp. 291–303). Brill Sense.

Riegger-Krause, W. (2014). *Health is in your hands: Jin Shin Jyutsu – practicing the art of self-healing (with 51 flash cards for the hands-on practice of Jin Shin Jyutsu.* Upper West Side Philosophers Inc.

Schwartz, J. (2017). Complementary approaches to wellness. In M. Powietrzyńska & K. Tobin (Eds.), *Weaving complementary knowledge systems and mindfulness to educate a literate citizenry for sustainable and healthy lives* (pp. 305–316). Sense. https://doi.org/10.1007/978-94-6351-182-7_19

Tobin, K., & Ansari, N. (2017). Complementary perspectives on the enigma of Diabetes Mellitus. In M. Powietrzyńska & K. Tobin (Eds.), *Weaving complementary knowledge systems and mindfulness to educate a literate citizenry for sustainable and healthy lives* (pp. 345–369). Sense. https://doi.org/10.1007/978-94-6351-182-7_22

CHAPTER 14

"How Are You Today?" A Narrative, Introspective Look at the Relationship of Knowing and Feeling

An (Inter)Personal Narrative

Andre Poole

Abstract

This chapter is primarily a narrative, introspective look at the relationship of knowing and feeling. It is a self-study/examination of wellness through the use of complementary health practices, predominately pranayama yoga. I explore what it means to be well versus being healthy, as I believe that a distinction can be made between the two. An unexpected health project emerges from the results and subsequent research and investigation. Ripple effects leading up to and transmitted from this research are also identified, and preliminary next steps explored.

Keywords

wellness – complementary medicine – pranayama yoga – mindfulness – teacher | researcher – authentic inquiry – ethnography – hypertension

1 A Beginning

I approached both writing this chapter and the activity it describes as an activity of personal inquiry. I want(ed) to know, examine, explore, and investigate my own wellness using complementary health practices. Much of this chapter is in the form of a dialogue, some of it to the page and others are an internal voice.

Understanding, or at least unpacking, what being well is versus being healthy lies at the foundation of this exploration. I did have some expectations for change during the use of pranayama yoga and Jin Shin Jyutsu in one manner or another, but I did not expect to find a hidden problem, or rather a new project, to be worked on.

 | DOI:10.1163/9789004527348_014

2 A Simple Question

How are you today? – Really, take a moment to truly determine how you are feeling today? My usual answer is "hanging in there." It is a phrase that frustrates some who receive my very boilerplate answer while placating the (often disingenuous but) polite query outright. However, if I were honest with you, the reader, I would admit that "hanging in" is the way I feel quite often. However, what does "hanging in" mean and is it a sufficient state in which to live? Essentially, after there are certain questions, you must ask yourself: what does it mean to be well, what does it mean to being healthy, and what do the answers to those question mean for you and your family?

Is there, as I believe, a distinction that can be made between being/doing well and being healthy? If so, how can that distinction begin to be investigated on an individual level?

This difference in distinction, while familiar to us all, is not a trivial thing to contemplate. I made a deliberate choice to make "How are you today?" the first four words of what you are reading. It is very possible that you, the reader, either asked this question of someone today or you were asked the question. My overarching challenge has been the ability to answer this fundamental question honestly. Many years ago, while doing research into emotions and how they are expressed I came across the idea of interoception. As defined, interoception is the awareness of the phenomenological and physiological condition (Craig, 2002) at the moment or, more simply, how you are feeling on a (literally) visceral level (Sherrington, 1906).

Do you know how you are feeling? Other than obvious things such as a grumbling stomach, a wave of dizziness, or a throbbing toe, can you (or do you) take notice of how things feel 'inside' and how they influence your decisions and the bidirectional relationship between emotions and sensation (Wiens, 2005)?

Don't let this moment pass. Take a moment and really feel.

Did you notice anything? Did you allow yourself to notice anything? Be honest about the moment with yourself.

I am not submitting this question or its answer as a form of judgment by you or of you. I submit it as a realization that I had to come to when asking myself the same question throughout each day, especially the most 'normal' ones. I am reminded of a recent experience I had in a school I visited where the principal had a large brass singing bowl. The bowl has large enough for an adult to stand in and had foot-shaped paper cutouts to guide the user to stand on. The principal commented to me that she uses the bowl as a therapeutic tool for some of her students when they are in crisis. During her explanation, and my subsequent trial moment in the bowl, she told me of one incident where a student expressed his gratitude for his experience standing in the bowl by stating that he was able to 'finally feel' himself.

So, is the question of how you are feeling a trivial thing? That may depend on your audience, which, includes the subject (in this case myself). When a physician asks the question, they are asking with interest but also professional distance. The question becomes a very literal inquiry rather than a socially polite question. Additionally, the 'how' is not solely the domain of the physical and tactile realm. Our mental and emotional states often play a significant role in how we are feeling as well. The physical, mental, and the emotional are not siloed, independent domains that seldom have interaction between each other. To the contrary, my emotions are often influenced by how I am feeling physically and vice versa.

Pain, in my experience, moves across these domains reasonably freely. The pain of some cognitive or emotional stress is often followed by some other physical manifestation of fatigue and discomfort or at least a lower tolerance for discomfort outside of the norm. Was something obscuring the aforementioned singing bowl student's feelings? Was that mask some pain that he could not articulate or explain temporarily suppressed or removed?

For example, the stress of academic writing, inclusive of what you are reading now, does cause strong emotions of fear, confusion, and to some degree, a feeling of loss (specifically of time and effort). The discomfort becomes comfortable and familiar, like an old childhood blanket that has a hint of the smell of holidays gone by.

3 Sick and Tired of Feeling Tired and Sick

With that, ask yourself if you feel 'well'? From the time we are children we often state that we "don't feel well." That phrase becomes a familiar refrain that is often heard and used but serves to keep the meaning of wellness synonymous with being healthy. What I now have come to accept is that these two terms, while related, are not equivalent; more adjacent or parallel.

I want to be healthy *and* well. I don't know what to expect or who it will affect but I anticipate, and hope, that something that I can use with those closest to me will emerge.

In turning thoughts and words into actions, complementary wellness systems will be personally explored over the next month. In the past, I have participated in Vindhya yoga classes to deal with issues I have had with flexibility and as a type of stress relief and I currently see an acupuncturist for pain and relaxation purposes. What is described throughout the rest of this chapter are primarily new experiences: pranayama yoga and Jin Shin Jyutsu (JSJ).

4 Who Am I ... Really?

Taken literally, I am many things simultaneously when using this question as a measure of the relationship between myself and the world around me. They are labels used to quickly explain vocation, education, gender, sexuality, race, socioeconomic status. In the general context of this piece, the best way to describe me would be as an African American, middle-aged mid-career teacher | researcher. Now, I do recognize that I could have taken the easy route and just defined myself as a teacher or, more generally, an educator. However, that would be an oversimplification of reality. I view myself as a child's brown paint: a fluid solution of various colors that was once a body of separate and apart components that has formed something new and now inseparable whole. The father does not end where the educator begins. The friend is the same figure as the student. The husband is indistinguishable from the son.

Ok, so what?

These roles compete for a limited set of resources and energy throughout each moment of social life. What energy is left for one last role: the first-person self-me? While trying to attend to the wellbeing of others how do I satisfy my need for being well? Is trying to help myself a selfish thing?

This question/conflict speaks to my inner confusion about balancing the need to help, and the gratification I get from that type of service, with the need to tend to my own issues Whom do I choose? Obviously, I cannot help others unless I am able to, from a health perspective.

The cumulative effect of teaching, including being a unicorn to some degree as an African-American male in an elementary school setting, much less living in a larger urban center such as New York, has taken its toll. As teachers, we are expected to match the energies that our students exhibit on a minute-to-minute basis. These energies could be physical, emotional, mental, and in my opinion, even spiritual. In an almost Freirean way, teachers bank these energies, for later withdrawal and use in the classroom. However, like any high traffic stretch of carpeting, teachers get worn out with this use-renewal-reuse cycle of energy. I, like many others, have fallen victim to this pattern during my career.

I was a burned-out teacher who had to leave the profession for a short time. Self-care before my resignation was not really something that I considered or contemplated to any substantial degree. I was fine with making it through the day so that I could make it to the next day. I thought of non-traditional Western health maintenance as the best way to address ill feelings. My experience with alternative systems of wellness was very limited and undeveloped, and my attitude towards such systems was mainly to view them as hippie hocus-pocus.

However, what I did not realize until after my resignation was that I was in pain. A pain that I didn't know was there until the discomfort was removed. The pain had become normal and comfortable. It was a way to know that I was useful and worthy. If I had no pain, then how could I know that I was functioning and functional.

5 A Common Language

What is your relationship with pain? That can be an interesting question, but one many of us do not ask ourselves often. So again, thoughtfully, ask yourself (as I have asked myself): What is my relationship with pain? Is pain a stain on the carpet; which I ignore for days at a time? Is that a bald spot that I try to obscure by teasing the hair around it? Is my pain a shining beacon that keeps me awake and aware of the world around me? Or is pain something I just wish I could transfer from someone else. As a matter of experience, there are very few things we may be able to agree on. Pain is one of the few exceptions. Every single person ever born has experience with pain. Pain knows no economic, social, racial, or age boundary. Pain is truly equal opportunity. What we feel as discomfort is a shared language and often is the main describing factor when discussing wellness (or the lack thereof).

I am often amazed at how people can discuss pain both freely and with great shame. Some wear pain as a great badge of honor. After all, pain is weakness leaving the body, isn't it?

Similarly, what is your relationship with wellness? Is wellness something warm and familiar as the emotions one may feel for a parent? Could wellness be fleeting like unrequited or unexperienced love? Or is wellness a battle akin to a rivalry between siblings? Do you allow wellness to enter your life and lifestyle willingly or do you find reasons to continue doing the familiar and rote activities that distract and distance us from being well (or just being)?

Science at its base nature is about structure. Structures that allow for dichotomies, dichotomies lead to categories, categories form divisions, divisions lead to greater questions, and questions lead to a desire to find order, or put another way: structure. Science is a cyclical business both in its theoretical aspects as well as its practical ones. Many would argue that science is all about the practical: how can I use this plant or how can I harness the power of the sun? We strive to understand, and to a lesser degree control, the world around us. But how well do we understand ourselves? How well do you know yourself? More literally, how well do you know *thyself*? What are you feeling right now? ... literally? Think about that for a moment. What do you feel?

While writing the first draft of this paper my feet felt hot. Hot in the same way the flu might make you feel hot and cold at the same time; feverish even. The soles of my feet often feel tight and sore due to metatarsalgia.

I have come to accept that I view much of my life through the lens of personal pain. I don't view this as a problem, or pessimism, or take a deficit perspective. Pain is just something that is present and truly is an in the moment phenomenon. I am not sure how I have come to this place intellectually or cognitively, but I do know that pain is something most of us want relief from. But not all sensations and pain are as tactile or easy to describe and pinpoint. Pain may be physical, emotional, psychological, and in some cases, pain may probably be imagined but is, nonetheless, experienced as pain. So how do we ameliorate or eliminate pain?

6 Situation and Situating

So why take this on? Simply put because I had to. I am forced to. What forced me was the desire to be better, to feel better, to live better, my biological determination for self-preservation. However, within that is the need to examine and understand more about what is happening, with some level of detail, as I try to make changes to my life(style).

From a physical/external, I chose to follow the precepts and theories surrounding event-oriented inquiry (EOI). Events, in general, are identified as Kenneth Tobin and Stephen Ritchie defined them as, "contradictions that arise as culture is enacted" (2012, p. 118). Contradictions, in turn, were identified through physiological data collected using fingertip pulse oximeters. Essentially, spikes or dips in the data were used as ways to identify events for further investigation. Either of the measures, heart rate (BPM) or blood oxygenation (SpO_2) could be used in the identification of an event. Egon Guba and Yvonna Lincoln's authenticity criteria (1989) are not only used and observed but are a crucial underpinning to what I want to do and learn as a result, in the ongoing sense not in the terminal sense, of this new health project. What this means specifically is to look at what happens, both immediately and over longer timeframes, and to interpret and learn from the experience in order to make and/or understand changes in my personal ontologies and epistemologies.

The internal/existential aspect of the 'doing' is to observe how my ongoing mindfulness practices alongside these new yogic practices (which are cataloged below) have changed physiological awareness, emotional awareness (Wiens, 2005) or interoception (Craig, 2002). Additionally, Ken Wilber's integral model and levels of consciousness development (Wilber, 2005) are considered and present but not in a dogmatic, tightly bound way.

But honestly, I am interested to see if anything changes from a measurable health perspective. I like looking at numbers and finding patterns.

Lastly, I also want this to be about my voice. The free-writing could be seen as following a narrative structure of one-part Van Maanen ethnography (2011), one-part stimulated recall (Lyle, 2003), and a rant or two mixed in occasionally for good measure. One first daily free-writing entry is done just after each morning session of Kapalbhati Pranayama (rhythmic rapid breathing) yoga, which is used as intervention and mediation. The second daily entry is done at any point during the day after some reflection or can begin as a note to be revisited later through (the aforementioned) stimulated recall. In part, this fits in very well with (my interpretation of) Wilber's first three AQAL (all quadrants, all levels) sections:

- quadrant I: the "I" – how am I feeling,
- quadrant II: the "it" – my "pains" or what ails me, and
- quadrant III: the "we" – my collective; my family – the ripple effects beyond personal practice.

My personal JSJ experiences, have to this point, primarily been guided sessions being led by Kenneth Tobin, a JSJ practitioner and professor at the CUNY Graduate Center. I have been very surprised at some of the experiences I have had with him during our sessions and have decided to try to integrate JSJ into my self-help regimen.

Hopefully, I hope that as you are reading this, my voice comes through. Within that voice are the struggle, pain, sarcasm, and hope. At times, the structure may be difficult to follow or seem disjointed. But I am choosing to write this as the thoughts emerge from me.

Not all, if any, of these things, are considered a strong part or path to good academic writing but honestly at this point I am not sure if I care. This has been a very hard and ongoing issue to deal with when writing or when I allow others to review what I write because of my own insecurities and opinions about what I find interesting or compelling.

What I do find interesting and compelling is finding complementary ways of handling issues with health and wellness. Western medicine has provided us with many wonders that help us feel better. So wondrous are some of these things that we get addicted to the high speed and low effort that is required to achieve a better feeling.

But I digress ...

7 Day Zero

So why do all of this? I really want to see what, if any, affect teaching has on me in the moment and if any changes over one month can be made to address health. The narrative serves to situate the data in the context of a relative and qualitative artifact of mood, activity, and interaction with students. Oximetry and/or the blood pressure serve as quantitative indicators through which a more traditional, analytical lens can be used to examine what is/was happening. In combination, this takes an approach that could be viewed as "human science research" (Van Manen, 2016, p. 38). This approach is both phenomenological, hence grounded in the lived experience, and hermeneutic, by attempting to interpret and determine the embodied meaning within the moments examined.

8 And So, It Begins ...

I figure that as this goes on, I will look back at the week that was. Occasionally taking a rooftop view of the situation helps to frame what has happened at ground level. Also, and honestly, this will also give me a chance to reflect, truly reflect, on what has been happening. Hopefully, reading the freewriting again and looking at the data will help me see what is often obscured and feel what is often unnoticeable.

There are no real expectations except educative ones. Can the root question be answered, at least in part? I welcome the experience.

I've decided to start by setting up a cushion on the floor on the night of Day 0 (which would be the evening before Day 1) and have a laptop out with the video downloaded and cued up ahead of time. Hopefully, the savings in time would allow for the first reading to be more related to my actual waking BP and BPM rather than something that may be a manifestation of setting up my (new) practice. I expect that as this goes on some of the conditions will be emergent and contingent based on need.

9 Week One: Reflection

This was an interesting experience. I am glad that I woke up at early in the days leading up to the first readings to see how I would feel at this hour as a 'dry run.' That aside I hope I did this correctly. My knees and hips hurt a little bit too. I haven't been in that sitting position for that long in a long time. My sides hurt during the yoga though. Just goes to show how weak my core is. I've had to sit with the arm of the couch up against my back just to keep tall and not slouch during the yoga. That really has me disappointed with my lifestyle. I need to do better. I am really surprised how much my sides hurt during ... Not terrible by any means but more than soreness would feel. I wonder how long it would take for this to pass. I expect not until the end of next week.

Also, this pressure level can't be a fluke if after 3 days it's still that high minutes after waking up. All I do is walk downstairs, grab the cuff sit, take a few breaths and take the reading.

I am conflicted as I write this wondering if my eagerness to please myself interfered with the meditative nature of the yoga. It was very hard to stay in the moment through each session as I was struggling with a bit of fatigue as well as trying to make sure that I leave the house on time to have a smooth commute.

This has been the most dedicated I've been to any health and wellness project in my adulthood. There is a sense of shame attached to that while simultaneously understanding the feelings of invincibility during my younger days. As a husband and father who is caring for a parent, health and wellness has suddenly become a very salient topic for me.

One interesting thing happened during the night of Day 8 while trying out JSJ main central vertical: my feet started to get very hot during the flow. I remember thinking that my feet feel confused and that I didn't get much restful sleep and was a distraction during the yoga. I needed to consult someone else with a more developed practice to see if he has ever had a similar experience. I don't know if that would account for anything in the readings for the following day (Day 9).

10 Week Two: Reflections

My focus was all over the place this week. I had a hard time feeling comfortable. Several thoughts kept entering my head in regards to the upcoming day at work, this research, my daughter, etc. I could not get comfortable. The experience reminded me about my troubles with sleep. Often when I want to go to sleep and I feel myself drifting, the act of noticing and being aware of the sensation of falling asleep happening, actually wakes me up. I was looking/listening for a sensation and that kept me out of the moment. I think that the best word for how I feel right now is 'insecure.' However, I am not sure why … I've had some interesting results from this so far. Specifically, I don't feel as hungry. That lack of hunger is an interesting thing especially since I probably burn more calories from the now extended amount of active time that I endure in a day.

Now looking at the BPM data from just now there was an increase. My thoughts must have put some stress into that. Probably went very far to undo the good of the yoga itself.

Starting the JSJ this week added a new wrinkle to this story. I don't like doing JSJ on my own and would prefer being guided through the practice or having it performed or practiced on me. Something similar to what Malgorzata experienced (Powietrzyńska, 2017) and the exposure that JP and I have had with JSJ in recent months (see chapter 11, this volume).

The yoga is becoming more comfortable and slowly making its way into a habit that I look forward to. I do also see the need to also be mindful of the amount of sleep I get in order to want to get out of my warm bed on a cold fall morning. But the yoga has become one of the best parts of my day. It is my only moment of peace. Yoga is my moment to feel like me – without the labels that define most of my social ties. No one is in need of me and so I can tend to myself. It is my own little 20-minute man cave …

From an evaluative perspective I believe, rather, I know that there have been some changes in my behavior and my tendencies. My eating habits and my energy maintenance have moderated during these last two weeks. I don't eat the same volume of food as I do not feel as hungry. There is evidence to support that a reduction of body mass index (BMI) can result from ongoing rapid-breath Kapalbhati yoga practice (Chauhan et al., 2017) but admittedly I did not take any BMI related measurements beforehand. Upon reflection, I do not think that this omission is a bad thing. Weight loss or changes in appetite were not amongst the effects I had considered as possible outcomes when planning these activities nor did I have any specific expectations other than a general change in habitual behavior with regards to wellness practices.

What has been unexpected has been the general downward trend in blood pressure readings. Systolic and diastolic measures have been declining, in general, from day one through the end of week two. I will have to chart the results to see if this continues. But I am concerned with some of the pre-yoga readings being so close to, or within, the prehypertension range (Weber et al., 2013): systolic pressures between 110- and 139-mm Hg (9 readings) and/or diastolic pressures between 80- and 89-mm Hg (5 readings). A few, specifically three, of my diastolic readings would fall under stage 1 hypertension (90 to 99 mm Hg).

Surprising and scary but hopefully the downward trend will continue over the coming days and weeks. I've been meaning to look up the research on nitric oxide and nasal breathing. I anticipate there will be a little gem in there to give me some insight on what I am doing. As of now, it is too early to tell what any of the data means so I really don't have any context at this point.

There was an interesting personal moment on Day 12. Just as I finished JP and I ran into each other at the top of the stairs. She wants to wish her grandfather a happy 80th birthday. What an interesting moment. A six-year-old with one missing and one very wobbly front tooth is eagerly anticipating greeting her now 80-year-old grandfather with an early morning hug and kiss. He is happy to have now outlived his own father. This is now giving me a goal. I need to have my grandchild greet me on the morning of my 80th. I'm am glad to have them both and be present for today. I recognize that I must do better to feel better to make this goal a reality. I am glad that my dad has reached 80 (years old). This was a big deal to him to outlive his father. He has mentioned it a few times since his cancer diagnosis. Other than regular walking and his early morning calisthenics he really doesn't do much to maintain his health. My mother died at 54 from ovarian cancer. Her youngest sister died from ovarian cancer as well. If I don't start taking a better look at my habits, health, and overall wellbeing my children won't be able to greet me on my eightieth birthday because that event will never come. I don't want to depend on pharmaceutical answers to health, but if I don't give my body the opportunity to take care of itself then 80 won't happen. Avoid problems by taking on projects. Health problems vs health projects.

11 Week Three: Reflections

This was an off-and-on week for me mentally. The first week was a time to start developing routines and a workflow. I think that I will try to wake up at 4:30 from now on. The hustle in the morning is a bit taxing and I don't want to come to resent the yoga as a result. The temptation of a warm bed on a chilly morning tends to be very seductive …

Get on up → get set up → get a reading → get all yoga'd → get it down → get on the road. The focus for week two contained more of the same while also trying to understand what is happening through examining the data while also trying out the JSJ main central flow on my own for the first time. I am more confident in my ability to conduct the research aspect of this health project, but I have occasionally shown real fatigue from and with this endeavor.

The fatigue doesn't really last into the day, but the evenings are rough, especially if I am teaching at the college. The next morning is just awful when that is the case.

I did more listening during the week; listening to my body that is. My appetite has been steady, and I find this new normal to be refreshing. I really appreciate not feeling as hungry even with the lower intake. This an interesting dichotomy.

Even with that said, I also feel like there is no quiet moment. Even now, with no one around, it isn't quiet. I have this symphony of fragmented thoughts bouncing off every corner of my head. The various aspects of my life that require my energy are all competing for my attention. It's like a class of students who all have something to say to their teacher. To each of them what they have to say is vitally emergent and important. But what about those students who say very little to nothing in class? They may have the most pressing needs but don't vocalize them out of shyness or fear. What thoughts and issues within the symphony need my attention but are too shy to come forth? A deafening silence would be nice from time to time but neither the yoga nor the JSJ seems to grant that wish … For now. One can continue to hope …

Also, at some point in the week, I changed sitting positions again. I don't remember when or why but I seem to recall that it may have something to do with the hardness or the chair. I've moved on to the couch with my back pressed firmly against the chair. My knees are bent with my feet on either side of the cushion. This position almost looks like someone huddling up to keep warm, but it is more comfortable.

12 Week Four: Reflections and Conclusion

After 31 sessions of recording my blood pressure (BP) before and after the pranayama yoga (over 37 days) has left me with a number of curiosities to unpack.

I had an opportunity to take some readings during acupuncture. I've been curious about this for a while, and I hope (my acupuncturist) Billy is on board with me using the oximeter. He's always expressed interest in some of what I've been researching in wellness, and we've talked about the research many times. I enjoy the talks about how alternative/complementary methods should complement work done by the person seeking change. None of this is meant to be a magic bullet but if treated that way only disappointment could follow.

I sit still for many minutes after – generally until my original alarm goes off. Grateful for the peace. I think that I might be too grateful for the peace I was mentioning earlier. I don't want to seem like I don't want to be around people, but I am around them all day except in the car and the bathroom ... While this is not an always a peaceful existence, I can't imagine that it is not different from other people. So why do I need this coping mechanism so much? Am I the outlier or does everyone else need these moments too and they just don't get to have that time for themselves?

I need to consider possibly bringing others into this practice. My aunt and father are awake at the times when I am doing the pranayama, but I don't know if they would be interested. Also, I don't know much of my aunt's medical history to really benefit or if there are any risks (hypertension, gastritis, etc.).

One question that came to my mind was to ask why my waking or pre-yoga BP was so high that first week (days 1–6). These initial readings would place me in the elevated range, but this was never something that presented itself during any routine physical examination.

While not in a danger range, I do know that systolic pressure over 130 could be a problem. It wasn't until much later on that I discovered that readings in that range are considered elevated and that high BP is likely to develop if steps are not taken (American Heart Association, 2017). This gave me a real sense of concern due to some family history with hypertension as well as the knowledge that morning hypertension was actually a thing to be concerned about. After all, who amongst us would even know that we were experiencing an early-hypertensive state during normal, everyday activities much less the first moments of your day.

Over this time, my mean pre-yoga systolic (see Figure 14.1) was 120.3 (SD = 8.4) ranging from 108 mm Hg to 138 mm Hg while pre-yoga diastolic was 82.7

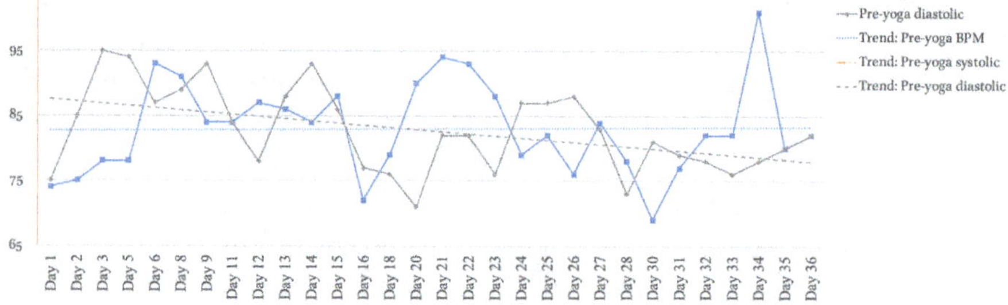

FIGURE 14.1 Pre-yoga measurements

(SD = 6.3) ranging from 71 mm Hg to 95 mm Hg. What is positive about this outcome is that, over the 37 days, the readings for both systolic and diastolic pressures showed an overall downward trend. Based on American Heart Association (AHA) recommendations (2017), the averages fit within the low elevated range, however, there were several individual days that would present themselves as stage 1 hypertension in either the systolic (4 days) or the diastolic (15 days). Stage 2 hypertensive readings were also present in the diastolic (mm Hg => 90) in another 4 days.

The same downward trend is present across the 37 days with the post-yoga readings (see Figure 14.2). The mean post-yoga systolic was (a more mentally comfortable) 114.9 (SD = 5.6) ranging from 106 to 128 mm Hg and the mean post-yoga diastolic was 75.7 (SD = 5.0) with a range from 68 to 88 mm Hg. The number of stage 1 hypertensive events were completely eliminated in the systolic (4 days to zero) and reduced significantly in the diastolic as well (from 15 days to 5) when compared to pre-yoga results. These readings are more in line with what I had expected in general based on my prior knowledge of my own health over many years.

The single-point data point BP baseline of 114/77, against which these results above could be compared against, come from my most recent physical examination completed four months prior to the start of this dataset.

It was comforting to see a general reduction or normalization in BP to something I (along with my loved ones, doctor and the AMA) could be more comfortable with. As noted within many of the log entries with elevated level, I was really concerned in the moment.

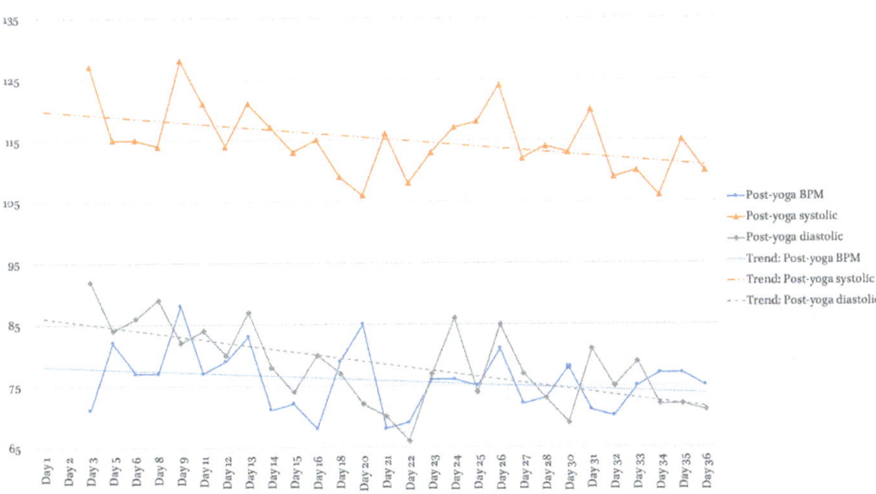

FIGURE 14.2 Post-yoga measurements

An additional question that could be raised based on the results would be if the reduction in blood pressure, and any other corresponding health measurement such as heart rate or $SpO_2\%$ in either average or trend, could be predicted or determined. It is my opinion that there could be some degree of that possibility occurring, but I would not say that the trend would be a direct or indirect correlation but more of a change in those readings due to a shift in mindset toward being more aware of the moment, essentially mindfulness rather than a change in fitness.

I did find that the time immediately after the yoga is best spent in quiet solitude. No note taking, no lunch prep, no conversation. Just sitting and being. The quiet time is very enjoyable.

I am generally feeling better. I was just reminiscing over the peaceful feeling from this morning after the yoga. The feeling informs me of something that may be missing in general: a sense of inner peace. I am very tired; physically, mentally, and emotionally.

13 Under the Context of Multiple Knowledge Systems

The experiences that have been presented could be described or categorized as falling under the lens of the traditional, data-driven, Western-medicine system understanding of health and wellness. They could also be seen through a more personal view of wellness rooted through Eastern systems, such as mindfulness or yoga. Either way these systems, either Eastern or Western traditions, should not be looked at as opposites or in competition with one another. Rather, these systems should be seen as complementary. Several hospitals/hospital systems, such as the Mayo Clinic (Mayo Clinic Staff, 2018) and Mount Sinai (Mount Sinai Hospital, 2018) have centers that provide these wellness systems as part of patient recovery techniques or offerings under the umbrella terms such as complementary therapies or integrative medicine. As a part of the movement toward making this type of treatment more accessible and a part of the traditional medical treatment, the Carol G. Simon Cancer Center of the Morristown (NJ) Medical Center integrative medicine program offers JSJ and other active-role healing techniques as a part of their treatment options for patients and their caregivers (Atlantic Health System, 2018).

By offering and making spaces for these practices to become part of not only mainstream treatment but also, and possibly more importantly, the mainstream conversation, yoga (asana, pranayama, etc.), JSJ, and other complementary systems become part of a larger tapestry within the possible avenues of care.

14 What May Follow

When considering where to go to next, I have two semi-overlapping standpoints. On one hand, I believe that nothing would benefit the community more than what I have experienced firsthand. However, I am not sure that I am, currently, well placed enough socially in order to expand the beneficence of what has taken place (Tobin & Ritchie, 2012, p. 119). The second sphere is more personal and intimate: expanding beneficence to those closest to me: my family. In this, however, I feel that I must tread lightly. I do not want to force what I believe may be beneficial onto them, specifically my children.

Also, I do believe the benefits I experienced are real and clearly measurable, but I have to take into account the various health conditions, ages and gender-specific issues that may arise with some of these practices. In my father's case, he received a colorectal cancer diagnosis at the beginning of the year. I admit to being fearful of what the next year may hold and although facilities such as Morristown Medical Center know how to integrate these complementary practices into lifestyle and wellness, I am not comfortable enough with my level of expertise to risk anything with his health (such as non-pharmaceutical blood pressure management through yoga).

While I would be proud to help and would like what I am experiencing to have some extra-personal effect, I recognize that I need to have a better understanding of the effects as a regular practitioner so that I may be a decent guide at the beginning of someone else's journey. I think of this as a series of possible, future-facing ripple effects – a bit of paying it forward (so to speak).

I have also continued with the early morning pranayama yoga practices albeit without the physiological data collection. There was a slight bit of pressure that I felt during the data collection, such as worrying about isolating variables and making sure that what I was doing made some sense, because I wanted the collection of data to go well. I didn't have expectations in the traditional sense of making a prediction. I did expect a certain amount of emergence and contingence to be present throughout. Using oximeters, by its very nature of showing the user moment-by-moment readings, may bring awareness but I would not call it pressure (and I've used them enough over my doctoral studies that I've come to a point of not even noticing them for the most part). The blood pressure cuff brings more of an interruption (if you allow it to) because of the nature of measuring BP. As a result, the act of sitting down, placing your arm in the right configuration, and waiting for the cuff to inflate then deflate could bring some anxiety into the equation depending on how it was utilized. I did not find this to be an issue because the readings that were collected here were either immediately before or after the yoga sessions.

15 The Beautiful Struggle

One of my favorite songs, "Get by" written and performed by fellow Brooklynite Talib Kweli (2002) goes as follows:

> Life is a beautiful struggle
> People search through the rubble for a suitable hustle
> Some people usin' the noodle, some people usin' the muscle
> Some people put it all together, make it fit like a puzzle

Many times, when I feel some adversity or some difficulty in my life I often seek out this song for motivation and renewed drive. Undertaking this investigation, ultimately, was meant to be an introspective, investigative, and educative process. One takeaway is that I have difficulty understanding how I am and embrace a relationship with wellness as the beautiful struggle.

There is risk, however. There are axiological, epistemological, and ontological shifts taking place as my exposure and comfort with knowing myself and feeling more 'well' (note: not better but well). However, I must ask myself if these modalities are palliative in nature? In an honest moment, and with any real reflection on how the modalities function, it is possible to also conclude that what a significant amount of traditional Western medicine does is also palliative. Over-the-counter medications don't treat the cold, they suppress the symptoms, for example, the body takes care of the rest. After watching my father undergo radiation and chemotherapy for his cancer treatments, I can say that those methods are intended to be more curative than palliative as they attack the cause (along with the healthy parts of the body unfortunately). At the core, I want to not only feel better because of a reduction in symptoms but I want to be well because of a reduction or elimination of causal factors.

Interpersonally, I am more interested in allowing someone else to be at ease either by comforting them through elevating their importance within the conversation or by diminishing my own importance by omitting or repressing my own state(s). I am also fearful of how this will be read by others along its various stages of sharing, editing, and eventual submission for publication. This is probably the most honest part of this self-investigation; I am full of fear and, as a result, try to mask the fear and its associated pain deep within my persona. I am not sure what the answer is because I am not fully sure that it matters. Wellness through knowing one's self should be painful to some degree – any growth is. But I also don't want my remedy to be something analgesic or topical. I want substantive change. Just as I am writing this very sentence, I recognize my bad posture and correct it to something more 'correct.'

It is a start …

References

American Heart Association. (2017, November 30). *Understanding blood pressure readings*. https://www.heart.org/en/health-topics/high-blood-pressure/understanding-blood-pressure-readings

Atlantic Health System. (2018). *Cancer integrative medicine programs*. https://www.atlantichealth.org/conditions-treatments/cancer-care/cancer-support-services/cancer-integrative-medicine-programs.html

Chauhan, A., Semwal, D. K., Mishra, S. P., & Semwal, R. B. (2017). Yoga practice improves the body mass index and blood pressure: A randomized controlled trial. *International Journal of Yoga, 10*(2), 103–106. https://doi.org/10.4103/ijoy.IJOY_46_16

Craig, A. D. (2002). How do you feel? Interoception: The sense of the physiological condition of the body. *Nature Reviews Neuroscience, 3*(8), 655–666. https://doi.org/10.1038/nrn894

Guba, E. G., & Lincoln, Y. S. (1989). *Fourth generation evaluation*. Sage Publications.

Kweli, T. (2002). Get By [Song]. On *quality* [Album]. Rawkus Entertainment.

Lyle, J. (2003). Stimulated recall: A report on its use in naturalistic research. *British Educational Research Journal, 29*(6), 861–878. https://doi.org/10.1080/01411920320000137349

Mayo Clinic Staff. (2018, January 26). *Hirschsprung's disease – Symptoms and causes*. https://www.mayoclinic.org/diseases-conditions/hirschsprung's-disease/symptoms-causes/syc-20351556

Mount Sinai Hospital-New York. (2018). *Complementary therapies*. https://www.mountsinai.org/patient-care/service-areas/pain-management/pain-management-services/integrative-medicine

Powietrzynska, M. (2017). Taking charge of our own wellness through complementary approaches. In M. Powietrzynska & K. Tobin (Eds.), *Weaving complementary knowledge systems and mindfulness to educate a literate citizenry for sustainable and healthy lives* (pp. 317–330). Sense Publishers. https://doi.org/10.1007/978-94-6351-182-7_20

Sherrington, C. (1906). *The integrative action of the nervous system* (Vol. 2). CUP Archive.

Tobin, K., & Ritchie, S. M. (2012). Multi-method, multi-theoretical, research in the learning sciences multi-level. *Asia-Pacific Education Researcher, 21*(1), 117–129.

Van Maanen, J. (2011). *Tales of the field: On writing ethnography* (2nd ed.). University of Chicago Press.

Van Manen, M. (2016). *Researching lived experience: Human science for an action sensitive pedagogy*. Routledge.

Weber, M. A., Schiffrin, E. L., White, W. B., Mann, S., Lindholm, L. H., Kenerson, J. G., Flack, J. M., Carter, B. L., Materson, B. J., Ram, C. V. S., Cohen, D. L., Cadet, J.-C., Jean-Charles, R. R., Taler, S., Kountz, D., Townsend, R. R., Chalmers, J., Ramirez, A.

J., Bakris, G. L., ... Harrap, S. B. (2014), Clinical practice guidelines for the management of hypertension in the community. *Journal of Clinical Hypertension, 16*, 14–26. https://doi.org/10.1111/jch.12237

Wiens, S. (2005). Interoception in emotional experience. *Current Opinion in Neurology, 18*(4).

Wilber, K. (2005). Introduction to integral theory and practice. *AQAL: Journal of Integral Theory and Practice, 1*(1).

CHAPTER 15

Taking Agency; Walking Away and Coming Home

How COVID-19 Changed My Relationship to My Job, My Emotional Wellbeing and Exploring Alternatives to Food as a Coping Mechanism

Corie A. McCallum

Abstract

In this chapter, I explore significant wellness challenges that I faced during the initial phases of COVID-19 in March, 2020 in the United States. Using contemplative practices and boundaries as forms of self-care, I discuss how I addressed negative coping mechanisms and improved my emotional wellbeing.

This work reflects my personal wellness research project that emerged soon after I learned I would not return to work for the remainder of 2020. It includes notes that I wrote for myself at varying times during the early spring and into the summer of 2020 as well as my reflections.

Keywords

emotions – boundaries – self-care – contemplative practices – negative coping mechanisms

1 Prologue

I know that my perceptions, both in relation to COVID-19 and in my educational experience, are laden with privilege. I acknowledge that what I say in this chapter may not be received well, especially by those who have felt the sting of COVID-19 directly through losing loved ones, losing their jobs, or facing trauma as an essential worker. This work is not meant to minimize or overshadow COVID-19's significance in anyone's life or to deflect from the racial and economic disparities the pandemic has amplified. Rather, by exploring my own challenges and triumphs in my health and wellness during the height of the COVID-19

 | DOI:10.1163/9789004527348_015

pandemic, I hope to offer an alternative discourse centering growth and positive change as part of exploring the emotional impacts of the pandemic.

2 Surprise! We're Going Home

Prior to COVID-19, I spent the majority of my days in a school. Whether working or actually attending classes, social interactions with students and colleagues were planned and purposeful. However, since the pandemic began in March 2020 until now (March 2021, as I am editing this chapter) students, faculty and administrators across the United States have spent their time in front of a screen rather than in person. This change's impact has been felt world-wide. From teachers scrambling to make online content for 2nd-graders, to college professors trying to make a physics lab work remotely, there has been a major effort to adjust rapidly to the new ways we both live and work. I argue though, that for some, this was a welcomed and needed shift away from the everyday monotony of school, work, repeat.

At the university where I currently work, walk-in or general help services at the Registrar, Financial Aid, and Student Affairs and Conduct offices must now be addressed by administrators from their home environment. This shift from home-as-a-respite to home-the-workplace has consequences. Each student-administrator service requires building or maintaining relationships via little black boxes or avatars, rather than face to face encounters. The logistical and technical gymnastics required to resituate our entire division of employees was daunting. However, connection issues were only a sliver of the larger concerns that arise from moving to a fully online service model in a matter of weeks. Did these consequences change our experiences for the better, or worse? Perhaps the better question is, *how* have they changed our experiences?

Personally, integrating my home and work environments elucidated serious obstacles for me especially around stress management and coping mechanisms. I hadn't given one thought to how this displacement could exacerbate poor wellness practices or highlight non-existent ones. Prior to COVID-19, I loosely managed (I use "managed" very lightly as you will soon read) my work-life balance and wellness practices, falsely believing there was a magical separation between my work life and my home life. In short, I needed to address two health projects that I had been avoiding by clinging to a false work/home dichotomy. The first of those was my relationship with food. The other was a lack of stress management which inspired my budding relationship with walking as a therapeutic exercise. What began as a national health crisis would eventually become the impetus for my personal transformation through a wellness-centered approach.

3 Quarantine Exposes My "Bad" Behaviors – My Work from Home Reality

I started social distancing approximately one week early *before* COVID-19 prompted New York City and NY State to shut down and transition to work-from-home policy for colleges and universities. I had recently returned from Colombia where I visited Medellin and Cartagena. On the plane home, I was riddled with sickness. Nausea, stomach cramps, profuse sweating and a fever were some of the symptoms I endured during the 6+ hour flight from Medellin to JFK airport in Queens. When I returned home, I went to work for about a week. I thought I had just picked up a bug from the airports, so I continued, *not* resting, even working from home while sick. The weekend immediately following, I went to an urgent care center and tested for multiple strains of the flu and oddly, strep throat. At that time, the first week of March, 2020 no COVID-19 tests were available to me. Although I had a 102-degree fever, I was negative on all other tests and I was sent home on March 9th. I have still not returned to the office. However, by storm, work came to me. And like many of my higher education colleagues, the work has not stopped coming.

At first, I did not believe that working from home would cause any major disruptions to my personal life. I considered myself lucky. I have no children to care for and I already had most of the technical equipment needed to setup a home office, even if it was in my living room. Missing, however, was a balance between work and home time as that boundary had been blurred. I would check emails and fix things late at night on my laptop when my insomnia lingered. As I have a work cell phone and a work laptop with VPN access that allowed me to access university systems, I would never disconnect. I responded to emails throughout the day and often at night as well. Though I am not a workaholic, I value being informed and responding quickly. It brings me joy, sometimes, to answer questions or deliver good news in the wee hours of the morning to unsuspecting students and or staff. In Student Conduct, a win is a win. And, if there is just one small thing I can do to make the process easier for students, and myself, I usually try to do that, regardless of the time or physical location. As time progressed throughout the quarantine though, I found that maintaining any work/home balance – between Zoom calls, emails, TEAMS meetings, and the regular ebb and flow of a workday – had become a significant challenge mentally.

In every room, I was accessible. When I wanted to walk away from job stresses, there was nowhere to go. I tried moving my "office" out of the living room into a corner of our guest room, so I could go downstairs (a luxury in and of itself) and put down the phone. However, I remained literally one buzz away from the next problem, crisis, or even innocuous email advertisement that viscerally impacted me until I actually checked it – and I HAD to check it. Finding balance was emerging as a priority for me even though I was unable to visualize it at the time. Guthrie et al.'s (2005) study found that, for student affairs administrators, finding balance in their personal and professional lives was "nuanced and extremely individualistic" (p. 124). They argue that, while there is no predetermined solution for student affairs administrators for finding balance, there are multiple considerations that can impact their ability to find it. Some of those challenges include personal alignment with institutional goals, their supervisor's management style and the level of control an administrator has in their position (Guthrie et al, 2005). In student conduct work, especially from home, finding balance and controlling how I manage my own time has been essential to addressing my emotions in a healthy way.

Work-from-home life is a double-edged sword. Though I can stop checking everything and go radio-silent, doing so produces a heightened level of anxiety, pressure to be "in-the know" and the inevitable feeling of guilt for not at least "checking in." The other option is to go *all-in*. Constantly checking and responding to emails, has its anxiety inducing factors, too though. Needing others to respond so I can move forward, waiting for those who *do* practice work-life balance to initiate their portion of the work becomes vital then. There are certainly some great advantages to going all-in, like knowing at all times what is happening, but, when I do that I can never relax. I had also been trying to write every day to finish my dissertation. Adjusting to life in quarantine was not easy, but it was easy to rely on coping mechanisms I had been using for years. I knew that I could not continue down that path much longer …

4 Admitting Some Hard Truths in Quarantine

I thought my experience at home would be vastly different than in my workplace, but it did not begin that way. When we began working remotely in March of 2020, I continued the same destructive behaviors that I had at work. However, at work, they had been present for so long that I was blinded to them. Now home, I was forced to watch my self-destruction manifest in what I thought was my sanctuary. My unconscious thoughts and even some unconscious actions became center stage events at home where I was alone with myself.

As Sewell (1999) explains, our culture and patterns of thin coherence are revealed in unsettled times. The pandemic was just one of many unsettling events that would unfold. As a country during 2020 we endured a pandemic, George Floyd's death at the hands of law enforcement, the continued unjust treatment of Black and Brown people, the Black Lives Matter movement, an unprecedented election season and an attempted coup. As those events unfolded with my husband back at work and me in my make-shift bedroom office, I was both alone with, and surrounded by, my poor health choices. Prior to quarantine, the separation of work and home allowed me to believe that I had/have a different home persona. I believed that at home I automatically made better, healthier decisions for myself – even though I rarely actually did. During quarantine as my work-home fields changed, the places where I enacted my habitus (Bourdieu, 1992) morphed and reformed before me. My old coping mechanisms did not work in this new environment.

In my physical workspace at the university, I was thoughtful about my personal practice as a student conduct administrator, but not about how I treated myself or allowed myself to be treated. Questioning certain rules, be they about student conduct regulations or whether I can skip what I know will be an unproductive meeting, was easy. However, before leaving campus I was struggling mentally and emotionally with changing my office's practices or creatively circumventing the rules. For example, within the confines of the college's disciplinary procedures I am limited in the kinds of interventions I can offer to students regarding infractions of college policies. Though I may personally believe one intervention would serve a student better, it is not always within my power to enact it. At times when my personal beliefs were in opposition with my job, I would become stressed and engage in comforting, but sometimes harmful behaviors. The separation from my physical campus environment and the transactional space of an office illuminated previously obscured practices (Tobin, 2012) embedded in my praxis of student conduct administration. Although I was unaware prior to the office exodus, Pierre Bourdieu's (1992) concepts of habitus and fields were (as always) at play. When I changed the field (on-campus office to home office) I discerned what habits I engaged in physically and emotionally to uphold the expectations about how "good" student affairs professionals think, work, and behave. Everything that I accepted as "the way it is" and my adept reproduction of the status quo at the college and of larger social structures transformed in a fully remote environment.

Being away from the physical space of the college, I considered the *how* and the *why* of what I was doing on a daily basis, both in the actual practice of student conduct and the way I performed the practice. Prior to COVID-19, I occasionally considered whether the interactions I was having with students were beneficial or harmful to them, or the College, or even the larger university system. Did the interactions benefit *me* in any way? While I routinely reviewed the manner in which I evaluated and investigated cases, and interacted with students to improve "outcomes," I rarely reflected upon my personal practice and the sociocultural contexts that impact how I perform student conduct work. Working from home fundamentally altered the *how* of what I do as a conduct administrator. Most poignantly, a new work stress had entered my home. My boss, staff, and anyone with my email address, and work phone number, had unprecedented access to me, in what I considered to be a "safe space," and my highly valued privacy was seriously compromised.

The week before COVID-19 shut down New York City in March, 2020, as I mentioned earlier, I had taken off work to recover, but did not hesitate to make myself available while home. Though I was very sick, I still felt guilty for taking time off. I monitored my temperature every day to see if it were possible for me to return to work. I checked emails regularly and even texted to check in with my office staff. In hindsight, it seems to me that unfettered access to me was okay, as long as I was the one initiating it. What had changed for me during COVID-19? And how did this change put me on the path to a *different* health project? What follows is how COVID-19 became a salient personal event that led to a change in my habitus and the structure of my world.

4.1 *Food – My Medicine and My Poison*

It is tedious and somewhat ironic to describe the way I use food as comfort, in print. When I write about how I did something in the past relating to food, it does not mean that I no longer engage in these behaviors. I simply mean that I am looking at my choices with a different lens. At work, and again when work became working at home, I used food as a coping mechanism for the myriad emotions I experienced in a day. I would go from happy, to stressed, to sad, to relieved sometimes within the span of an hour. To control those emotions, I would eat something. That process did not change while working from home. Emails I could have easily let sit in my inbox until the next day while working on campus suddenly became urgent, as if I had to justify every moment not spent working, which led to my grabbing a quick snack before diving back into the chaos. Months ago, I would have described my coping strategies around emotional eating and lack of work life balance as "bad" or "negative." However, I have learned that putting value judgments on my choices, and how I talk to and about myself only intensifies a circular, emotional response of guilt, shame, and despondency. I needed to reframe my thinking and change my judgmental lenses for ones that helped me see clearer.

My lens now is health-centered and focused on my overall emotional and physical health. I no longer focus solely on food, or how food contributes to my feelings, and ultimately, my weight. I try to avoid obsessing over weight-based indicators like clothing sizes, my actual weight in pounds, as definitive measures for how I *feel*. Even as I recall my past practices around food, I feel anxious and embarrassed to admit that, sometimes, yes, a brownie did and does make me feel better. But, for me the difference is that I can recognize how and why that brownie works (or does not work) to alleviate stress or give me joy. Again, it is difficult to delineate my past uses of food from the present way I view or use food, especially in writing, because I have not exactly *changed the what* of my actions, but have drastically changed the *why* of them. Yes, I will still eat a brownie sometimes when I am stressed, but I do so with the knowledge that this is a temporary fix (if a fix at all) and that there is something more I need to address that the brownie may represent. Still, for me, the lines between now and then are blurred. This story, my story, is messy. My habits around food are in flux, but my interrogation of them is steadfast. I'm no longer on autopilot, mindlessly eating and expecting to feel better. Another difference for me is how I am choosing to reframe food choices. I take agency over them and my actions. If I am eating, I am checking in with myself to see if I am hungry or eating to relieve some other issue. I perpetually and emphatically manage the urge to slip back into food oblivion where I do not have to think or feel, but just consume. As difficult emotions arise, checking in with myself and my emotions becomes integral to my wellness.

My desire to eat as a coping mechanism for managing my feelings fueled both positive and negative emotional states for me. I also learned that not only *negative* emotions fueled, as positive states did as well. Celebrating, relaxing, accomplishing something great was as much a trigger as arguing with my husband or being stressed with difficult conduct cases. Things both in and outside of my control all contributed to my eating any and everything that I wanted in hopes of feeling better, even though I often got sick because of it. For me, my primary tool for comfort has always been and honestly still is, food. I have known for a long time that I needed help and if I am honest, I had it. I had years' worth of exposure to Jin Shin Jyutsu (Tobin, 2017), meditation (Kabat-Zinn, 2014), breathing meditation (Alexakos, 2015), heuristics (Tobin & Alexakos, 2020) [which I still use and wholeheartedly believe in!], and finally, therapy. In hindsight, I was not ready to receive those gifts. I did not know how to work towards healing especially in regards to body acceptance and some identity issues. I had not come to the point where I could deal with being a fat, Black woman in higher education *and* address how everything, especially my work, impacted my emotions around food. The intersection of those facets of my life were too much to bear at once. What I thought was just a coping mechanism for dealing with my emotions and experiences with my multitude of identities, was actually harming my body.

I would like to pause here for a moment to nuance my perspective. I am not shaming, belittling, or chastising myself for my previous actions. I recognize that I saw food as a tool to give me comfort and I have no shame about that. If I am honest, it did work sometimes and I do not believe I or anyone else should be shamed for admitting their truth. While shame is a powerful emotion, capable of creating and shaping social norms (Turner, 2009) it is not the only – or the most effective – impetus for changing habits or seeking help to do so. Healing, too, is a motivator for change and alleviating shameful feelings, though it would take the experience of working from home in isolation to recognize that what I actually needed was to heal.

4.2 *Food – A Part of My Community*

During New York's initial quarantine period, I decided to reconsider how eating, was shaping and shifting who I was as a person. At work, my consumption issues were rampant. Any excuse, even excuses I did not know I was making, led to my using food as a comfort and a crutch for what I would learn was a toxic work environment and job burnout. For example, there was a specific group of people I had lunch with regularly. Our "lunch with the crew" times were awesome. They provided all of the benefits of social fellowship. We were great at building solidarity; we would share positive emotional energy (EE) as colleagues and friends (Collins, 2004). The group also helped alleviate stress and the effects of strong emotions that impeded my ability to work on a particularly tough day. I would feel at peace being with my in-group. We looked like a 1990s diversity poster. Someone from every "walk of life" – people with disabilities, racial/ethnic minorities, LGBTQ folks, old and young – was a part of our group. However, we rarely ate without one of us being on a fad diet, limiting one food group or another, or sometimes "not eating that day," but everyone helping polish off a fresh bag of Wise potato chips, a group favorite! I look back upon those times with nostalgia and a longing to return to them, but only for the social interaction. As Collins (2004) asserts, successful rituals are energizing and build up our in-group solidarity. Unsuccessful rituals, or failed interactions, drain us. They deplete our emotional energy (Collins, 2004). Because our lunch crew was replete with positive and affirming relationships, I relished those interactions even though they too exacerbated my issues with food.

In recalling my on-campus experiences prior to the quarantine and how I have presented them in multiple iterations of this work, there is a reflexive quality to what I write or recall about my experiences in the present. When I return to each section of this work to address edits or commentary, I am drawn to the ways in which I describe/d myself, my emotions, how this work benefits me and the potential for it to benefit, or harm others. The editing process also allows me to engage with past thinking which informs how I proceed with writing and living going forward. Each section I engage mediates and is mediated by the other (Alexakos, 2015). Similarly, as I engage with comments of others, that process too mediates and is mediated by me. But not all of my experiences are dialectically related. Sometimes, I am just looking back with "rose-colored glasses." Although I can see how that statement is not "true" either, I cannot disconnect to just "look back." As I review this work, time and again, I am reminded to remain resolute in the interrogation of my choices and actions as they relate to how I view food and my emotions, as well as how I present them in writing.

I am hesitant in writing this section where I reveal some common refrains I told myself to alleviate the cycle of guilt and shame. As I am only a few months out of a practice that I participated in for years, it feels raw to share them here even months after writing and editing this work on several occasions. I made excuses and told myself stories that soothed my guilt-binge-shame cycle, memories of which sometimes still torture me. When I reflect upon my past habits, it is as if I am watching a stranger and feeling sad for her. But then the fog clears and I recognize myself. In earlier iterations of this work, I wrote that I was ashamed and anxious, but that I was relieved. I still feel those ways, but there is more under my surface. I also feel a sense of agency, power, and ownership. I do not have to carry the weight of it all in secret anymore. And hopefully, I never will again.

4.3 *Food – My Poison and My Medicine*

> *In the mornings I wake up thinking about food, but wait until I can savor a hot breakfast at work.*
>
> *In the afternoons I feel tired from the heavy lunch I eat and need a "pick me up" of caffeine and chocolate from a vending machine or a stash of candy I regularly keep in the office.*
>
> *In the evenings, I tell myself I worked hard all day and I deserve a nice meal to relax with, one I do not personally have to prepare.*
>
> *On weekends, I say that I had a stressful week. I am "allowed" to binge drink on the weekends and "calories don't count" at celebratory brunches or parties.*
>
> *Some days, I say I am going to stop.*

The above justifications I created for myself are still embedded in my thoughts. It is only through active engagement with my emotions that I can treat myself well now, without even a morsel of food involved. I have discussed at length how eating was a crutch for my emotions, but, I would be remiss if I did not address how so much consumption hindered me physically in addition to the ways my emotional pain manifested. Being home with myself for months forced me to *really see me*. Before COVID-19, my personal appearance was not my priority. I have been a larger-bodied person since I can remember, so I knew how to dress the part well enough to avoid blatant criticism. Similarly, I also know my ability to think critically and reproduce the acceptable values and successful interactions in the workplace were and still are the traits that are valued in my work. Frankly, nobody was booking me as a model so I thought that as long as I looked professional enough and suppressed the nagging feelings that something more was happening with me, I was fine. Although, in my heart I felt I was far from fine. At home in my endless rotation of sweatpants and no-longer oversized tee shirts, looking professional and acting unbothered by it became even less important. Combined with the distress of my declining physical condition, (backaches, plantar fasciitis, trouble breathing, etc.), I could not shake the feeling that what I was doing was not only hurting me physically, but "eating my emotions" as a coping strategy for stress stopped working, *totally*. No matter what I ate to make myself feel better, feel less stressed, I still woke up daily to an unrecognizably rounder face, a harder time getting up in the morning, and a weakened immune system. I had nearly every complicating factor that intensifies the impacts of COVID-19 and I was scared.

5 Walking Away from It All

The excitement of ordering takeout yet again had begun to wane a month into the lockdown. I had run out of excuses about why I needed to have this food or that food. I had also started to recognize that we were likely quarantined for a long-haul, though I never expected to still be in it a year later. I was feeling sick. Sick of the sluggish feeling I had each morning, dreading going to work, even though work was in the next room and I was miles away from any angry students, demanding colleagues or an hour-long commute each way. There was no way I should have been feeling worse when I was significantly distanced from all of the things that I thought made me eat my emotions. I knew I had to make a change.

Through isolation and physical distance, I learned how to distinguish between my emotions and the emotions of others. Work stressors have not disappeared while home, but I have a distance-based security blanket. No matter what the incident, I do not have to interact with students, faculty or staff *in person* and therefore I am not directly exposed to their emotions. At home, as soon as the call or Zoom meeting ends, I literally turn off the screen and feel relief. I do not have to explain anything or debrief with other office staff if I do not wish to do so. The complex social interaction that I previously experienced in the office, led to extreme emotional drain, which I used food to alleviate.

6 Emotional Distance

To explain my experiences with engaging the emotional energy of others in my daily work, I return to theorist Randall Collins (2004) and his work on Interaction Ritual Chains. Interaction rituals (IR), the mechanisms by which we interact and engage with daily social life have four major components or "ingredients" that combine to produce four major outcomes that impact individuals. When present, the components help provide mutual focus and entrainment, both of which are integral to successful social interactions. Successful IRs are those that are energy producing and unsuccessful or failed interactions are those that are energy draining. Think about the lunch crew I discussed previously versus having an angry student lashing out at me. The outcomes of successful IRs center around four major experiences: creating group solidarity; producing emotional energy (EE), the feeling of excitement or potential to act within the individuals of a group; creating symbols that serve as representation of the group and act as group markers; and finally, producing "feelings of morality" or a protective feeling toward the group and the emblems or symbols that represent it. The experiences I had with my lunch crew regularly produced successful interaction ritual chains. As a member of that group, I felt solidarity with the other members, we had symbols that represented us, like our favorite restaurant or our favorite table in the conference room. In contrast though, my experiences with on campus meetings with students, faculty, or staff represent examples of failed rituals or unsuccessful rituals, which had draining effects on my emotions.

On campus, I struggled to disconnect personally from student issues. The faking of smiles and engagement with students who had behaved inappropriately with blatant disdain for our interaction, the meetings with faculty that resulted in unmet expectations and failed IRs all worked to deplete my emotional energy. Again, the physical separation from students and colleagues as a result of COVID-19 has shown me just how emotionally involved I was, and personally I took each and every interaction with a disgruntled student. I built up all kinds of emotional energy based on my interactions with students and seemed to mirror their emotions. I did not guard myself. I had virtually no boundaries. Every statement about the quality of their college experience or that they felt wronged I considered a personal affront. At home however, there was no opportunity for me to change students' environments or to alleviate their concerns, which made the stress worse.

7 Walking on Broken Glass

Acknowledging my emotional eating was my first step toward healing. Gradually, I would take additional steps toward building awareness around my triggers and eventually take agency over the healing process. I had to learn to make different choices with wellness, not just food issues, as my priority. Just as the idea of ordering food began to wane in April, 2020, I decided that so too did binge-scrolling Instagram, avoiding work emails, and saying yes to nearly every request for a meeting or call after "work hours." It was as if I had taken one step in a different direction than the day before, and very slowly, I kept going. As I mentioned previously, I had plenty of offers of assistance and even tried therapy, but for reasons both known and unknown, at that time, I could not accept help – I had to be ready to seek it for myself.

A few years back in 2017, I walked and did some group fitness classes. At that time, I had an older model Fitbit lying around the house somewhere that I used for weight loss purposes. I defined success regarding my health as weight loss back then but thought maybe this time, I could just walk for the sake of walking. Walking was free and something that did not require interacting with folks too closely. Initially, I was tempted to recharge my FitBit to track my steps, but decided on an alternative tactic. I knew right away that if I began walking as an "exercise," I would falter with it under the slightest inconvenience. Too windy, too rainy, too cloudy or any other weather-related excuse would be in my back pocket and then there were the unspoken weight-related measures that I wanted to avoid. I did not want to begin negotiating what I ate (chocolate!) as rewards for steps-taken. I reframed walking as holistic exercise instead of physical fitness and began using it as a way to forget about chocolate. Finally, I decided to just get going. In April, I walked 16 out of 30 days. In May, I walked 24 out of 31 days. By October, I had walked an average of 28 days a month.

The daily walks I took were nothing special, so I thought. I would throw on whatever sweatpants were near, grab a mask, and I would come back when I felt alright. Those little bastions of peace soon became indispensable parts of my days. I walked when I was upset. I walked when I was unsure how to solve a student concern. I walked to clear my mind. I walked to cry. I walked to feel good. I walked to process whatever my emotions were at the time or not – and that is how the walks became my solace. When chicken parmesan, still my favorite dish, no longer made me feel relieved or comfortable, I just went for a walk. When I felt stuck, trapped in the house with so many screens, I walked to relieve the stress. When I received good news, I went on longer walks to celebrate. At the risk of sounding like an influencer-turned-health-guru, walking helped me transform the relationship between my emotions and food in many ways. By Christmas time, I had built a reflexive practice that changed not only how I coped with job stress, but also how I viewed my position in the world as agential and powerful.

8 Walking To – A New Practice

A reflexive practice is one that allows for the possibility of becoming aware of the unaware (Bourdieu, 1992). Like breathing meditation or a heuristic for mindfulness, I allowed my thoughts and emotions to flow freely and without judgment while walking. I continued to focus on the walks themselves, how the air felt, what the trees looked like as the leaves first budded, grew into full leaves, and then bloomed. When emotions arose, I noted them and allowed them to become unstuck. I began to explore the possibilities of daily movement as a part of a repertoire of self-care, but also a way to engage awareness and growth. In her study of heuristics as tools for mindfulness in education, Malgorzata Powietrzynska (2015), asserts that a significant part of mindfulness is the interconnection of emotions and our actual conduct. On my walks, I allowed my emotions to arise, but I also began to parse out what, if any steps or action I could take to ameliorate them *outside* of my walks. I was not cured, but I had found a process, a practice, that grounded me, solidified much needed boundaries, and lifted the weight of being fat and Black and a woman navigating higher education. My identity as a fat, Black, woman has been a point of contention for me in the past as discrimination and prejudice from others shapes some of my lived experience. I have had to learn how to differentiate between my own beliefs about my identities and projections of others' beliefs that I may have triggered. I have had to reclaim my own agency and reject those projections. Walking gave me the space and the opportunity to investigate those projections without judgement.

Doctor and psychiatrist Bessel Van der Kolk (2015) states that the brain-disease model of mental health conditions removes agency from patients and transfers the power of healing to doctors, pharmacists, and insurance companies. In my experience, I knew that therapy would be and had been helpful to me in the past, but only through *my choice* to engage it. Further, my agentic involvement in a healing activity, walking and engaging in reflexive practice while doing so, is what I believe assisted me in recovering from emotional eating and traumatic experiences I suffered from previously.

These walks illuminated hidden possibilities that I was blinded to by the confines of my office suite. On campus it seemed like I had no options for reprieve from stress, but that was a fallacy. Being home allowed me to walk away from a situation after a tough conversation or interaction. Being home allowed me to go outside at any time of the day or night and breathe fresh air. Being home afforded me the chance to take calls and video conferences outside. I could see the sun and experience it throughout the day, rather than when I stopped working. I can focus at night and lurk on my laptop in the late hours to get writing done and still make it on time for work the next day. Even as I write this now, I am reflective about why I believed I could not do these things prior to COVID-19. Of course, nothing was actually stopping me, but my awareness that these were viable options was obscured to me at the time. I could not see the potential for what a meditative practice like walking could do for me personally. Rather, I saw what those practices could do for others, but I did not believe they would work for me. In Lori Gottlieb's book, *Maybe You Should Talk to Someone*, she recalls her therapist, Wendell, reminding her of a cartoon that showed a prisoner behind the bars of a jail cell, but the other sides of the cell were wide open. As her therapist explained, "we feel completely stuck, trapped in our emotional jail cells, but there's a way out – as long as we're willing to see it" (p. 152). I can *finally* see around the bars.

9 Quarantine Exposes *Their* Behavior

It is imperative, I believe, to incorporate how my personal changes interact with and are impacted by the larger, macro and meso-level structural changes we have experienced as a society as a result of COVID-19. Will we evolve into a nation that values remote work in the same ways that we celebrate landing 9 to 5 corporate jobs? What disparities among school-aged children arose because of leaving the classroom for months on end? How could we have stopped women from being forced to leave the workforce in droves in 2020 because they needed to care for their children? These questions frame my thinking about the larger structures in play, but also how changes in my direct community on the meso level (college) and micro level (my office specifically) can act as starting points for sustained systemic changes.

On the micro-level, COVID-19 forced me into a deep exploration of my axiology and epistemological stances. The simultaneous experience of isolation and over-stimulation by current events, and changes in higher education overall, set the scene for an examination of culture and its enactment within higher education. In considering culture, I employ Sewell (2010) and Randall Collins' (2004) Interaction Rituals as foundations for examining the events that have ultimately transformed the structure of higher education through the pandemic. For the first time since the last pandemic over 100 years ago, the United States is forced to consider how education and the culture around which we enact education itself has been impacted as a result of COVID-19. This pandemic has illuminated glaring discrepancies and inequalities among class, race, gender, and many other groups/subgroups by which we classify and categorize students and ourselves. As The Steve Fund reports, some of those discrepancies, especially around anxiety and depression impacted Blacks and Latinos at significantly higher rates (2020). Not only has the pandemic highlighted outdated ideas about the culture of education, once again people of color are more vulnerable to the negative impacts of it.

As an educator and student affairs professional I am in constant conversation with myself about what kinds of knowledge and ways of knowing I value (Alexakos, 2015). I believe that incorporating emotional wellness as a part of education, especially for racialized students would improve education for many. I believe our greater society is grappling with the need for more inclusive education as so many colleges and universities have shifted to online coursework. Without the context of a grassy quad, fancy computer labs, and regal-looking brick residence halls – a student is sitting in front of a screen engaging with Zoom as the platform whether they attend an R1-research university, an Ivy League college or a community college. While there are certainly differences in the quality of education one may or may not receive in an online environment, I am curious just how much the physical environment, social interactions and an emotions-friendly curriculum could shape new educational experiences, and whether previous practices are worth saving.

10 The Living at Work Reality

While care is an important concept, personal wellness is often overlooked in higher education (Anderson et al., 2020). The priority of care or concern was geared toward students when the pandemic began and though that was certainly warranted, I argue that care for our colleagues and administrators is of value, too. It allows them to extend caring to those they interact and work with, like students, on a regular basis. Before we understood that we would be home for an extended period of time, I was instructed to create a work-from-home contract with my staff. We did not know how long we would be working remotely, yet we were instructed to create a plan as if we were gracefully allowing staff to work from home, rather than it being imposed. I was concerned because everyone around me, my boss especially, seemed to be focused on making sure people were actually at home and *working*. The school administration needed to justify paying people to be at home and wanted staff to continue working at the same capacity as on campus. I understood that concern, albeit tragically capitalistic, but maintaining a level of normalcy for students was important – though we were all adjusting. It seemed that the strings of control were snipped away by being home and we were grasping at anything to maintain it. Again, I understood this perspective in some ways. There were some risks in sending an entire division of employees home and paying them to be there. But this perspective did not take into consideration the positive impacts working from home could elicit. With just a bit of concern and care for staff wellbeing prior to the pandemic, we might have been more prepared to be "successful" at working from home sooner. In the absence of face-to-face interaction, care may be what rebuilds a socially-distanced community.

While social distancing is a relatively new catchphrase, it certainly is not new in describing the relationship between academic and student affairs divisions at my college. There is a striking similarity between faculty members' experiences and the experiences of administrators and staff, but the pandemic has seemingly strained the relationship. Faculty have been rethinking their expectations of students in light of this pandemic, including changing their communication styles and curating online spaces for class interaction (Pryal, 2020). Similarly, administrators have been managing their homes as work spaces while addressing the increased emotional labor both women faculty and administrators are managing as a result of COVID-19 (Costa, 2020). In conjunction with new practices that require faculty and administration to work together more effectively, we are all suffering. Loss of resources has also played a significant role for everyone to work effectively from home. Higher education has suffered record-breaking job loss since the onslaught of COVID-19 (Douglas-Gabriel & Fowers, n.d.). Working together to pool resources and support our areas respectively would be beneficial for all in this circumstance, but the added stress of the pandemic has further isolated us. In my experience, creating new and completely virtual business practices and everyday functions has been tumultuous. It requires collaboration and creativity that is difficult to conjure in these times.

In May 2021, after living through the consequences of the first iteration of COVID-19 in the early part of 2020, it is easier to quantify just how the virus impacted the greater workforce, including both post-secondary and primary education. In my experience, and others, the stress of working from home illuminated not only my own problematic coping skills, but highlighted my institution's lack of preparation. Similarly, my lack of boundaries, both those I constructed for my own protection and those of others, were and sometimes still are a challenge for me to maintain and recognize. Transitioning from an on-campus, walk-ins-welcome-office to an appointment only, physically-distanced, virtual campus model illuminates hidden facets of social and cultural norms that I had previously adopted categorically. I never turned anyone away without an appointment. I would reprioritize my schedule to incorporate impromptu meetings or student concerns into the day before finishing my own work. I would come early to catchup on work I missed from accommodating others. I was not alone in those practices, but that does not make them acceptable or even sustainable. I accepted these practices and reproduced them regularly. However, I am hopeful that this work will give voice to other student affairs administrators, and nuance the experience of working from home during COVID-19 and the ripple effects it created.

11 2021 – It's Still Not Over …

Now, it is June of 2021, and as I revisit this chapter in preparation for its publication, I am wrought with fear. I have admitted some hard truths about myself and revealed some deeply personal flaws. Despite my fear of embarrassment though, I have had the opportunity to overhaul my thinking and my actions and to document those changes so that they are beneficial to me and potentially (hopefully!) others. However, I must also consider that this work could do harm as well. I do not want this chapter specifically to come across as a neoliberal viewpoint of meditative practice or mindfulness practices that serve to uplift "internal regulation" or "individualist responsibility" as a means for healing and overall wellness (Forbes, 2017, p. 149).

I am very conscious of larger social structures and institutional inequalities, especially highlighted by the pandemic. The incessant mantras of "do more, with less," "do better," and "always do your best" are the artifacts of many forms of social control that I have internalized over the years. Ironically, I credit contemplative practices like walking, free writing, and heuristics (Tobin & Alexakos, 2021a) with drawing my awareness to the bootstrap mentality and other cultural norms that had become so embedded in my life. I am not healthier because I finally laced up my tennis shoes and got to walking. Instead, when freed from a routinely harmful environment, I learned that I could carry it with me. I became desperate when I believed that in my own home I still could not accept my authentic self without food and overworking as coping mechanisms. In turn, I sought practices that allowed *me* to control how far, how deep, and how much I could change and this assisted me in recognizing what was outside my locus of control.

I can say that now that I am better because I have learned how to deal with challenges in a way that does not personally harm me, as much, anymore. I'm healing myself so I can fight harder against the inequities that shaped how I got to where I was in the first place. I was, and still am sometimes, conditioned to look internally for a problem's resolution, regardless of the issue's root causes, but the difference now is that I know to zoom out – search for and then interrogate the bigger picture. There are macro, meso, and micro-level structures that act in concert with my own insecurities. My willingness to engage with those difficult interactions is what spurs me forward. Even as I write this, it seems like I have taken a dark turn away from my original point and it almost seems like I am angry, but I am not. I want to be critical. I want to challenge the notion that "knowing thyself" is the *only way* to change. Knowing myself is now a part of my repertoire, an intentional way of being that continually develops as a part of and as a reaction to our social world.

Even after acknowledging some difficult ideas about my growth, I can confidently say that I have drastically improved my health and wellness, both mentally and physically. After an ongoing year of separation from the social and cultural norms of my daily commute, physical workspace, interactions with hostile students, and the constant push to do more with less, I have gained valuable life lessons. For me, the pandemic was the impetus for significant changes around the way I viewed food and exercise, but it was also so much more. This pandemic ultimately led me to the interrogation and examination of why I developed those coping mechanisms at all.

Having documented my personal changes as I undertook this process, I have reflected on the past 18 months to set new goals and intentions for when I do finally return to my physical work space. Moving forward, boundaries have become essential to my wellness and I intend to enact them within the workspace. Measuring "success" with task lists and meetings held or other administrative to-dos is also something that no longer serves me or the students/colleagues I work with effectively. I am working now to reduce those measures as much as possible and focus on building relationships and partnerships rather than just directing and performing acts as an administrator. I know that these steps will be difficult and steep and, in some cases, task-lists and performative interactions will be unavoidable. However, recognizing and maintaining a constant awareness of how I am managing my boundaries (or not) is ongoing. I will make mistakes, forget to check-in with myself, but I will know that I can walk away and come home, again.

References

Alexakos, K. (2015). *Being a teacher | researcher: A primer on doing authentic inquiry research on teaching and learning.* Sense. 10.1007/978-94-6300-295-0

Anderson, V., Rabello, R., Wass, R., Golding, C., Rangi, A., Eteuati, E., Bristowe, Z., & Waller, A. (2020). Good teaching as care in higher education. *Higher Education* (00181560), *79*(1), 1–19. https://doi-org.ezproxy.gc.cuny.edu/10.1007/s10734-019-00392-6

Bourdieu, P. (1992). The practice of reflexive sociology (The Paris workshop). In P. Bourdieu & L. J. D. Wacquant (Eds.), *An invitation to reflexive sociology* (pp. 216–260). The University of Chicago Press.

Costa, K. (2020). Women's emotional labor in higher ed and the COVID-19 crisis. *Women in Higher Education, 29*(5), 13–15. https://doi.org/10.1002/whe.20849

Douglas-Gabriel, D., & Fowers, A. (2020, November 17). The lowest-paid workers in higher education are suffering the highest job losses. *Washington Post.* Retrieved February 17, 2021, from https://www.washingtonpost.com/education/2020/11/17/higher-ed-job-loss/

Forbes, D. (2017). Mindfulness and Neoliberal education. In M. Powietrzyńska & K. Tobin (Eds.), *Weaving complementary knowledge systems and mindfulness to educate a literate citizenry for sustainable and healthy lives* (pp. 145–158). Sense Publishers. https://doi-org.ezproxy.gc.cuny.edu/10.1007/978-94-6351-182-7_10

Guthrie, V. L., Woods, E., Cusker, C., & Gregory, M. (2005). A portrait of balance: Personal and professional balance among student affairs educators. *College Student Affairs Journal, 24*(2), 110–127.

Kabat-Zinn, J. (2014). *Wherever you go, there you are: Mindfulness meditation in everyday life.* Hachette Books.

Powietrzynska, M. (2015). Heuristics for mindfulness in education and beyond. In C. Milne, K. Tobin, & D. DeGennaro (Eds.), *Sociocultural studies and implications for science education: The experiential and the virtual* (pp. 59–80). Springer Netherlands. https://doi.org/10.1007/978-94-007-4240-6_3

Pryal, K. G. R. (2020). The bad and the great: Another COVID semester. *Women in Higher Education, 29*(11), 6–14. https://doi.org/10.1002/whe.20912

Sewell, W. (1999). The concept(s) of culture. In V. E. Bonnell & L. Hunt (Eds.), *Beyond the cultural turn: New directions in the study of society and culture* (pp. 35–58). University of California Press.

The Steve Fund. (2020). *Adapting and innovating to promote mental health and emotional wellbeing of young people of color: COVID-19 and beyond.* The Steve Fund. https://www.stevefund.org/wp-content/uploads/2020/09/CRISIS-RESPONSE-TASK-FORCE-STEVE-FUND-REPORT.pdf

Tobin, K. (2017). Researching mindfulness and wellness. In M. Powietrzyńska & K. Tobin (Eds.), *Weaving complementary knowledge systems and mindfulness to educate a literate citizenry for sustainable and healthy lives* (pp. 1–18). Sense Publishers. https://doi.org/10.1007/978-94-6351-182-7_1

Tobin, K., & Alexakos, K. (2021a). *Transforming learning and teaching: Heuristics for educative and responsible practices.* Brill | Sense.

Tobin, K., & Alexakos, K. (2021b). *Doing Authentic Inquiry to improve learning and teaching.* Brill | Sense. https://doi.org/10.1163/9789004446885

Turner, J. H. (2009). The sociology of emotions: Basic theoretical arguments. *Emotion Review, 1*(4), 340–354. https://doi.org/10.1177%2F1754073909338305

Van der Kolk, B. (2015). *The body keeps the score: Brain, mind, and body in the healing of trauma.* Penguin Books.

CHAPTER 16

Wellness during Illness

Improving the Quality of Life through Health Literacy in Mexican Children and Adolescents with Chronic Kidney Disease

Beatriz Verónica Panduro Espinoza and S. Lizette Ramos de Robles

Abstract

We consider this chapter to be polyphonic because we share a series of approaches, reflections and experiences regarding the health-disease processes experienced by children and adolescents with chronic kidney disease through several sociocultural lenses: polyphony, narratives and lived experiences. The ensuing narratives are an attempt to capture and understand the realities of the experiences of children and adolescents and their mothers as they endure the health-disease process of chronic kidney failure. We came to realize that emotions play a critical role in coping with this disease. For example, sadness, hopelessness, anger, and discouragement towards living are the most recurring emotions in these children and adolescents. The emotions of the mothers were expressed in the form of sadness and fear and the realization of the possible death of their child. We propose that health literacy strategies be developed to address the reality of the existence of health-disease situations such as those we present in this chapter.

Keywords

wellness – illness – chronic kidney disease – emotions – health literacy

1 Preamble

Lizette: When one imagines a research methodology class within a doctorate in education, one imagines that students would define a study that corresponds to a field in education. Curiosity about areas of scholarship such as curriculum, the teaching-learning process, educational policies, models for teacher education, among others are what come to mind. For more than 10 years that I have taught graduate classes, these have been the themes that my students and I

 | DOI:10.1163/9789004527348_016

have researched. However, in one of the research methods classes, I remember Beatriz, an MD, whose specialty was pediatrics, explaining that she wanted to look at education through the lens of children and adolescents with Chronic Kidney Disease (CKD) so that she could understand the reality of children and adolescents who, due to their illness, drop out of school and spend most of their time in a hospital or at home. She was also curious as to why the mothers of her patients with CKD took on the main responsibility for caring for their son or daughter. Beatriz wanted to understand the sociocultural realities of her patients which represented a challenge for her as a trained physician.

When Beatriz realized she needed to situate herself and her patients as human beings and not just patients she asked me to help her in the research project. This immediately posed many questions in our minds which we needed to discuss. For me, I did not fully understand how to guide such research. For both of us, what could the field of education offer? To what extent can we understand the reality of her patients with CKD and intervene? What socio-cultural frameworks could I recommend for her study which would have to be situated within two worlds: medicine and education?

Beatriz invited me to visit the hospital. In my initial visit, I met children and adolescents living with different stages of CKD. Some were optimistic and even smiling, many had elusive and indifferent looks, and others seemed angry. Looking at these children and adolescents I became sad. When I left the hospital, I cried. Their images came to my mind frequently (they still do) and I knew that this project was more than important. It became a commitment from me to work with Beatriz, and to continue working with her, to help in any way possible with the lives of these children and adolescents even though we knew that in most cases death was inevitable for many of them.

Beatriz: Working as a physician and a medical practitioner has led me to discover through the eyes of children something more than a disease. It is possible to make visible not the sick, but small children and adolescents who are not only ill, but with a personal story, perhaps short in time but intense in experiences. Similarly, beings cannot be seen as isolated, but as members in a close relationship with their family. My search for care strategies is to complement my professional training as a physician in order to approach caring for a patient from a multidisciplinary approach. Doing research with an ethical sense to contribute to the resolution of a problem from the specific area of health education leads to knowing and having a deep understanding of other realities.

What I seek through literacy for health and during illness is to educate not only the children but also their mothers and through them their families and their peers so that they can have, more dignified ways of life and with less cost to the patient. However, this experience also leads to discovering that isolated and local efforts are not enough. Education strategies must be institutionalized and enforced and even then, they are not enough because it is not just about a disease. The hidden side of the impact of chronic kidney disease on children and their families is also related to medical coverage and services provided by health and social institutions, with public policies, support networks, and collective awareness.

What we share today is a part of the project that has as its main purpose to understand the experiences of children and adolescents with CKD and their mothers as main caregivers, and to identify educational strategies that could be designed to alleviate their challenges and suffering.

2 Education and Health Are a Universal Right

The right to an education and good health are enshrined both in the Universal Declaration of Human Rights and in the constitutions of different countries (United Nations, 1984). The importance of receiving an education and being healthy lies in the recognition that education and health have the potential to serve society as a catalyst for sustainable development and as an instrument to empower a population so that people may improve their quality of life. In México, these two rights are reflected in Articles 3 and 4 of the Constitution (Diario Oficial de la Federación, 2016). We suggest that a society's maximum enjoyment of health should be construed as indispensable to protect life, ensure the development of all people including children, promote peace, security and the development of prosperous societies.

We consider México's constitutional establishment of compulsory and tuition free public education and guaranteed health protection to be a debt to its citizens in which repayment is determined by how accessible it is to all of society. By a debt to citizens we specifically mean that once free public education and being healthy are constitutionally guaranteed then the Mexican state must also create the necessary societal conditions so that all people can avail themselves of these social benefits. However, this is not the case. For instance, compulsory basic education covers the ages of 3 to 18 years old. It is calculated that coverage at the primary level is 96%, however this decreases progressively at levels beyond primary. For example, only 66% of the 15 to 18 years old student population attend the secondary level (INEE, 2018). It is important to note that at the primary level even though most children attend school, it should not be assumed that they finish and go on to the next sequence. The high dropout rate has economic consequences. For example, the Household Educational Poverty Index, which is a measure of the educational levels attained within Mexican households, indicates that 57% of households have not completed their education at the educación básica (preschool, primary and middle school) levels thus further contributing to the poverty level of Mexicans (INEE, 2016).

Another contributing factor of failing to reach all of society is child labor and the violation of minors' human rights. The Consejo Nacional de Evaluación de la Política de Desarrollo Social (2018) reports that 4 out of every 10 children between the ages of 12 and 14, while attending school, have jobs outside of the home which may be full or part-time. In rural agricultural areas, the situation is graver because many students must work the fields for months at a time, thus missing large numbers of school days. Illiteracy is 4% of the entire population of México (INEA, 2018). At first look this number does not seem high, perhaps even admirable, until it is realized that 6 out of every 100 females over 15 years of age cannot read or write, which is equivalent to 6% of the population or 7,679,000 women (INEGI, 2015). The situation is such that regardless of what guarantees a population has, there are sociocultural contextual factors that mitigate not only the law (Gallard, Pitts, Brkich et al., 2018), but also its spirit and intent (Gallard & Antrop Gonzalez, 2013).

In the case of the right to health we note that, according to UNICEF (2017), the child mortality rate is an indicator of well-being, given that the majority of child deaths are avoidable. In the case of México, despite the actions of the Secretaría de Salud (Ministry of Health) that are directed towards guaranteeing the right to health, many children and adolescents live in conditions of high marginalization, disempowerment, and vulnerability that limit their access to health services. According to UNICEF-CONEVAL (2014), in Mexico 51% of children and adolescents live in poverty of which 20% are in extreme poverty. The impoverished living conditions of girls, boys, and adolescents severely diminish their ability to take advantage of the Health for Childhood and Adolescence Act of 2013–2018, whose main objective is the reduction of mortality of the population that is under 19 years of age (Secretaría de Salud, 2014). Today the mortality rate in children under five years of age in México is 13%. While this is a decrease from a rate of 20% in 1990, it still remains a critical issue.

One of the critical issues contributing to the mortality rate of children under five years of age and adolescents is kidney failure. Chronic Kidney Disease (CKD) is a health project that affects the study group of this chapter. CKD is the tenth highest cause of mortality in children under one year of age and sixth highest in the group of 15 to 24 years old (INEGI, 2016). In pediatric patients with CKD, the highest mortality rate is found in the 15- to 19-year-old group

(127 deaths per 100,000 inhabitants) and is followed by 10 to 14 years (38 deaths per 100,000 inhabitants) (Secretaría de Salud, 2018).

For pediatric patients, food is essential not only for their health, but for proper growth and social development. Unhealthy eating habits alone do not cause chronic kidney disease in children. However, a healthy diet is critical in that it can determine the progression of kidney damage. For example, one of the pillars of treatment for patients with CKD is adherence to a diet that enhances the nutritional, water and electrolyte balance while reducing the possibility of presenting comorbidities while adjusting fluids, protein, reducing sodium, potassium and phosphorus. Non-nutritional habits, such as large amounts of sugar consumption, have been a public health problem, and are a contributing factor for multiple diseases. Unfortunately, in México a high consumption of sugars and fats contribute to a high rate of obesity, and an increase in diseases such as diabetes mainly in children. Exacerbating the issue of non-nutritional habits, is the recent emergence of the pandemic caused by the SARS-CoV-2 virus. The health and medical communities are currently trying to understand how the SARS-CoV-2 virus has affected the eating patterns of México's population.

In recent months the government approved a law for products that are high in fat and sugar – that producers must include nutritional information on the product's label. Even though this is a step in the right direction, we recognize that societal changes in consumption patterns are habitual, culturally rooted, and are slow to progress. Change not only is slow but also requires the sum of efforts from all of society.

3 Our Study

For the purposes of this study when we refer to health education we are also referring to science education. This is because in the case of México's public education system, health education falls under the domain of science education in the national curriculum for basic education. México's national curriculum includes standards for both basic education and teacher training. Despite recent efforts at reform, health education continues to be integrated in the standards for science education. For example, in primary education the topic of health is part of the Knowledge of the Environment standards (SEP, 2019) and within teacher training health is part of the standards found within the Introduction to the Nature of Science (SEP, 2018). The experiences of Lizette, a co-author of this chapter, as a primary school teacher, and other anecdotal evidence she has accumulated through years of experience, indicate that health education as a content field is virtually ignored both in basic education and teacher training. One of the implications of this neglect is that the development of health literacy is also ignored. In this study, we came to recognize that health literacy is of fundamental importance, as it is one of the most important determinants of health, and that it may be superior to other factors such as age, level of education, type of employment and income (Fisher-Wilson, 2003). We do not deny that the content of health can also be considered science, but that is not our concern. We focus more on the idea that by integrating health into science education, health literacy can be made invisible or it can be ignored, depending on how it is situated/emphasized within the national standards of México.

Our study analyzes how social debts to society, in the form of governmental guarantees to an education and good health, affect vulnerable groups such as children and adolescents with CKD. Universally, CKD is a growing global public health problem that leads to significant deterioration of the quality of life and the risk of premature death and high cost (Hill, Fatoba, Oke, et al., 2016; National Kidney Foundation, 2002). When CKD disease occurs in children or adolescents, it usually results in high patient school dropout and/or a lack of educational grade-level advancement.

Additionally, the disease, in its last treatment phases, further hinders school performance through disproportionate absences due to an excess of days of hospitalization. Even though young people with CKD are guaranteed a public education, their formal education is limited, postponed or suspended due to the Secretaría de Educación Pública's [SEP] (Ministry of Education) infrastructure that is not inclusive of students with chronic and terminal diseases. This lack of accommodation within the educational infrastructure that SEP has established necessitates that formal/informal education is left to the family, mainly mothers, as well as health and medical professionals to deal with. In an attempt to give continuity to formal education and reduce falling behind in their studies, patients with prolonged or frequent hospital stays, continue their formal education in a hospital classroom with non-certified volunteers. Educating the patient about their care during the disease and ensuring treatment fidelity, is the responsibility of the health team which includes medical, nursing, psychology and social work personnel.

It is within the above context that we developed this study, which was to document the experiences of children and adolescents who are suffering from CKD. Initially, we started this study to understand the realities of children and adolescents with CKD. However, as we gathered data, we became acutely aware of the experiences and roles of the patients' mothers who became the primary caretakers. We suggest that mothers assuming the role of the majority caretaker may be related to gender situated sociocultural conditions, specifically associated with gender roles. For example, in México it is mostly the men who are responsible to work outside of the home supporting the family, while women take care of their children at least during the first years prior to entering school. It should be noted that in some cases both men and women work but when a child is diagnosed with CKD, it is the mother who quits work and dedicates herself to caring for her child. We found that only in rare instances the dominant caretakers are men.

3.1 *Looking at Their Reality through Multiple Sociocultural Lenses*

We start the discussion of our research from the idea that a sociocultural framework offers us a more complex way to interpret data. Through sociocultural lenses we can recognize that science education, which in this case is inclusive of health education, is a form of cultural enactment (Tobin, 2006). This implies that embedded within each sociocultural situation are issues of culture, politics, ethnicity, gender, race, socio-economic status, and power. Calabrese Barton (1998) suggests that we can think of science and science education in a dynamic way in which science knowledge is perceived as connected to the learners and their lived experiences. The sociocultural perspectives that all knowing is situated by culture, politics, ethnicity, socio-economic status and power, and cannot be disconnected from the learner, we believe applies to the field of health education also. Additionally, we believe that the concept of social fields is critical because within each social space are systems which are constantly in a state of dynamic fluidity. Social fields and accompanying social spaces are forms of cultural production that situate their dynamic compositions such as space, time, goals, individuals, and material, as well as other social categories such as age, gender, race, and class among their components (Tobin, 2009). Thus, if we take the notion of connected entities, as advocated by Levitt and Schiller (2004), we understand that when health education leads to health literacy, a form of empowerment for the pursuit of personal and collective well-being is developed.

Using these theoretical frameworks, we are mindful that our research is a process of constant co-construction where knowledge emerges from the dialogue of the participants, and where the researcher is one of the co-constructors of multiple situated realities (Sisto, 2008). Accordingly, we used narratives, interviews and focus groups to achieve a dialogical construction of reality through the eyes of the patients and their mothers in which meaning was negotiated with us. This required us to underscore the idea that from an interpretive and hermeneutic perspective, we needed to value the voices of the patients and their mothers regarding the experiences during their CKD treatment and the resulting diminished quality of life.

Narrative is defined as a different form of dialogue, a retrospective (re)construction of meanings and a way of understanding one's own actions and those of others. Narrative communicates the narrator's point of view by revealing our private thinking that is loaded with emotions, thoughts and individual interpretations of reality (Eisner, 1994; Chase, 2008). Narrations facilitate the appropriation of diverse cultural knowledge and provide a framework for the dialogue between emotions, reason, and experience (Egan, 1994). To arrive at meanings regarding the experience of children and adolescents with CKD, patients were asked to write narratives about what CKD has represented in their lives. With the written narrative exercise, children and adolescents had the opportunity to give voice to their lives, which are often silenced (Chase, 2015).

Focus groups and interviews were also implemented with the mothers of the patients in which they discussed the experiences of having a child with CKD. Focus groups and interviews were developed around two key concepts: (a) dialogism and (b) reading-awareness of the world as proposed by Freire (1998). Interviews were of a semi-structured type whose main topics were related to the meaning of diseases, demands for children's attention as related to the disease, support networks, impact on personal life, and impact on family life and education. In total, nine narratives were written by patients who had an average age of 14 years. Twelve individual interviews or oral narratives were also conducted with six mothers, whose average age was 42 years and seven focus group sessions with both patients and mothers lasting three hours each. Human interactions and their meanings are what allow for the understanding of the object(s) of research. Likewise, there are no structures of meaning independent of their interpretation, since the narration made by each individual establishes a way to understand the meaning of their world and their experiences. As products of the narratives, written texts were analyzed under the guidelines of content analysis, in which units of meaning were identified as "the self-interpretation that the subjects report in the first person, where the temporal and biographical dimension occupies a central position" (Bolívar, 2002, p. 4).

The voices of the patients and their mothers about their experiences with CKD enabled us to develop text(s) that are polyphonic. In this polyphony of voices, it is possible to find multiple intersecting discourses, whose richness does not imply the fusion or mixture of one sense into the other, but the enrichment and unity of meaning that is sought. Bajtín (Bahktin in English, 1999) raises the link between dialogue and otherness, which come together in a process in which "sense discovers its depths by meeting and touching another sense, an alien sense" (p. 352). Children and adolescents' voices are referred to as Patient 1, 2, 3 … (P1), those of mothers as Mother 1, 2, 3 …, (M1), narratives and interviews as N and IN, respectively. Similarly, the wording, spelling and diction used in each of them are faithfully respected. The voices of the authors also open a space in order to share the sensations experienced during the development of the studio.

Our work is situated within a hospital in Guadalajara, (Jalisco) México that offers its services to a socioeconomically and culturally vulnerable population. Participants of this study are pediatric patients in phase V of CKD which means that their kidneys are functioning at the most minimal of levels. Phase V patients are on dialysis or hemodialysis.

3.2 *What They Had to Say*

Using a polyphonic text method, we present the experiences of children and adolescents with CKD, as well as that of their mothers. The voices of children and mothers intersect, contradict each other, become accomplices and intertwine to narrate and signify a fragment of their reality. While children and adolescents are directly involved, mothers are the ones who shared the most experiences. We believe that this is because, in the focus groups, the mothers found a safe and empathetic space. We suggest that another motivating factor is that all of the mothers were going through a similar but distinctively difficult personal situation. Accordingly, listening to different individual experiences with similar patterns created support links between them and they were able to identify and empathize with other mothers. Additionally, we consider that in a moment of suffering, being heard can represent a therapeutic moment.

3.2.1 Voices of Children and Adolescents

Analysis of the written narratives indicated the following topics or themes:
- The change of meaning of everyday life and self-concept
- Impact of CKD on their personal-family life
- Living with CKD

Analysis of the written narratives indicated the following topics or themes.

3.2.1.1 *The Change of Meaning of Everyday Life and Self-Concept*

CKD makes a marked difference between children who experience it and those who live healthy lives. Life changes for the worse in the face of this illness: "I am not like my cousins, friends … I just want a normal life" (P5N5). "I see this disease as a disability." (P9N9). According to Bakr, Amr, Sarhan, et al., (2007), children with CKD suffer from stunted growth and secondary sexual characteristics development, bone deformities and stigmas due to invasive medical procedures that disfigure them. This affects their image and perception with respect to their peers.

3.2.1.2 *Impact of CKD on Their Personal-Family Life*

This chronic renal disease does not only afflict or effect patients but also the rest of the family: "Well, but not only me and my mother have changed but also my brothers because they must get used to my new style of living ..." (P2N2). In this regard, Bakr, Amr, Sarhan et al. recognize that CKD impacts the lives of children and their families, which also predisposes them to develop psychiatric disorders. For example, the most transcendental changes in the life of a patient (P10N10) are related to three aspects:

a. Compliance with the dietetic prescription: "My illness has changed my life because I do not eat the same. All the food has no salt, and the water must be measured" (P10N10).

   Most patients agree with this opinion since sodium and water restriction is a recurring complaint. Adherence to a prescribed diet is difficult for them. They display a series of emotions and feelings, among which is anger, despair and sadness. Patients who repeatedly fail to comply with the dietary indications, even knowing that it will have effects on the deterioration of their health status, represent self-injurious and even suicidal behaviors that must be addressed (Blum, Álvarez & Gordillo, 2009).

b. Limitations associated with the game and fun: "I do not play the same games ... I do not have fun as it is" (P5N5).

   These types of limitations are associated with the presence of dialysis and hemodialysis catheters, heart disease, as well as osteodystrophy, malnutrition and water overload. The children remember nostalgically what they have stopped doing: "I can no longer be riding on the bikes" (P4N4), "I can no longer ... get into the pools" (P10N10), "I can no longer play in the street" (P3N3), "I don't play the same" (P5N5), "I don't have fun as it is" (P5N5). Playing games such as soccer and riding bicycles are a priority and satisfactory aspects of childhood. Losing this aspect of childhood constitutes one of the greatest yearnings and sorrows experienced.

c. School absences: In half of the narratives children report that CKD has severely affected their studies, with many dropping out of school "The disease has changed my life because I do not go to school anymore" (P3N3).

School and social life are altered by the need to reorganize daily life and projects, depending on hospital care and treatments (Blum, Álvarez & Gordillo, 2009).

3.2.1.3 *Living with* CKD

In the case of children and adolescents, living with CKD triggers a series of emotions and feelings such as depression and sadness, followed by anger, despair and boredom. Expressions of sadness are associated with performing peritoneal dialysis: "I have three months of dialysis and ... sometimes I get sad" (P8N8); and the lack of family support: "I feel a little sad ... after I have hemodialysis the truth my family has supported me less" (P8N8). This process translates into moments of disappointment and the appearance of desires to abandon treatment: "I feel sad and not wanting to continue" (P8N8). Sadness and prolonged pain lead to depression, which is linked in large part to dissatisfaction with their limited recreation. Desires to die arise when they feel alone and without family support: "Sometimes I think of dying because I feel that nobody supports me" (P8N8). The hospital stays produce anger: "I don't like the hospital, they do a lot of studies" (P3N3) and boredom: "Something else happened to me, my catheter was blocked, I am hospitalized, Bored without doing anything just lying down, sitting" (P5N5). Despair is also present in the face of the disparity of demands due to illness and available resources, both tangible and intangible, which include materials, economic, time, and support networks: "also for her [for the mother] it is difficult because sometimes she gets stressed and we both despair a lot" (P2N2). According to Blum, Álvarez and Gordillo (2009), depression and anguish are the most frequent psychological disorders and are determined by organic damage, invasive treatments, impaired self-image, identity and self-esteem. In addition to anxiety and depression, children develop feelings of sadness, hopelessness, shame and guilt.

Lizette: In imagining the analysis of data for a study in educational research, we think of videos of interactions in classrooms, interviews, curricular and policy analysis, to mention a few. Through this experience, I have learned that there is always a fair amount of distancing by the researcher from the data as well as how it was collected. This observation has nothing to do with being objective or subjective but more one's emotions that come into play or not.

Studying Beatriz's data though, I felt like my emotions were being violently shaken. I was unnerved so much that if being stoic was my goal, I would and could not reach it. How could I escape the images of these children and adolescents with CKD when analyzing their narratives, the interviews and field notes from the focus groups with the patients and their mothers? How could I avoid being emotionally shaken to the core reading the texts in which there was so much sadness, anger, despair on the one hand and the desire to die as a way to end suffering on the other. These emotions became more profound when coupled with the reality of knowing that as the research progressed, children and adolescents would die while others arrived as new patients. This realization was one of the most difficult parts of this study for me because the emotions of the participants were mixed with my own. It is precisely this experience of emotions that we should know how to let happen and be included in the research. By doing so, the research then becomes a part of caring necessary to help alleviate suffering and even acceptance of death, not only for them but also for me.

3.2.2 Voice of Mothers

For pediatric patients, the participation of their parents is a fundamental aspect. As explained earlier, in the cases we analyzed it is the mothers who assume the responsibility of providing care and attention both at home and during hospital stays. These mothers report various difficulties in the care and adherence to treatment of their children, especially in the following areas: a) feeding, b) water restriction, c) pharmacological treatment and d) aggressive and anxiety behaviors of their children.

Our data indicated the following emerging themes:

- Care for the sick child and abandonment of themselves
- The expectation of death or life expectancy

3.2.2.1 *Care for the Sick Child and Abandonment of Themselves*

The mothers are mostly housewives, but since their son or daughter has been diagnosed with CKD they have had to dedicate much time attending to the personal and medical needs of their child, which includes going back and forth from home to the hospital and vice versa: "I bring him here and there more than anything, right "(M6IN11). When the illness has reached a point in which long-term hospital stays are necessary the hospital becomes like a second home: "Always, with him, all his life, all his life, all the life … we have been here in the Hospital. Look, Doctor, so long …" (M11N1). The few mothers who had a job have had to reduce their hours or leave it: "I can't work the same" (M6IN11). An increase of medical expenses is an economic aspect of the disease, increasing this burden is the accompanying reduction of household income.

Another dimension affecting the mothers is that of family and social relationships, as well as personal time: "one is no longer with friends, because there is no time" (M2IN3); "I am not the same, you lock yourself more in your world with your girl, or you dedicate yourself more to her than to you" (M5IN9), "one does not leave because one has to be aware of him" (M2IN3).

Given the living conditions of the mothers, it is common that their health is affected: "They are my knees, and this ... I feel unable to walk anywhere, because, to be able to help [her sick son] more, this ... go to one place and then to another and thus seek support, help ..." (M1IN1).

3.2.2.2 *The Expectation of Death or Life Expectancy*

The death of children is a hot topic and difficult for mothers to deal with. According to Gómez (1999), the death of a child is likely to cause more pain than any other death. Mothers are aware that it will happen prematurely and sometimes unexpectedly: "Yes, we would like it never to come, and, but ... I am aware, that this can happen Doctor, that can happen maybe at any time" (M1IN1).

The anguish and fear of loss and loneliness are present: "Let me go, well yes, because she is my only child, she is my only baby that I have in my house and then to stay alone I don't ..." (M4IN7); "[I'm afraid] well, that I die ..." (M7IN12); "But I have seen other moms who lose their children and I would not like to see myself at that time ... but I imagine how I see the other moms" (M1IN1). In short, just thinking about the death of one's children leads to evoke the death of the mothers: "And I say and I say no to him, I should die, no, no, I am very sincere" (M4IN8).

Children perceive their own death with less fear than their mothers, they seem to understand it better: "do not think I am afraid of death I am not one of those who says no" (M4IN7); and they may even want it: "They get angry, they get mad at life and think many things such as it would be better to die, all children think like that, those I know about kidney failure think the same" (M1IN2).

Beatriz: The polyphony of voices, obtained through diverse instruments and agents, leads to a better understanding of the reality of children and their families. Unique realities, but each one is lived by a person and their history. Insights into the sociocultural aspects of a patient lead to a better understanding of a disease such as chronic kidney disease and general literacy strategies, but also specifics for each of the family members. As an educational and medical researcher, a holistic witnessing of these experiences from the realities of the patient and family changes the conception and appreciation of life. The congruence of emotions such as sensitization and commitment lead to a type of research that forced me to act accordingly and not stay on the sidelines.

4 Towards the Construction of a Strategy That Improves the Quality of Life during the Disease Process in Children and Adolescents with CKD

In summary, the polyphony of both children with CKD and their mothers allows us to recognize new demands for health literacy, demands that are not always considered within the current approaches to this disease. Guzys, Kenny, Dickson-Swift et al. (2015) too argue that conceptual approaches to health literacy have attempted to move towards more critical positions, but the instruments used for evaluation of health literacy gains remain stagnant in the application of individual assessment instruments and are also limited in clinical care spaces. We believe that this parallels what happens in the field of science education where visions prevail that privilege mastering the content over the specific needs ignoring the sociocultural, economic, political conditions of the people in question (Roberts, 2012).

We raise the need for both the educational and medical fields to think differently when addressing wellness | disease issues. We suggest, that the design of a literacy strategy for a case like ours must start from recognition of the sociocultural conditions of the context and the knowledge of the agents involved in order to design a health literacy strategy to improve their quality of life. In our case, the main stakeholders, besides sick children and adolescents, and mothers, are physicians, professors, thanatologists, and dieticians, amongst others. We recognize that the sociocultural capital and the professional training of the aforementioned agents does not guarantee their total attention to the sociocultural conditions of their patients with CKD. Consequently, we propose the need for a health literacy model that should be dynamic and assist in developing a holistic understanding of CKD by considering these agents as members of a community that integrates sociocultural, health and medical knowledge regarding CKD.

A health education strategy must start from a critical pedagogical approach that promotes awareness, especially with multivulnerable groups. Multivulnerable groups need to have the tools necessary to increase their agency and attend to their wellbeing. We would be remiss if we did not consider the social spaces where the educational process and care during the illness unfold. Social spaces for educational purposes should not be limited to public schools but can include the home, and hospital so that children with CKD can be better informed about the progressive nature of their disease. Specifically, we consider that a health literacy strategy to attend children and adolescents with CKD should at least consider the aspects as shown in Figure 16.1.

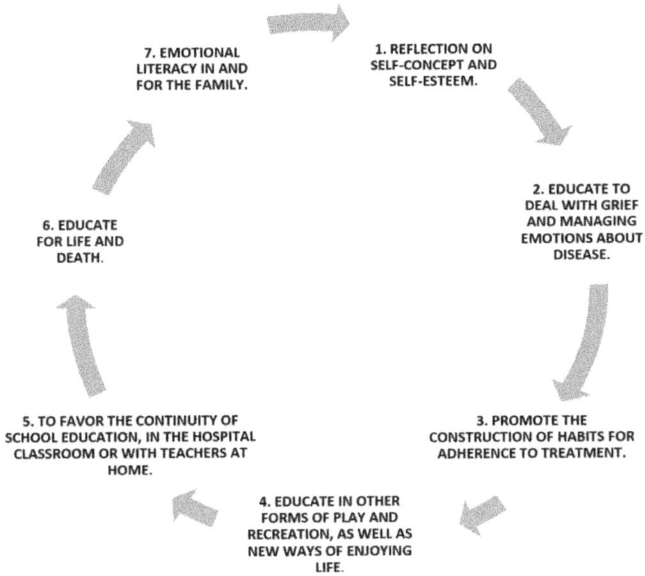

FIGURE 16.1 Health literacy strategies

While designing a health literacy strategy, we should not presume that people need a homogenous health education plan. Not all of us need the same knowledge. For example, in our cases the health education needs should be focused on the care of the renal disease, where knowledge is associated with medical treatment and a prescribed diet. This need implies a health education strategy that intersects with science, health and medical education. Having said this, there are other critical knowledge needs that deal with emotions such as anger, frustration, sadness, despair, among others, which are associated with the understanding and acceptance of the disease and death in the case of terminal diseases.

In general, for both fields of science and health education we propose a sociocultural approach and a critical perspective which helps both children and mothers and other stakeholders involved in the treatment of CKD to make informed decisions. We believe that the strategies to be followed could be sustained from critical pedagogy which according to Kincheloe (2011), its fundamental purpose would be to develop critical thinking of individuals through "an active process which encourages individuals to examine contextually the meaning of the information encountered so as to better understand the world and to contribute to the control of their own lives" (p. 15). We assume that a holistic analysis of the situation of children and adolescents with CKD in which they are socio-economically and culturally vulnerable, will enable us to help these patients empower themselves to understand cultural norms in such depth that the assumptions or doxas which undergird them may be exposed and if necessary refuted. That is, the patients will be able to understand the social, political, religious, ethnic, economic, and educational forces which positioned him or her and play a part in the medical treatment they receive. Only through contextual analysis, which is an act basic to critical thinking, can one accomplish that liberation which comes from an understanding of personal situatedness (Kincheloe, 2011).

5 Not Our Final, But Where We Are with Our Thoughts

We consider that the voices and experiences gathered so far pose serious challenges to the field of health and medical education as currently constructed in México. These challenges at least should lead to rethinking and restructuring the aims of science education in general and health education in particular as well as the medical curriculum. Restructuring and rethinking the national curriculum does not necessarily refer to specific knowledge of concepts, laws or theories, nor proper patient management but to the pedagogical implications of health science and health literate citizens and patient care. Zeyer (2012) recognizes that a part of health literacy is based on knowledge, but this should be developed based on the links between the field of science and health. Additionally, Zeyer raises the need to recognize the health/disease binomial, in which health literacy plays a role, not only in the promotion and prevention of diseases, but in the care of acute or chronic diseases and in therapeutic and palliative care. Specifically, aspects related to identifying emotions, understanding illnesses and death are aspects that are neglected in Western culture and little is said about them; much less educate around them (Podsiadlik, 2020). Consequently, these aspects constitute main challenges to restructuring the function of science and health education.

It is also necessary to understand the political aspects of education in general to overcome the structural barriers of health education in educational communities (Nutbeam, 2000). Health that leads to health literacy, especially from a collective and critical approach, can raise awareness and empower people to promote economic and social changes that include the coverage of their health rights, the management of health services and resources. However, there is a political cost and backdrop to the creation of public policies that improve their collective health because transformation of the institutions of society can create a backlash of resistance.

In order to gradually achieve a change in culture in which healthy nutrition is prioritized, we believe that health education, should begin at the prenatal period. But eating nutritionally should be accompanied by physical and recreational activities that take place in contexts that favor mental health, self-discipline and self-care. Studies have demonstrated that health literacy or health education is one of the most important determinants of health status, higher than others such as age, educational level, type of employment and salary (Fisher-Wilson, 2003).

There is an urgency for moral obligations, ethics, religious beliefs and spiritual aspects to come together in understanding the finitude of life. Much of the suffering we noticed is tied to a feeling of loss, but there are other ways of understanding the life cycle. It is also important to recognize that once guaranteed, the educational debt to society in health maintenance and care during illness – should be a function of the State towards its citizens. In México, it seems that everything points to massive health illiteracy that positions citizens in a vulnerable situation. We believe that part of the problem lies in how health education is represented in the national curriculum in that it is subsumed under science education. In order to assist in promoting heath literacy we propose that there is a need to generate initiatives based on research such as this, that serve small groups and that instill in them a critical awareness of health-disease, as well as the ability to fight for their right to a decent life.

References

Bajtín, M. (1999). *Estética de la creación verbal.* Siglo XXI.

Bakr, A., Amr, M., Sarhan, A., Hammad, A., Ragab, M., El-Refaey, A., & El-Mougy, A. (2007). Psychiatric disorders in children with chronic renal failure. *Pediatric Nephrology, 22*(1), 128–131. doi:10.1007/s00467-006-0298-9

Barton, A. C. (1998). Teaching science with homeless children: Pedagogy, representation, and identity. *Journal of Research in Science Teaching, 35*, 379–394. https://doi.org/10.1002/(SICI)1098-2736(199804)35:4<379::AID-TEA8>3.0.CO;2-N

Blum, B., Álvarez, A., & Gordillo, G. (2009). Psiconefrología. In G. Gordillo, R. Exeni, & J. De la Cruz (Eds.), *Nefrología Pediátrica* (pp. 753–771). Elsevier.

Bolívar, A. (2002). "De nobis ipsis silemus?": Epistemología de la investigación biográfico-narrativa en educación. *Revista Electrónica de Investigación Educativa, 4*(1), 1–26.

Chase, S. (2008). Narrative inquiry: Multiple lenses, approaches, voices. In N. Denzin & Y. Lincoln (Eds.), *The landscape of qualitative research. Theories and issues* (pp. 57–94). Sage Publications.

Chase, S. (2015). Investigación Narrativa. In N. Denzin & Y. Lincoln (Eds.), *Métodos de recolección y análisis de datos* (pp. 58–112). Gedisa.

Consejo Nacional de Evaluación de la Política de Desarrollo Social. (2018). *Estudio diagnóstico del derecho a la educación 2018.* CONEVAL.

Diario Oficial de la Federación. (2016). *Constitución Política de los Estados Unidos Mexicanos.* http://www.ordenjuridico.gob.mx/Constitucion/cn16.pdf

Eisner, E. (1994). Formas de representación. In E. Eisner (Ed.), *Cognición y currículum: una visión nueva* (pp. 65–92). Amorrortu.

Egan, K. (1994). *Fantasía e imaginación su poder en la enseñanza.* Morata.

Fisher-Wilson, J. (2003). The crucial link between literacy and health. *Annals of Internal Medicine, 139*(10), 875–878. doi:10.7326/0003-4819-139-10-200311180-00038

Freire, P. (1998). *Teachers as cultural workers.* Westview Press.

Gallard Martínez, A. J., & Antrop-González, A. (2013). The use of de jure to maintain a de facto status quo. *Cultural Studies of Science Education, 3*, 991–996. doi:10.1007/s11422-013-9523-6

Gallard Martínez, A. J., Pitts, W., Brkich, K., et al. (2018). How does one recognize Contextual Mitigating Factors (CMFs) as a basis to understand and arrive at better approaches to research designs? *Cultural Studies of Science Education.* https://doi.org/10.1007/s11422-018-9872-2

Gómez, M. (1999). Los niños y la muerte. In M. Gómez (Ed.), *Medicina paliativa en la cultura latina* (pp. 1133–1157). Arán.

Guzys, D., Kenny, A., Dickson-Swift, V., & Threlkeld, G. (2015). A critical review of population health literacy assessment. *BMC Public Health, 15*(215). doi:10.1186/s12889-015-1551-6

Hill, N. R., Fatoba, S. T., Oke, J. L., Hirst, J. A., O'Callaghan, C. A., Lasserson, D. S., & Hobbs, R. (2016). Global prevalence of chronic kidney disease – A systematic review and meta-analysis. *PLoS One*, 1–18. https://doi.org/10.1371/journal.pone.0158765

Insituto Nacional para la Evaluación de la Educación (INEE). (2016). *Panorama educativo de México. Indicadores del sistema educativo nacional 2015.* Retrieved January 18, 2020, from http://publicaciones.inee.edu.mx/buscadorPub/P1/B/114/P1B114.pdf

Insituto Nacional para la Evaluación de la Educación (INEE). (2018). *Panorama educativo de México. Indicadores del sistema educativo nacional 2017. Educación básica y media superior.* Retrieved September 18, 2018, from http://publicaciones.inee.edu.mx/buscadorPub/P1/B/116/ P1B116.pdf

Instituto Nacional de Geografía y Estadística (INEGI). (2015). *Población/Educación/Analfabetismo.* http://cuentame.inegi.org.mx/poblacion/analfabeta.aspx?tema=P

Instituto Nacional de Geografía y Estadística (INEGI). (2016). *Mortalidad.* http://www.inegi.org.mx/est/contenidos/proyectos/registros/vitales/mortalidad/tabulados/ConsultaMortalidad.asp

Instituto Nacional para la Educación de los Adultos (INEA). (2018). *México llega al día internacional de la alfabetización 2018 con un índice de 4.17%.* https://www.gob.mx/inea/prensa/mexico-llega-al-dia-internacional-de-la-alfabetizacion-2018-con-un-indice-de-4-17?idiom=es

Kincheloe, J. (2011). Exposing the technocratic perversion of education. In K. Hayes, S. Steinberg, & K. Tobin (Eds.), *Key works in critical pedagogy* (pp. 1–19). Sense Publishers.

Levitt, P., & Schiller, N. G. (2004). Conceptualizing simultaneity: A transnational social field perspective on society. *International Migration Review, 38*(145), 595–629. https://doi.org/10.1111/j.1747-7379.2004.tb00227.x

National Kidney Foundation. (2002). *Clinical K/DOQI practice guidelines for chronic kidney disease: Evaluation, classification and stratification.* https://www.kidney.org/sites/default/files/docs/ckd_evaluation_classification_stratification.pdf

Nutbeam, D. (2000). Health literacy as a public health goal: A challenge for contemporary health education and communication strategies into the 21st Century. *Health Promotion International, 15*(3), 259–267. doi:10.1093/heapro/15.3.259

Podsiadlik, E. (2020). *Grieving as a teacher's curriculum. Relevant prose and postscripts.* Brill Sense.

Roberts, D. (2007). Scientific literacy/Science literacy. In S. A. Abell & N. G. Lederman (Eds.), *Handbook of research on science education* (pp. 729–781), Lawrence Erlbaum.

Secretaría de Educación Pública, SEP. (2018). *Licenciatura en educación primaria. Plan de estudios 2018.* SEP. https://www.cevie-dgespe.com/documentos/1105b.pdf

Secretaría de Educación Pública, SEP. (2019). *Planes y programas de estudio para la educación básica. Educación primaria.* SEP. https://www.planyprogramasdestudio.sep.gob.mx/prim-intro-explora-conocimiento2019.html

Secretaría de Salud. (2014). *Programa de acción específico: salud para la infancia y la adolescencia 2013–2018.* Retrieved September 30, 2019, from https://www.gob.mx/cms/uploads/attachment/file/314995/PAE_Salud_para_la_Infancia_y_la_Adolescencia.pdf

Secretaría de Salud. (2018). *Perfil epidemiológico de enfermedad renal crónica en México.* http://187.191.75.115/gobmx/salud/documentos/perfiles-epid/enf-renal-cronica/perfilepid-enfrenalcronica2018.pdf

Sisto, V. (2008). La investigación como una aventura de producción dialógica: la relación con el otro y los criterios de validación en la metodología cualitativa contemporánea. *Psicoperspectivas, VII,* 114–136.

Tobin, K. (2006). Aligning the cultures of teaching and learning science in urban high schools. *Cultural Studies of Science Education, 1,* 219–252. https://doi.org/10.1007/s11422-005-9008-3

Tobin, K. (2009). *Sociocultural perspectives on science and science education* [Keynote address]. The 8th international congress on science teaching and learning, Barcelona, Spain.

UNICEF. (2017). *Levels & trends in child mortality.* Report 2017. USA: United Nations Children's Fund, World Health Organization, World Bank Group and the United

Nations Population Division. https://www.unicef.org/publications/files/Child_Mortality_Report_2017.pdf

UNICEF-CONEVAL. (2014). *Pobreza y derechos sociales de niñas, niños y adolescentes en México.* https://www.unicef.org/mexico/pol%C3%ADtica-social-e-inversión-en-la-infancia

United Nations. (1984). *The universal declaration of human rights.* United Nations.

Zarcadolas, C., Pleasant, A., & Greer, D. (2006). *Advancing health literacy. A framework for understanding and action.* Jossey-Bass.

CHAPTER 17

Practicing Mindful Living as a Professional Learning Community in a Thai Elementary School

Yau Yan Wong

Abstract

Teachers' mental health and their interactions with students have a strong influence on the students' learning and wellbeing. However, teachers are rarely given the tools to become aware of and manage their own emotions. In this study, I adopt a hermeneutic phenomenological approach to describe the journey of a group of like-minded teachers, who set up a professional learning community (PLC) to cultivate mindfulness in their personal lives and teaching practices. Through participating and leading weekly meetings, retreats, and workshops, this group of teachers gradually transformed their worldviews, beliefs, and way of being in their classrooms. Their work triggered ripple effects in their school community. A final session is a critical reflection of the PLC about their teaching experiences through practicing deep listening and loving speech. I conclude that mindfulness practice, if being taught and modelled properly, could improve students' wellbeing by enhancing self-awareness, reducing bullying problems, and improving focus. I share insights about the tips and challenges of teaching mindfulness in a K-12 school setting from the professional learning community's authentic inquiry with other educators.

Keywords

mindfulness – teachers' wellbeing – professional learning community

1 Waking up from an Unsustainable Lifestyle

Teaching is one of the most demanding occupations in the world because it is a highly people-oriented job that involves interactions with multiple parties daily. For example, teachers are supposed to provide a nurturing learning environment, be responsive to students, parents, colleagues, prepare students for tests, coach students through conflicts with peers, and handle disruptive

 | DOI:10.1163/9789004527348_017

behavioral problems in class (Jennings, 2009). The problem is teachers rarely receive training or resources for any of the above duties and how to manage stress at work. Quite often, teachers continue to work after school hours, and this affects their health and the quality of their family lives.

My parents were both secondary school English teachers in Hong Kong. I remember watching them grade piles of homework after work until 9 to 10 PM every day. Besides grading, they also had many administrative duties to do, including distributing notices, collecting money from students for field trips, supervising new teachers, and organizing extracurricular activities after work. My parents rarely got enough sleep. My mother was suffering from a range of health issues, like allergies and insomnia. Quite often my mother had angry outbursts at home due to the stress from work. As a result, our family rarely spent quality time together. I think this is a common condition that many teachers in Hong Kong have been facing until now.

Although I know from my parents that being a teacher is a very stressful job, I have high respect for this occupation. My parents sometimes took on the role of surrogate parents of their students and took care of their emotional as well as social needs. I saw that my parents had a strong influence on their students' lives. Many former students would visit my parents frequently and expressed their gratitude towards my parents. I believed that my parents were making an important contribution to society by taking good care of their students. Hence, after graduation, I followed in my parents' footsteps and became a teacher.

Since 2006, I have been working as an elementary school teacher. The working condition of teachers in Hong Kong had not changed much. I worked for long hours from 5 AM to 6 PM every day. After work, I carried piles of workbooks with me and spent hours on grading. Because I have a master's degree, I was promoted to the management level very quickly. I still remembered that I barely had time to use the restroom or drink water at work. My hair turned yellow, and I suffered from severe skin allergies. Sometimes I lost my voice because I had been teaching for too long. Because of lack of sleep, I became very irritable and depressed. Sometimes, I had angry outbursts in the classroom, and I felt ashamed after that. I used to resent my mother whenever she acted out of temper, and I made a promise to myself that I would never do that to my students or child. However, I followed the same behavioral pattern of my mother, and I began to understand better what got her in that angry emotional space. I thought if I continued this path, I would probably have mental health problems. I knew this kind of life was not sustainable. Teaching should not make me sick.

Teachers' emotional wellbeing has a strong influence on classroom learning atmosphere and students' emotional wellbeing because students see their teachers as their role models of emotional regulation, and they spend a long time learning together every day. I noticed that when I felt stressed and angry, my students would mirror my emotions. Children are very sensitive to the emotions of adults. I decided to look for ways to manage my emotions so that I would not hurt myself or my students. In the beginning, I coped with my stress by visiting spas more frequently and buying more stuff. However, the effect was not long-lasting. Fortunately, in 2009, I learned about mindfulness practice after moving to Thailand. Mindfulness practice has completely changed my worldview and overall wellbeing.

2 Understanding Mindfulness

I learned about mindfulness practice from my Thai husband, Chaw. He grew up in a Buddhist family. He felt worried about my poor health condition and suggested I try meditation. I heard about it in the past while I was studying psychology in college. But I had no idea how to meditate. I became curious about it because Chaw said meditation helped him reduce stress. I joined a half-day retreat at the Thai Plum Village International Meditation Centre in Kaoyai. I learned that mindfulness means 'remembering' in the sense of constantly bringing the mind back to the present moment (Hanh, 1999). Thich Nhat Hanh, the founder of the Plum Village, was leading the retreat. Hahn was a peace activist and an advocate for integrating mindfulness into daily life activities. In his talk, he explained that mindfulness can be practiced in our daily life while we are breathing, walking, or eating. With mindfulness, compassion and happiness become possible. I was hooked by Hanh's talk because I wanted to become a compassionate and happy teacher like him.

After the retreat, I began to study Hanh's books. His book called Planting seeds – practicing mindfulness with children (Hanh, 2011) had a strong influence on my teaching practice. He said teachers need to take care of themselves first. If they do not know how to be happy, they cannot teach children how to be happy. I began to adopt Hanh's mindfulness practices in my daily life. I slowed down and examined my life deeply. I cut out the activities that were not value-added or were depleting my energy. I took deep breaths or a short walk whenever I felt irritated. My skin allergies started to disappear. I practiced smiling meditation while I was teaching, even though I did not feel particularly happy. Gradually, I felt there was a change in my overall mood. My students responded to such a change, and they smiled more too. They felt less fearful towards me.

As I felt more energized, I spent more time talking with my students outside the classroom. At first, students told me little stories like how they spent their weekends. Later, they told me more personal problems. For example, a few students shared with me that their parents often yelled at them angrily or beat them up. One day, a grade 4 student showed me the bruises on her arms and legs. She asked me what she should do to feel less afraid of her parents. Some students asked me to help them when they got bullied. I recognized that children faced a lot of stress from home and at school, and they needed support to handle problems in their social lives. I also noticed that students with family problems often had difficulty focusing on their studies.

I decided to teach my students some simple mindfulness practices to help them alleviate their stress. Regarding the problem with domestic abuse, I thought it was not enough to just help students cope with the stress alone. I consulted the school counselor about this issue, but she said in Thai culture, it is taboo to teach other parents how to raise their kids and she did not want to cause any problem. So, I talked to the students' parents and shared my experiences in mindfulness practice. I talked about the importance of nonviolence and happiness in a family. In the beginning, I was not very skillful in communicating with parents and some parents got angry with me sometimes. My co-teachers did not understand why I had to approach difficult parents and got myself into trouble. But I could not simply ignore the suffering of my students and did nothing to help. I strongly believe that the wellbeing and happiness of children should be the priority in education. I thought teachers play an important role in promoting children's mental health.

3 Classroom Research on Mindfulness

In order to raise the awareness of teachers and parents on children's wellbeing and promote mindfulness practice, I conducted research projects in my classroom with two researchers from Thammasart University (Chongpaisal, Raweewan & Wong, 2012). Later, another researcher, Voranij Vasuratna, from Bangkok University, joined the research squad and we published another conference paper (Jarutawai, et al., 2014). These projects aimed to enhance children's emotional intelligence through mindfulness training programs. According to the students' self-report questionnaires, they felt a higher level of self-awareness, peace, concentration, and emotional stability. From 2015 to 2019, I conducted a few action research studies independently and explored other effects of mindfulness (Wong, 2019). In 2016, I presented the findings from the above research in a staff meeting. Later, a few like-minded colleagues decided to join this project and formed a professional learning community (PLC).

In this hermeneutic phenomenological study, I describe my journey in organizing a mindfulness PLC with my colleagues for promoting the wellbeing of students and teachers in an international program of a public school in Thailand from June 2016 to March 2019. PLCs in schools are inclusive, reflective, mutually supportive, and collaborative groups of people who find ways inside and outside their immediate community to investigate and learn more about their practice in order to improve the learning of teachers and students (Stoll, et al., 2006). The mindfulness PLC aimed to help its members develop a healthier lifestyle and improve the quality of teaching and learning through mindfulness practice. It had nine core members that were teachers from different grade levels and subjects. Each of the members in the PLC has their own perspective and application of mindfulness in their daily life and teaching practices. Besides meeting regularly, the PLC members also collaborated in conducting research through designing and implementing the curriculum, lesson studies, surveys, and interviews.

The research project conducted by the PLC adopts the framework of authentic inquiry, in which a group of teachers applied what they have learned to improve their practices in an event-oriented, polysemic, polyphonic, and collaborative manner. An authentic inquiry is a multilogical research methodology that seeks to address the needs of all stakeholders through engaging in reflexive practices and facilitating individual and collective changes (Tobin, 2015). It aims to bring about meaningful personal and social change through attaining the goals of educational, ontological, tactical, and catalytical authenticity (Tobin & Alexakos, 2021). The work of the mindfulness PLC described here is an authentic inquiry because it unfolded in an emergent and contingent way and responded to the salient needs and events in their surrounding community. Through participating in weekly practices, professional development workshops, and retreats, the PLC members gradually transformed their own worldviews and being and led to rippling effects for their students, coworkers, and school administrator.

4 Hallway Talk

The mindfulness PLC originated from a talk that I had with Karl (pseudonym), who was a grade 3 teacher and a keen meditator, in the hallway about a few bullying cases in our classrooms. We shared our frustrations about the stickiness of bullying issues. Identification of bullying cases is usually tricky because bullying happens mainly outside of the classrooms when teachers are not around. The victims are often too intimidated to inform their teachers. Moreover, when we noticed the bullying problem and began our investigation through interviewing students and parents, the interviewees became very sensitive and emotional. Sometimes, despite of our best effort, the parents of the victims decided to take their children out of our school.

We began to explore the root causes of bullying problems. Karl believed that the lack of compassion and lack of tolerance towards differences among children were the causes of bullying. He said the current education system in Thailand focused mainly on the development of cognitive skills and academic performance, but invested little time on cultivating self-awareness, compassion, and social responsibility. As a result, most of our students and their parents put too much emphasis on getting good grades, certificates, and awards, but they did not know themselves and why they need to learn. In addition, many students did not have sufficient emotional and social skills to negotiate with their peers during conflicts or face some major life challenges, like parental divorce and domestic violence. We thought the bullying problem was possibly a systemic problem.

Both Karl and I have been practicing meditation for several years and experienced some benefits of the practice, like enhanced concentration, calmness, awareness, equanimity, and happiness. We hypothesized that mindfulness practice could help reduce the number of bullying cases in our school. Karl learned from the staff meeting that I had been practicing mindfulness with my students in grade 4 for quite a few years. Hence, he borrowed the mindfulness lessons that I had been developing and then implemented them in his classroom. Later, a few like-minded colleagues began to share ideas with us regularly, about how to cultivate mindfulness and compassion among our students.

5 Introducing Mindfulness to Teachers

In 2016, our school appointed a new principal, Pranee Potisook, who was a keen meditator and showed interest in our mindfulness project. Hence, she asked us to organize a workshop about mindfulness practice for all teachers in the school. We invited one of the trainers from the Mindfulness in Schools Project (MiSP), Siri Chandler, to conduct a half-day workshop in our school. MiSP is a non-profit making organization based in Wales[1] and its courses are widely implemented in England as well as many other European countries. The purposes of the workshop were to explain what mindfulness is, and why mindfulness is important for the wellbeing of teachers and practice. In the workshop, Siri introduced some simple mindfulness practices that teachers could do in daily life. She explained that mindfulness is about "being" but not "doing," "responding" but not "reacting." Siri also said mindfulness is about observing, noticing, exploring, investigating, being with, and turning towards the present experience.

After the workshop, many teachers approached Siri, Karl, and I for more information. About 14 teachers expressed interest in learning more about mindfulness according to the after-intervention survey. As a result, from December 2015 to January 2016, I invited Siri again to conduct an eight-week mindfulness training course, called .b Foundations for educators to this group of teachers.

After the training course, the participants gave us some positive feedback. Below is a comment from Gary (pseudonym), a kindergarten teacher:

> I think I sensed some small changes happening in my life after the course. I used to react to my anger immediately and snapped at my family. However, lately, I was able to pause sometimes and recollect myself. I've become a more pleasant person after the training. (Feedback from a survey, Sep 11th, 2016)

One physical education teacher, Nat (pseudonym), gave the following comment:

> I like the mindful movements the most in this course. I can easily integrate it with my lessons. I think mindfulness is so important for young people because they are always on their phones and forget about their bodies. Mindful movements can enhance their bodily awareness and wellbeing. (Feedback from a survey, Sep 11th, 2016)

6 Developing a Professional Learning Community

After the training, about six other teachers showed interest to practice mindfulness with Karl and I on a weekly basis. They wanted to learn how to cultivate a personal practice and how to teach mindfulness to their students. In June 2016, the school principal suggested I put together a PLC. The mindfulness PLC was made up of eight teachers from different grade levels and subjects. Karl was an American grade 3 teacher, who was a long-time yogi and Vipassana practitioner. Kim (pseudonym), who was an American coteacher with Karl, also was an experienced yogi. Betty (pseudonym), an American grade 2 homeroom teacher, was a self-described beginner in mindfulness practice. Jessie (pseudonym), an American middle school English teacher, was interested in integrating her writing lessons with some reflective exercises. Gary (pseudonym) was a British kindergarten teacher, who was experiencing a lot of stress at work and was interested in learning how to better cope with stress. Jenny (pseudonym) was an American-Thai high school biology teacher who wanted to explore if mindfulness can enhance my students' pro-environmental awareness. Annie (pseudonym) was a Hungarian high school music teacher and would like to know how mindfulness helps students focus better. Pranee was the supervisor of the PLC, who participated in our activities occasionally.

The PLC members met every Monday afternoon and did various contemplative activities, such as sharing books, breathing exercises, deep relaxation, mindful movements, yoga, mindful communication, lesson study, etc. We also signed up for a six-week mindfulness training course for educators, called *Mindful Educator Essentials* by Mindful Schools. Through the course, we gained many useful teaching materials that can be implemented in a K-12 school. We taught this curriculum in our classrooms from kindergarten up to grade 7 during the morning homeroom sessions.

Gradually, this PLC became a close family. Not only did we share our teaching experiences, but we also practiced mindfulness together and helped each other solve daily life problems through the lens of mindfulness. Our weekly meetings acted as reminders for all of us to practice mindfulness regularly inside and outside of classrooms. In the beginning, I was the main facilitator of the activities. Later, more members took turns leading mindfulness-based activities. The mindfulness PLC incorporated polysemia (multiple worldviews), polyphonia (acceptance of different voices), and collaboration. For example, Jessie, a middle school English teacher, was concerned about the influence of social media on teenagers' self-identity and mental health. Hence, she shared my lesson plans on mindful communications and how to get unplugged. Another member, Jenny, was a biology teacher in high school and she had been advocating for a plastic-free society in my research work. In my session, she talked about the awareness of the human impact on the aquatic ecosystem and how we can replace plastic with other substitutes. Karl and Kim were our yoga teachers because they believed that cultivating harmony within the body was vital for the wellness and wellbeing of their students. Betty usually led the gratitude practices, which she felt had helped her manage negative emotions tremendously. Annie joined the PLC later than the others and had never joined any formal mindfulness training. Hence, she just wanted to participate and did not want to lead any activity. Sometimes, the PLC members invited their friends to join the meetings and the community was growing bigger.

7 Mindful Living at the Plum Village

Four of the PLC members, including me, joined the Mindful Living programme at Thai Plum Village in December 2016, where we lived with the monastics and lay practitioners for 5 days. We joined the retreat with the intention to deepen our understanding of mindfulness and learn some practices that can be implemented in our classrooms.

Upon arrival in the afternoon on Friday, we were welcomed by a female monk, and she told us briefly about the rules of the center. There were some specific rules in the monastery. For example, male and female practitioners lived separately in different dorms. Every morning, we woke up at 5 am and upheld the noble silence after 9 pm. Mondays were lazy days, which means, we learned to stop working and take a rest. During those five days of Mindful Living, we learned to slow down all our daily activities and bring a bit more awareness to every moment. We could see *gathas* (i.e., short poems) posted in many places, such as toilets, water faucets, dining areas, and bedrooms as gentle reminders of being mindful of every daily life activity. Most of the gathas were about how to conserve resources and energy for other living things. Every day we began our practice with morning chanting of the Five Mindfulness Trainings. The Five Mindfulness Trainings originated from the Buddhist Five Precepts, which include "do not kill," "do not steal," "do not lie," "do not have sexual misconduct" and "do not take alcohol or intoxicants." Hanh modified these traditional Buddhist precepts into a modern version, which becomes reverence for life, true happiness, true love, loving speech and deep listening, and nourishment and healing. The Five Mindfulness Trainings are the guidelines for practitioners on how to live a moral life.

After chanting, we would practice sitting meditation for 30 minutes. During the sitting meditation, we paid attention to the in and out-breaths without forcing. Then we practiced walking meditation around the beautiful mountains. We learned to synchronize the breaths with each step. Following walking meditation, we listened to a dhamma talk and practiced Sharing in a Circle, in which we sat together and took turns to talk about our practices.

7.1 *Mindful Eating*

All the meals in the Plum Village were vegan. We practiced food contemplation before we ate, such as thinking about the origin of the food, the hard work that had been put into the production of the food and sending gratitude to those beings that had sacrificed their lives for our survival. On the first day, I put a lot of food in my bowl, and I ate my lunch very quickly. I was always the first to finish my lunch. I was not aware of my habit until Sister Azera, Thich Nhat Hanh's long-time student, talked to me about this problem. Sister Azera is Vietnamese and worked in the U.S.A. before. She has been a dedicated dhamma teacher in the Plum Village for decades.

Sister Azera approached me at night while I was practicing walking meditation. She said, "Rhoda, why are you working so hard?" I said, "I want to make good use of my time here to practice." She smiled and said, "Mindfulness practice is not about working hard to achieve anything. It is about learning how to just be. I noticed that you are always the first to finish your meal. Do you always eat at your desk at work?" I felt surprised and said, "Yes! How do you know?" She laughed and said, "I know from my observation. You need to slow down, to enjoy every bite of your food slowly. Otherwise, you are going to have depression." I replied with confidence, "I studied psychology before. I don't think I will have depression." Sister Azera said, "No. Depression does not choose. It can happen to anyone. It does not matter if you are a psychologist or not. We cannot control the mind. If you continue to live in this way, you are being violent to your body. You will have mental illness later." I sensed strong compassion from Sister Azera, so I promised her that I would take good care of myself.

On the second day, I still put a lot of food in my bowl, but I ate much slower than the first day. Interestingly, I felt full faster. Moreover, eating slowly allowed me to savor the food more. I could taste the subtle sweetness and freshness in the vegetables. I gradually reduced the amount of food I ate for the following days because I became full faster. I believe that mindful eating may have the co-benefit of good health and sustainable development.

7.2 *Mindful Walking*

After lunch, we practiced working meditation with the monks for about an hour. Then we could choose one of the chores, such as cooking, washing dishes, doing laundry, cleaning the toilets, tidying up the beds, or gardening. When we were doing chores, we brought awareness to the task on-hand and restrained from talking too much. I helped to do laundry and make the beds for others because my mind usually wandered a lot when I did these tasks at home. It would be great training for me to learn to be present in these tasks. Interestingly, doing these chores with a bit more awareness made the whole process more enjoyable.

In Plum Village, Mondays are called the Lazy Days. We learned to practice "nowhere to go, nothing to do." My friends went to go hiking in the mountains. As for me, I'd like to spend some quiet time alone. So, I decided to volunteer to clean the toilets. Then I swept the floor of our bedroom. I felt exhausted, but I still wanted to do something. So, I went to the meditation hall to practice walking and sitting meditation for an hour. However, a few young monks came in and started playing the piano. I left the meditation hall and asked myself, "What do I enjoy doing the most?" I decided to just walk around the mountains and took some pictures. I really enjoyed walking like this without a destination or a purpose. When I walked back to the dormitory, I felt quite mindful. The joy of mindful walking remained for a few days even after I left the retreat. I learned that the energy of mindfulness arises automatically when I enjoy the practice.

On Monday night, Sister Azera talked to me again. She asked, "You did not join our hiking trip this morning. What did you do today?" I said, "I have done so much today. I cleaned the toilets and the bathrooms. I swept the floor. Then I practiced sitting meditation. And …" She laughed and said, "That means instead of being lazy, you worked very hard again." I laughed, "Well, yes. I guess it is my habit." She said, "There is a lot of doing energy in you indeed. It will take you some time to transform that energy."

Karl asked Sister Azera about his sitting meditation. He asked, "I had a lot of pain around my knees while practicing sitting meditation. Am I allowed to sit on a chair instead?" Sister Azera said, "Of course, you can. You should not torture your body while practicing mindfulness. We should practice in a way that is good for our body. I knew an old woman who practiced sitting meditation with folded legs for hours in a very strict retreat. She had some problems with her knee joints before. After the practice, she could not walk again. So, it is very dangerous to torture ourselves. You can practice in the most comfortable position." I learned from Sister Azera that being kind to our body is an important part of mindfulness practice.

In the next three days, for hours every day, I practiced walking meditation around the mountains. I walked slowly and paused to take a few pictures along the way. My passion for walking meditation became contagious and more friends joined the practice. We walked together, sometimes in silence, and sometimes we talked about our lives.

7.3 *Sharing in a Circle*

On the fourth day afternoon, I joined the Sharing in a Circle practice with Karl in a meditation room for male practitioners. After the practice, Karl took me to the patio and pointed to the balcony of another room. Thich Nhat Hanh was sitting there in his wheelchair. He was partially paralyzed after a stroke in 2014. However, at that moment, I did not see any suffering in him. He looked peaceful, radiant, and bright. I felt happy to see him and sent him my loving-kindness from my heart.

During the Sharing in a Circle, several practitioners talked about what brought them to the Plum Village. An American gentleman said he just lost his father and his brother last year. He suffered immensely and wanted to understand life and death better. One of Hanh's dhamma talks about dealing with the death of loved ones inspired him to come here. Hanh said a cloud never dies, meaning that we were never born or die. We just keep transforming from one form to the next. So, he believed that his father and his brother still existed in him and around him. This realization gave him a lot of comforts. There were other practitioners, who went through depression, domestic abuse, or wars, shared their stories from their hearts. No one gave any suggestions. We just sat in silence and listened attentively. Then we bowed to each other every time a speaker finished talking. The sangha is a safe place for sharing and healing.

In the last evening, we practiced Sharing in a Circle with all other practitioners and female monks again. The facilitator put a fresh flower in the center of the circle and lit some candles. The fresh flower represents the Buddha nature in all of us. We practiced deep listening and loving speech together. We took turns to talk about our most memorable experiences in Mindful Living. As the speaker was talking, other members remained silent and listen attentively. I said my most memorable lessons were learning how to slow down, enjoy my food, and enjoy walking.

At the end of the conversation, we practiced hugging meditation. At first, I was worried that I would feel awkward. But when Sister Azera hugged me, I felt very comforted. She said, "Remember to hug your daughter and your husband in the same way. They will love it!" Finally, I asked Sister Azera, "Is it okay if I did not mention Buddha when I am teaching mindfulness? Is it a sin for Buddhism if I do not acknowledge Buddha's effort?" Sister Azera answered, "If you intend to help people, it does not matter whether you acknowledge Buddha or not. Dhamma belongs to the world. It does not belong to anyone."

8 Returning from the Plum Village

Annie said she noticed a change in us after we returned. She said we seemed calmer and happier. I stopped eating at my office desk and instead ate in the canteen with other colleagues. Moreover, I began to explore a plant-based diet. Although I did not become a full-on vegan, I ate a lot less meat than before. Eating more vegetables and fruits made me feel lighter and energized. I also became more aware of my body movements throughout the day, especially when I was walking from one place to another. That helped me release some stress in-between lessons.

Karl, Jessie, Betty, and I shared our experiences in Mindful Living with other teachers in a staff meeting after returning from the Plum Village. Then we talked about how teachers could use the Plum Village practices as tools to enhance mindfulness of themselves and their students throughout the day. In December 2016, Pranee invited the mindfulness PLC to demonstrate some mindfulness activities in a professional development workshop. Each of us focused on different aspects of mindfulness. For example, I enjoyed walking meditation the most and decided to lead it in the workshop. Kim and Karl who had strong yoga backgrounds led the mindful movements. Jessie used to work in the business marketing industry and focused on mindful communication and social media. Betty joined the mindfulness training during a difficult time in her life and found gratitude exercise very useful for improving the outlook of her life. So, she led the Gratitude Stick exercise. Gary is a kindergarten teacher, who is very lighthearted and fun-loving. He decided to play a mindfulness game called Smile Please with other teachers. And finally, Jenny talked about the mindful consumption of plastics and sustainability. She got a doctoral degree in biology and her thesis was about cultivating environmental awareness among the youth to reduce plastic use. Siri and her friend, Mary (pseudonym), a school counselor from Concordian International School, also joined the workshop. They were impressed by the diversity of voices at the workshop and the enthusiasm of participants.

9 Scaffolding in Other Classrooms

In the academic year 2018 to 2019, the Mindfulness PLC designed and implemented an eight-week mindfulness training program from kindergarten up to grade 6. This program aimed to enhance students' emotional intelligence and wellbeing through mindfulness practice. We decided to take a polysemic approach in our teaching practices by synthesizing secular mindfulness practices with Buddhist mindfulness practices. We used the Mind-up curriculum designed by Hawn's Foundation as the backbone and synthesized with some Paws.b lessons and the Plum Village lessons. We called this curriculum the Mindful Learners because our students, their parents, and the teachers were learning how to be mindful together and mindfulness practice is about learning about ourselves. The whole curriculum adopted the competency-based model of emotional intelligence created by the Department of Mental Health, the Ministry of Public Health, Thailand in 2000. The structure of the model includes three components namely virtue (conduct), competence (wisdom), and happiness (peace) (Department of Mental Health, 2000). Each lesson targeted one of the sub-components (competencies) in the model. The curricula of different grade levels have a similar structure (Table 17.1). However, the

TABLE 17.1 The Mindful Learners syllabus for grade 3

EI components	EI competencies	Week	Activities
Virtue	Self-awareness, Emotional self-control	1	Mindfulness Bell (Mindful Schools) and Yoga (Joyful breathing, standing poses)
	Empathy	2	Befriending Practice (.b Foundations)
	Responsibility	3	Mindful Consumption (Snack Contemplation)
Competence	Self-efficacy	4	Weeble-Wooble Exercise (Paws.b)
	Interpersonal relationships, problem solving	5	Deep Listening and loving speech in pairs (Plum Village)
Happiness	Peace, relaxation	6	Getting through the storm (Body-Scan from Plum Village)
	Gratitude, Life satisfaction	7	Ten-Finger Gratitude Exercise (.b Foundations)
	Self-esteem, Life satisfaction	8	Happiness Toolkit & Painting a Happy Picture (Paws.b)

vocabulary and exercises were adjusted according to the students' abilities in different age groups. We created PowerPoint slides and worksheets for each class. I demonstrated a few lessons in each homeroom and observed the rest of the lessons conducted by other PLC members and colleagues.

During an evaluation meeting, the PLC members reported that they felt other colleagues who had never joined any workshop before did not feel confident in teaching mindfulness. But the benefit of scaffolding the teaching in the whole elementary program is that more teachers were exposed to the practice. From my experience, I noticed several challenges when I rotated through various classrooms. First, not every homeroom teacher welcomed the practice because it was a top-down command from the principal. Some teachers were intimidated by the potential religious association of mindfulness and mentioned they were not comfortable being around when I was teaching. Second, even though some teachers were interested in mindfulness practice, they did not feel confident to teach after watching my classroom demonstrations. After the implementation of the mindfulness program, the PLC members and I continued to teach mindfulness in our classrooms, but teachers in other classrooms did not. Hence, we felt that ongoing training should be provided for interested teachers to enhance their self-efficacy in teaching mindfulness. Moreover, the training should be voluntary rather than compulsory for all staff so that teachers who do not feel comfortable teaching mindfulness do not feel ostracized.

10 The Practice of Deep Listening

After the implementation of the mindfulness program, the PLC was discontinued because most members already understood the basic principles and the application of mindfulness practice. We decided to keep in touch on an informal basis. In our last meeting, Karl, Betty, Annie, and I had a group discussion about the implications of mindfulness in the wellbeing of our school community. During the conversation, we adopted the practice of loving speech and deep listening from the Plum Village. Loving speech and deep listening are part of the Five Mindfulness Trainings in the Plum Village. It is the practice of becoming aware of the suffering caused by unmindful speech and the inability to listen to others (Hanh, 2009). The qualities of deep listening include "not interrupting the other, listening from the heart, without any judgment or comparison, quieting the inner chatter and commentary about what the other person is saying, so that we become a clear mirror for them, reflecting back on what we are hearing" (Hanh, 2011, p. 196).

Similar practices, such as radical listening, have been implemented in classrooms for cultivating a supportive and safe space for discussions. For example, In the Mindful Speaking and Listening Heuristics developed and implemented by Kenneth Tobin and Konstantinos Alexakos (2022), developed and implemented the Mindful Speaking and Mindful Listening Heuristics among university students to help them become present and self-aware, being able to take multiple perspectives, acknowledging deep emotions without getting stuck, and being compassionate during communication. Alexakos et al. (2016) implemented radical listening, heuristics, and other mindfulness practices to facilitate several cogenerative dialogues about some sensitive sociocultural topics among students and teachers at the Brooklyn College, New York. These practices have been shown to promote authenticity and wellness among those involved in the conversations.

In the following conversation, I adopted the role of a facilitator of the practice of deep listening and allowed the other members to express their feelings and opinions openly. The goal of the discussion was to contemplate what we learned so far about mindfulness as a community and how we could move forward from where we were. (The transcripts below are from an audio recording, Mar 28, 2019.)

1. Does mindfulness practice enhance students' learning?

Betty: For me, it depends on the student. If the student actually absorbs the ideas and tries to put in effort in the practice, then it can. But for some kids, it might not really click with them. So, if they are really doing it in a sincere way, it works. So, it depends on the student.

Yau Yan: Yes. That's a good point. For those students who genuinely practice, do you think mindfulness enhances their learning skills, like critical thinking skills or how they interact with others in group work?

Betty: Yes. I think those students who would do or get mindfulness practice are generally more self-aware. So, I think having that awareness translates to any of the subjects that they are doing that require them to think in a more critical way. And so, I don't know if it's the type of students or the type of individuals who are already able to have these skills to be aware. I am not sure if mindfulness enhances their skills or just the type of person they are.

Karl: Some students may be inherently more aware than others. It's just about their personality or where they are brought up. Some students might be not focusing on anything because of how they are raised. I think that second-grade level is kind of young and we can't really tell yet. Maybe in some students, we can, but if they do it continuously and when they get older, we can see it. Right now, it is kind of so young. Your question was does it benefit their academics? Or student learning? Definitely yes.

Yau Yan: Learning can be academics or the emotional side of learning too, like the motivation side. They are more curious, also can be more compassionate towards the other students.

Karl: Yes. I think it can benefit that, because they slow down, and they think about whether they are learning more, and they are aware of that. Or if they're showing their emotions, they are not going to distract other people because they are thinking about maybe I shouldn't distract other people and I should listen, instead of distracting. That'll be mindfulness. Like John (pseudonym) for example, he usually just shouts out. But with mindfulness, he can focus instead. He can learn better, and other people can learn better because he doesn't shout out anymore. For me, that will be using mindfulness.

2. Can mindfulness help reduce bullying problems in school?

Betty: We have students that didn't really improve. But I think there were students that became more aware. And one thing that we did was mindfulness. But we also talked directly about bullying. So, there were a few different approaches that we took. And there was a student like Joe (pseudonym) who doesn't seem to have any effect on like he doesn't seem to have heightened awareness. But other students like Mike (pseudonym) who at least seemed to know he was doing it, but he couldn't control it. He does seem to be able to control his emotions more. So maybe he acted out less to other students. But it doesn't work across the board. For some students, it could be helpful.

Karl: Maybe it will take more than one year to see any difference. It's not going to change someone overnight. But if they continue with mindfulness practice for a few years ... a couple of years, we'll then see the change. For example, Nathan (pseudonym) got a lot better.

Betty: Yes, he got a lot better.

Karl: But I don't know if it is because of mindfulness or not. But it might be.

Yau Yan: It's quite hard to isolate mindfulness from other measures that you've used to improve students' behaviors. Besides mindfulness, you also talked directly to students about their behaviors or did some other activities that may not be mindfulness-based.

Karl: Like the bullying lessons we did. They are not called mindfulness, but there is mindfulness in those lessons. Like think about what you do before you do with somebody else. Would you want them to do it back to you? That's mindfulness because they stop and think first. I think all the bullying lessons that we did are pretty much mindfulness lessons.

Betty: Yes. True.

3. When and in what subjects can teachers introduce mindfulness?

Karl: For me, it'll be social studies, like when we talk about cultures and people and different things like that. But it is inherent in every subject. I wonder how mindfulness fits in music lessons because they are trying to feel their notes and feel the pitch and how it is different. I think mindfulness will work for music, especially. But for science in particular, I haven't noticed anything. They are just inquisitive already, so much that I cannot figure out if it is mindfulness or not. They are already like that. What about music?

Annie: In the younger students, they don't do mindfulness or things like that. And it's too late to start for high school students.

Yau Yan: So, when is the best time to introduce mindfulness to students? For me, I float in-between different classrooms this year. And I feel like ... it seems like IP3 (i.e., grade 3) start to be responsive to the lessons or more ideas to share about mindfulness. IP2 (e.g., grade 2) also have some but it's the beginning of awareness. But grade 1 or younger don't really have much self-awareness.

Betty: Yes, maybe there is some scientific explanation of that, like when the metacognitive development begins. But I think you are probably right, about grade 3 when I can see that they become more self-aware.

Karl: About what age level would be good to begin teaching mindfulness? I think the earlier the better. I mean just because grade 2 didn't talk about it ... They are probably just not able to express themselves at their English level. At grade 3 level, they are expressing more because they have better English. I think the earlier the better. For parents, even before they go to school for sure, or right away when they were born.

Betty: Well, maybe too early.

Karl: No, never too early.

4. Can mindfulness practice enhance students' ability to handle destructive emotions?

Karl: Yes, for sure. Like Mike gets mad fast. And if he uses mindfulness, he will be able to control more and not to act on it. Maybe Nathan did that too. He used to disrespect everybody and teachers, but he improved a lot towards the end of the year. He still does things, but ...

Betty: Yes, I think his awareness is being increased a lot, not only because of mindfulness, but he had a lot of serious consequences after what happened. So, it caused him to have to be more aware. He will think more before he acts.

Yau Yan: That's a good point that not only teaching mindfulness, but kids need consequences to improve.

5. Should mindfulness practice be included in a formal school curriculum?

Betty: I would disagree just because I think it's conditional. I would agree if there were someone who is able to teach it and model it because it's not a good idea to just ... maybe just the curriculum tells the teachers this is what you need to do, but then if it is not actually modeled, it is not going to be effective.

Yau Yan: That's a good point.

Karl: I think it definitely has to be secular mindfulness to be included in the formal curriculum. But no religious connotation. For me, or for people who are a little bit older or teachers, it might be when you hear mindfulness, you think of Buddhism. But for young kids, when they learn about mindfulness, they may not get the impression that it is Buddhism. So, if it's not a religion, they won't feel bad about it. As long as it is secular, it is safe because otherwise, people might have a wrong impression about it. If you tell them that it comes from Buddha, or said Buddha did this and that, they might relate too much to him and that they shouldn't be doing it or get scared of it. I think fear ... I think some people are just scared about it because of the history of it. They don't want to associate themselves with Buddhism or Eastern religion where it kind of came from. When it really ... it's not something that is religious about it. It's just about being aware of yourself.

Yau Yan: Yes. It's about self-awareness ...

Annie: Yes, I said yes because mindfulness is already included in many schools in England. So, what I see from my point of view that today you have a huge number of ADHD students and it's really good for them. This practice can guide them. Like if they practice in the morning, they will be calmer and pay more attention. And if you study it from a psychologist point of view, now it is already part of the psychology in the secular part, not the religious part.

Betty: Basically, I disagreed previously. But I do agree that it doesn't have to be called mindfulness. But I think there should be some kind of social emotional learning in school, whatever you call it. That should be part of the curriculum because it's critical for their development.

Yau Yan: Yes, that's a good point. The vice-principal also asked me to call mindfulness something else because of the religious connotations. But he also thinks teaching students social emotional skills is a good thing. I think it's about the labeling issue. I also agree with Betty that the top-down approach will not work, like forcing every teacher to do this won't work. It depends on teachers' willingness to do it and modeling mindfulness correctly.

6. Is mindfulness an important quality of a teacher?

Everyone: Yes, definitely. Every profession.

Betty: The best teachers are very reflective on their practice. All that you call it, mindfulness, awareness, or reflectiveness is just really important for whatever you do. But for teachers, you always have to be noticing how things are working and what could be improved. So yes, it just requires a lot of mindfulness.

Karl: When you are teaching, your emotions are very important. If you let it go and are not aware of your emotion, you get out of hand very fast. You will get angry at the students. Even I used to do that a long time ago when I wasn't into mindfulness because I was not aware of my emotion, and I said something mean to them or I was too strict. I didn't know what the consequence was of myself being too strict because I was not being mindful. So yes, being a better teacher is being mindful.

Yau Yan: Yes. I agree too. For me, it's not mainly on the cognitive side. But when I started practicing mindfulness, I became more aware of my emotions. It is easier to notice when I get angry, than noticing when I am thinking when I am not thinking. So, I am more aware of my anger and how it affects the way I talk to my students and my attitude towards them. And then later, I am aware of my thinking. Like I have some judgments about some of my students and I become aware of that.

Annie: I think I rarely get angry with them. I think because my subject is not optional, especially for high school and they all have to do it. So, if someone doesn't want to participate or does some mean things, I use some tools to deal with them. I got angry with one girl this year, but I hope I didn't act on it. Ha ha ... I just told her that at this point you have two options, either start participating or go back to your classroom. Otherwise, I will give her a low grade and I am fine with it.

Yau Yan: I think you talked about a good point here is whether we act on it or not. It's not like when we practice mindfulness, there won't be anger. You probably notice more anger than not having mindfulness. It's okay to be angry. I remember when I joined Luangpor Pramote's (revered elder in Thai Forest sect of Theravada Buddhism) retreat, Ajahn (teacher in Thai) Prasan said you are controlling your mind and suppressing your mind, like I tried to force myself not to be angry or greedy or any afflictive emotion. But that's not the point. The point is just to know. You can do anything in your mind, but just don't act it out. And if I do, just know so.

11 It's Time to Change

The story of the mindfulness PLC showed the power of authentic inquiry in initiating and implementing systemic change for promoting the wellbeing of the school community. The formation of PLC originated from the intention of a group of like-minded teachers to solve the bullying issues in their classrooms through practicing mindfulness together. Hence, the activities in the PLC are event-oriented, responding to the salient needs of the students. The weekly meetings gave plenty of opportunities for the PLC members to experiment with new ideas and receive feedback from their peers. In addition, when teachers practice mindfulness together as a community, they constructed new knowledge and influenced each other's worldviews. Therefore, the actions of the PLC have both educational and ontological authenticity.

Nevertheless, going against the mainstream attainment-oriented and forward-planning trend of modern education has not been easy for us. In Thailand, most teachers and parents believe that giving a lot of homework and exams to students is beneficial for students' development. Quite often, students need to spend hours on after-school tutoring and cannot sleep until late at night. The situation got worse during the COVID-19 pandemic. After sitting in front of the computer for over 7 hours for online lessons, many students need to do more homework and more tutoring than before. The following research finding from Thai UNICEF's website about Thai youth's mental health condition is worrying:

> A recent mental health assessment among adolescents in Thailand found that 28 percent of adolescents experience high levels of stress, while 32 percent are at risk of depression and 22 percent are at risk of committing suicide, according to DMH's Mental Health Check-in, an online mental health evaluation platform which collected data from 183,974 adolescents during the 18-month of COVID-19 pandemic from 1 January 2020 to 30 September 2021. (UNICEF, 2021)

Not only students but also teachers are facing many new challenges. Many teachers like me are practicing concurrent teaching, that is, teaching online and onsite simultaneously. I often felt mentally and physically drained after teaching. The turnover rate of teachers during the pandemic is increasing because many teachers could not cope with the pressure from the hybrid mode (Ali, 2020). The attainment-oriented and forward-planning focus of modern education are the causes of this mental health epidemic in our youth.

In Asia, there is a common belief that a curriculum is rigorous if it includes hours of lecturing, difficult content, a huge number of challenging assessments. However, many children's passion for learning has been killed throughout this painful learning process. As a result, by the time students graduate, they have rarely learned about themselves or how to enjoy life. Taking away our youth's childhood, their love of learning, or even their joy of life, is a form of abuse. It is time to stop this violence against our youth, to redefine what success means and what true happiness means. The goal of this study is to show that it is vital for teachers and parents to critically contemplate the meaning of education, what our children really need right now to have healthy bodies and minds, and how to steer education towards a more balanced and sustainable direction.

Mindfulness is an important quality of teachers, but mindfulness alone cannot bring about meaningful personal or social change. The effectiveness of mindfulness practice depends on whether the teacher of mindfulness embodies and exudes kindness. I came across many teachers who said they did not have time to fit in any mindfulness lessons. However, mindfulness practice is not an activity that requires a whole lot of extra time to do. When teachers are aware of their own emotions, when they refrain from hurting the students, and when they are being kind to their students, they are practicing and teaching mindfulness already. Mindfulness practice is a mindset, a shift in consciousness, and a lifestyle that aims to free our minds from difficult emotions so that we will not cause harm to ourselves and others.

Certainly, not everyone is open to mindfulness practice. However, the goal of introducing mindfulness into a school community is not about imposing a set of beliefs as truths. Instead, it should be about presenting an alternative lifestyle that is different from the mainstream modern lifestyle, which often puts too much emphasis on attainment, accumulation of materials, and fast results. Mindful living is another life template or lens that people can try to adopt in their daily life and see if a simpler and more conscious way of living can bring more joy, more meaning, and more calmness to their lives. Hence, no one should be forced to practice. Students should be offered the freedom to do alternative activities if they did not want to join the group practice. And teachers need to be given the agency to decide how to nurture students' wellbeing. But I as well as other PLC members believe that giving an opportunity to our fellow students and teachers to learn another way of thinking, being, and living is essential for the overall sustainability and wellbeing of the global community.

Meaningful and genuine systemic change in a society comes from the accumulation of smaller changes that are based on patience, perseverance, and compassion. Important change may just begin from a hallway talk. However, when teachers find their own voices and pull their resources together, their actions will trigger rippling effects.

Note

1 https://mindfulnessinschools.org/

References

Alexakos, K., Pride, L. D., Amat, A., Tsetsakos, P., Lee, K. J., Paylor-Smith, C., Zapata, C., Wright, S., & Smith, T. (2016). Mindfulness and discussing "thorny" issues in the classroom. *Cultural Studies of Science Education, 11,* 741–769. doi:10.1007/s11422-015-9718-0

Ali, S. S. (2020, October 8). Educators teaching online and in-person at the same time feel burned out: The Covid-19 pandemic has led many schools to offer both classroom and virtual instruction, but teachers say doing both concurrently is exhausting. *NBC News.* https://www.nbcnews.com/news/us-news/educators-teaching-online-person-same-time-feel-burned-out-n1243296

Chongpaisai, P., Raveewan, M., & Wong, Y. Y. (2012). *Development of emotional intelligence with meditation-based curriculum in a primary school in Thailand* [Paper]. BAI international conference 2012, Hokkaido, Japan.

Department of Mental Health. (2000). *Research report: The development of Thai Emotional Intelligence Screening Test for ages 12 to 60.* Ministry of Public Health, Thailand.

Hanh, T. N. (1999). *The heart of the Buddha's teaching*. Broadway Books.

Hanh, T. N. (2009). *Happiness: Essential mindfulness practices.* Parallax Press.

Hanh, T. N. (2011). *Planting seeds: Practicing mindfulness with children.* Parallax Press.

Jarutawai, N., Lowsuwansiri, A., Taechamaneesathid, P., Tangsangob, N., Chongphaisal, P., & Wong, Y. Y. (2014). Mindfulness training at schools in Thailand: An experimental approach. *International Journal of Information and Education Technology, 4,* 123–126.

Jennings, P. A., & Greenberg, M. T. (2009). The prosocial classroom: Teacher social and emotional competence in relation to student and classroom outcomes. *Review of Educational Research, 79*, 491–525. https://doi.org/10.3102/0034654308325693.

Stoll, L., Bolam, R., McMahon, A., Wallace, M., & Thomas, S. (2006). Professional learning communities: A review of the literature. *Journal of Educational Change, 7*(4), 221–258. https://doi:10.1007/s10833-006-0001-8

Tobin, K., & Alexakos, K. (2021). Doing authentic inquiry. In K. Tobin & K. Alexakos (Eds.), *Doing authentic inquiry to improve learning and teaching* (pp. 21–42). Brill | Sense.

Tobin, K., & Alexakos, K. (2022). Expanding the horizons of cogenerative dialogue. In K. Tobin & K. Alexakos (Eds.), *Transforming learning and teaching: Heuristics for educative and responsible practices* (pp. 39–66). Brill. https://doi.org/https://doi.org/10.1163/9789004507609_003

UNICEF. (2021, October 18). *COVID-19 pandemic continues to drive poor mental health among children and young people- UNICEF and Department of Mental Health caution on World Mental Health Day.* UNICEF, Thailand. https://www.unicef.org/thailand/press-releases/covid-19-pandemic-continues-drive-poor-mental-health-among-children-and-young-people

Wong, Y. Y. (2019). The enhancement of elementary students' emotional intelligence through mindfulness training. *Panyaphiwat Journal, 11*, 2–13.

CHAPTER 18

Total Involvement with Life

Being-in-the-Flow

Wolff-Michael Roth

Abstract

In this chapter, I describe and theorize a phenomenon related to one known in the popular literature and psychology as *flow*, a concept used to refer to a particular state of being associated with positive affect. Unlike existing, overly psychological views and conceptualizations of the phenomenon, my own descriptions emphasize aspects that only an event-based ontology appropriately captures. Working from my many, daily experiences of being-in-the-flow and drawing on phenomenological and pragmatic literature, I develop a way of approaching the experience of being-in-the-flow that is not marked by rationalism. Importantly, my approach abandons classical conceptions of the individual subject opposed to objects and world that are the goals of the former's intentional activity.

Keywords

flow – experience – experience of experience – consciousness – passivity – evental ontology – transaction – absorbed coping

1 From Persistent Cogitation to Absorbed Coping

> "I" am riding the bicycle for quite some time already and all of a sudden realize that a period of time has gone without "my" "noticing" "the environs" or "the time" "passing" – "I" can provoke the falling away of presence by focusing, for example, on the repetitive movement of my legs and feet pushing on the pedals;
>
> I sit at my desk, writing … until I suddenly realize that the morning has passed without that "I" have gotten up once. Although 'I' have written more than 6,000 words, "I" "have not been aware of" "time," "myself," or "my surroundings" – though there has been perhaps a dim sense of a process of "writing." (Roth, 2012, p. 124)

 | DOI:10.1163/9789004527348_018

This chapter centrally is concerned with a phenomenon associated with wellbeing: the total involvement in life in a form of happening referred to here as *being-in-the-flow*. The descriptions of experience in the opening quotation share some common features characteristic of a particular way of being-in-the-world related to what psychologists have named *flow* (Csikszentmihalyi, 1990). The latter concept has been defined as "the state in which people are so involved in an activity that nothing else seems to matter; the experience itself is so enjoyable that people will do it even at great cost, for the sheer sake of doing it" (p. 4). But there are issues to be considered both in the definition and in my own rendering of those activities that so engross a person that they lose themselves in and to them. Thus, the amply appearing quotation marks suggest that the English language, as Western languages generally, is ill-suited for "capturing" those experiences that, as such, are not (consciously) present to ourselves other than in some dim sense. The "I" appearing in these descriptions is unable, in the state of being-absorbed, to think an "I" separate from what is happening. Doing and thinking are part of the happening but are not experienced as issuing from a separate subject. Entitative things common to everyday talk, including time, surroundings, environs, and verbs expressing transitive relations with the world of things are precisely not what characterizes the experience of being-in-the-flow with which I am concerned here.

Both my opening paragraph and the psychological definition use the word *experience*, a term that may connote to some that the person engrossed in activity somehow represented to themselves whatever affect is occurring during the duration of absorption. But this is not so. Indeed, the preceding definition of flow refers to the experience of joy, which is an emotion, and emotions are, as shown below, external to the happening. Thus, each of my two descriptions intimate the slipping away of conscious awareness. Moreover, this slipping away itself generally is unavailable to consciousness in its entirety (just as we are unable to be consciously aware falling asleep). The transition from a consciously aware state to being-in-the-flow has syncopal quality because parts of the event belong to two very different and mutually exclusive states: conscious awareness and non-awareness. Finally, the objective (clock) time that has passed between the slipping away and returning of conscious awareness is not at all experienced as such. It is not captured by language in the way that we normally intend it. What happened between getting into the flow and coming out of it is unavailable – contrary to what psychological explanations may lead us to think – precisely because it is characterized by the absence of conscious awareness of things, the experience of experience.

The most important aspect of the phenomenon of being-in-the-flow in the context of the present volume is its contribution to wellbeing. The conscious awareness of being (feeling) well is characteristic of the moments following the period of having been in the state of being-in-the-flow. But that feeling of wellbeing has its origin precisely in that period in which the "I," the doing, objects, and the environment have not stood out. Instead, the feeling of wellbeing is associated with a sense of resonance, an echo, the origin of which dates back to the period of being-in-the-flow when the presence was not made present (Roth, 2012). Here, resonance "means that something else reaches into the present in the form of an echo, but precisely because there is an echo, something else has been, which itself is not accessible in the way the echo is" (p. 127). That is, the state of being-in-the-flow comes with a form of affect that in the period following it is felt and understood as contributing to wellbeing.

In this chapter I draw on weeding as an aspect of gardening, which, though it may appear mundane and a mere chore, in my case is just one of those activities that allows me to get into the state of being-in-the-flow. Indeed, a recent study showed that gardening, as cycling or walking, is an excellent context conducive to wellbeing (Ambrose et al., 2020). Gardening appears to be a form of activity amenable to being-in-the-flow and the resulting feeling of wellbeing.

2 Biographical Context

The topic of this chapter and the conceptualizations of the phenomenon at its core are strongly rooted in my own biography. I did not always have the forms of experiences described in the introductory quotations. Indeed, as a teenager, attending a university-oriented stream of schools (Ger. Gymnasium) where we were indoctrinated to the belief in the superiority of the thinking over mundane activity, I came to believe that the mind was everything and the body a necessary evil and nuisance. I could not relate to other people without having that homunculus in my ear checking on and monitoring what I was doing. Before responding (naturally) in social situations, my mind was spinning in high gear to evaluate what would happen if … I said this or did that. It may not surprise hearing (reading) that by the time I was 19 or 20 years old, I periodically suffered from serious depression. I was reading short stories featuring people who committed suicide, and I eventually set out to travel to India to seek salvation – though I never did make it there because, after having crossed several countries, I decided to return and finish the college-level year that completed pre-university education.

By the time there was a space in a psychological group therapy program that my parents had enrolled me in, it made no longer sense for me to participate because I already had changed too much and developed too far. I had started a form of meditation associated with a relaxation technique referred to as *autogenic training*, which I was adapting for my own needs. The method includes six standard aspects: (a) muscular relaxation in the different parts of the body, felt has heaviness; (b) generation of the feeling of warmth of body parts in (a); (c) influence on cardiac activity based on a mantra of "my heart beats slowly and regularly"; (d) passive experiencing of breathing – "there is breathing" rather than "I breathe"; (e) feeling of radiation from the solar plexus area; and (f) generation of coolness of the forehead. I was also reading a lot about Zen and its fundamental rejection of the body–mind dualism, which I recognized to be the basis of my earlier experience.

Autogenic training and the readings allowed me to evolve to the point that I could engage in many types of activities without having the homunculus appear in my ear watching over me and telling me what to do. I was developing a high degree of spontaneity to act and talk. In days when I still worried about naming, I referred to what was happening in terms of Zen (Masciotra et al., 2007). Indeed, much of what I do – including academic writing, gardening (such as pulling weeds), exercising, tending to bees, and cooking – now takes me into a state of being-in-the-flow, a "process of total involvement with life" (Csikszentmihalyi, 1990, p. VII). That is, even the most mundane aspect of life, considered by many as doing chores (e.g., pulling weeds), take me into a state of complete absorption and optimal performing. These are associated with positive affect and, as the following phenomenological description shows, to the disappearance of an "I" who, self-consciously, acts on and toward external things in an external world, including other people. While doing research or writing a text, "I" am so absorbed that my wife can enter and leave the office without my taking note of it. Just as Heidegger (1977) described using hammering as an example, in absorbed coping there is no (intellectual and thematic) grasping of things. Instead, in absorbed coping, concern and care are subordinate to the "in-order-to" constitutive of the happening (e.g., academic writing, gardening, exercising, tending to bees, and cooking).

For three and a half decades, I have been involved in research on knowing and learning. A central theme of my life in research has been that of seeking coherence, between (a) different theoretical frameworks and (b) theories of knowing and learning and my own life (cf. Roth, 2007a). From the beginning, I realized that in the theories bandied about in the research communities – e.g., cognitivist or (social, socio-cultural) constructivist theories – the forms experiences described here (being-in-the-flow) had no place. These theories had the same cognitive bias that characterized my teenage years, treating thinking, to paraphrase Vygotsky (1997), as if it were the thinker of thoughts. After I started classroom research on learning around 1990, I became interested in understanding the whole person, including those aspects that were at or beyond the limits of any constructivist metaphor for understanding how we act and learn in the various walks of life (e.g., Roth, 2011). The most outstanding and least addressed phenomenon I investigated concerns that of wellbeing arising from the immediate experiences during instances of being-in-the-flow.

3 Phenomenology of Being-in-the-Flow

3.1 *The Subject of Activity*

Being-in-the-flow has been an integral part of my life for a long time, and certainly was present while being a world class rower. But more than the rowing, an event related to my academic work comes to mind as an example when I was in that state. I had collected the data for my dissertation and all I needed to do was using the university's mainframe computer that had the required capacity for doing the preferred analyses. I entered the computer lab when it opened at 8 am. I do not remember any details, having gotten completely absorbed into the activity of running different tests. And despite this absorption, I apparently coped with all the challenges that the statistical analysis of a complex dataset poses. I sort of became consciously aware of the world again when I was asked to leave. It was midnight. I realized that I had not (knowingly) been to the bathroom, or eaten, or had a drink – i.e., I had not felt any needs. I had spent 16 hours completely absorbed in doing the different analyses, printing results, and running other, alternative analyses. (At the end of the workday when I was writing this paragraph, I realized that the glass of herbal tea I had prepared 3 hours earlier was still standing untouched about 5 inches to the left of the keyboard. On another day, I only noticed my wife's presence when she laid her hand upon my shoulder.) The following day unfolded in much the same way but for the fact that I accomplished with what I needed to do for the dissertation (which I completed during the subsequent three weeks). I remember a deep sense of satisfaction that arose from the realization of how much I had accomplished.

In this, admittedly extreme situation, all sense of self or needs had disappeared. It was as if only the activity itself existed; and it existed for itself, as the subject "I" had disappeared. After leaving the computer lab on both days, I had no recollection on who else had been present, how many other individuals had been present, or what else had happened. I became aware of myself when the lab instructor's request to leave knocked me out of the state of being-in-the-flow. The psychological concept of flow often is encountered in the context of description of special activities, for example, by players of videogames, athletes involved in high level sports (karate, climbing), accomplished artists, and the likes (cf. Findlay, 2019). But, as seen in the quotation opening this chapter, being-in-the-flow also characterizes many other, rather common activities that constitute my life, including cycling and writing academic texts, or, as in the following quotation, something as mundane as doing weeding.

> I have gone into the garden to weed. I pull a weed, pull a weed, pull a weed … and all of a sudden, I realize that two hours have passed without "my" "noticing" the situation, that "I" "have been pulling" "weeds," where "I" "have been pulling" "the weeds," not even of an "I" that has been the subject of the weeding. (Roth, 2012, p. 124)

This account of pulling weeds show that mundane tasks, too, may be accomplished in complete absorption with all the positive effects on wellbeing that characterize immediate experiencing in special situations associated with high-level performance. Indeed, it has been suggested that the impediment to flow experience at work is due to the fact that "when it comes to work, people do not heed the evidence of their senses. They disregard the quality of immediate experience, and base their motivation instead on the strongly rooted cultural stereotype of what work is *supposed* to be like" (Csikszentmihalyi, 1990, p. 160). Again, this author takes an overly psychological view, for, while being-in-the-flow, there is no "heeding of evidence," a predicate that requires a subject over and against which it stands.

In the opening phrase of the account of weeding, I note: "I have gone into the garden to weed." But, as the following statements make clear, "I," "weeds," and "pulling" are placed in quotation marks, because in the immediate experience, these aspects of the situation do not stand out as entitative things. They are not represented. Most importantly, the subject ("I") does not experience itself as subject, with specific identity, needs, or thoughts. Doing so, for example, by thinking about one's identity, would require making the self the content of the ongoing experience, which is antithetical to being concerned with whatever the activity is to achieve (e.g., pulling weeds, writing a scholarly article). The problem with writing about being-in-the-flow in terms of the subject referring to itself as "I" is that it is plagued by a fundamental problem of Western ontology: it accounts for activities in terms of agents and their activities that result from their intentions (e.g., Bergson, 1908; Nietzsche, 1922). The underlying mythology, according to Nietzsche, is that of the belief that there is an agential cause to every change. The activity is posited twice: activity and subject. The subject is something constant and different from becoming. (There are some indigenous languages that do not make such reductions, so that animals, for example, bear the name of a typical activity to which they are associated, see Roth, 2019.) Bergson and Nietzsche recommend changing from agent-centered statements to ones in which the event is central to the ontology. In the present instance, therefore, the immediate experience is more consistent with the statement, "There is weeding," "There is cycling," or "There is academic writing." Weeding, for example, is concerned with getting the weeds out and away from the plants that the gardener is caring for and tending. The subject (identity) so dear to social scientists, characterized by its own and others' constructions, only reappears when the event (weeding, cycling, or academic writing) is reduced to entitative things.

When we use phrases such as "There is weeding," on the other hand, any statement about an entitative subject (I), object (weed), and intentional action (pulling) then relates to the happening as a photograph relates to a lived situation. Weeding, as the event in which absorbed coping occurs, constitutes being-in-the-flow in a form in which neither subject, nor its activity, nor the transitive object of activity are standing out because they have been made present again in the present.

3.2 *Tools and Objects*

My favorite tool for weeding is a painter's spatula that in my hands is much more useful and efficient than the tools specifically sold for weeding. It easily enters even some hardened soil, and lends itself to lifting and loosening a short stretch of the ground, enough so that the roots are removed together with the leafy part held between the pinched fingers of the left hand. The spatula is not used all of the time in weeding but whenever circumspect activity anticipates the particular weed at hand to break upon being pulled.

This account of the tool "I" use in weeding has a problem. This is so because it appears as if I were somehow representing the tool or the weeds in my mind and then, having figured out what to do next (e.g., whether to use it or whether to just pull the weed), put it to use. But this is far from what actually is occurring. The spatula does not stand out in my mind as a thing; nor do the pinching, the soil, the individual weed, and so on. In the way I described it for other tools – including signs or the keyboard used for writing academic texts (Roth, 2003; Roth & Jornet, 2017) – the tool is transparent in proficient and effective use. It disappears in use, just as the keyboard I am using to write this text disappears in writing. Indeed, over time I have become so proficient with the keyboard that words spill out onto the page in a way similar to their spilling out from my mouth. There is no prior cogitation, thinking of a word that then somehow has to be gotten onto the page. The only time that the spatula stands out is when it is not there and I have to look for it or when something goes wrong – as if it were when it broke. But then there no longer is being-in-the-flow.

In philosophy, this relation between absorption and the fundamental ways of being in the world of gardening has been theorized as an "unthematic, circumspect absorption in the references that constitute the handiness of the totality of useful things. Taking care always already is what it is on the basis of a familiarity with the world. Dasein can lose itself in what it encounters in the familiarity and can be numbed by it" (Heidegger, 1977, p. 76). That is, unlike in constructivist accounts of activity, being-in-the-flow is not characterized by entitative subjects, who make objects, self, and activity present to themselves (by means of representation) as a basis on which to engage in further action.

My description of being-in-the-flow makes apparent that during the event, the spatula (tool) does not exist in the manner that it might when described in the catalogue of a hardware or garden store, that is, in the way that it gives itself to the scientific gaze. As a result, the world of weeding does not "consist" of a collection (addition) of entitative things, something people seeing through a scientific lens would use to populate a Cartesian space where no two things can be in the same location. Instead, as apparent in my description of the spatula, in absorbed weeding and the event of being-in-the-flow, the tool loses what the objective (scientific) gaze reveals; and it gives itself in a specific mode characteristic of the weeding. It does what it is to do without any other representation and, subject and subjected to the event of weeding, it becomes transparent in use. In such transparent use, the tool no longer stands between subject and the object operated on, as third entity entering between and bridging the original entitative things (Roth, 2007b; Roth & Jornet, 2019). Instead, it constitutes an extension of the subject into and intersecting the world together with which it evolves.

The foregoing does not mean that while being-in-the-flow I am not relating to the world. An objective gaze would reveal that I am not trampling the plants under my care while weeding, I continue staying on the road while cycling, I drink without spilling from a cocktail glass while conversing, and I use the keyboard without a thought while writing these lines. The point is that while being-in-the-flow, the related experiencing itself is not an object of reflective consciousness. Any knowing of tools and objects is *immanent* in and transparent to activity rather than transcendent. While being-in-the-flow, there is absorption into doing and there exists nothing apart from this doing, no tool, subject, or object that withdraws itself into itself to be standing over and against me.

3.3 *Getting into and Falling out of the Flow*

After an event of being-in-the-flow has ended, I find myself in a state of well-being and positive emotions. I am pleased with what has been accomplished and the progress that has been made. Consciously trying to get into the flow may actually be antithetical to achieving the intended state. The experience has been made by many in the Buddhist or Zen tradition, where beginners, because they try hard, fail to become enlightened. The more we are waiting for something – e.g., the end of a lesson, the coming of Christmas morning, the end of the workday, or the beginning of sleep – the more time stands out and the slower it seems to move. As a result, the waiting becomes even longer. Many athletes, too, have had a related experience: when they are thinking about their game because they want to change it, their level of performance decreases. Indeed, they are not in the flow of the activity because their concern and care no longer is the activity itself but its improvement. Thinking about the implement (e.g., golfers think about clubs, angles of impact, or position of the ball) inherently goes with the subject as separate from the activity, tool, object (ball), etc.

Bearing an essential quality of passivity, getting into the flow bears similarity with falling asleep. I begin with the intention to weed, much as I lie down with the intention to sleep. Initially there is still some chatter in my mind, thought chasing thought as the internal dialogue goes on. In those instances when I actually will have experienced being-in-the-flow of weeding, I become aware of it after the fact – much in the way that I will become aware of having slept (and thus fallen asleep) upon awaking. Just as in other instances when I experience being-in-the-flow – writing academic texts, cycling, building a garden shed – there is an initial focus on the activity accompanied by a readiness to abandon oneself to it while performing it. Indeed, I know how to set up favorable conditions for getting into the flow. For example, even though I might feel tired and little inclined to exercise, if I only begin cycling focusing on finding a rhythm, I will later find that being-in-the-flow has occurred. Even though I might not really feel up to continuing on an academic text, I know that just sitting down and writing something unrelated, will eventually set me up to turn to the text and get into the flow. (On the morning when I wrote this phrase, exactly that same phenomenon had occurred: After a rocky start because of a night with poor sleep, I eventually found myself having experienced flow.) In the case of writing, the location, too, is important, as I will not get into the flow if I write on my laptop in the kitchen or elsewhere than at my desk. In academic writing, as in cycling, it appears to be the rhythmic movement of the fingers, finding their ways on the keyboard, until I get to the point that I no longer have to cogitate for words to emerge from the movements of fingers and hands across the keyboard. Readers might have had the experience of not really wanting to engage in a conversation – e.g., with the neighbor on an airplane. But, after beginning with some resistance, you may eventually have found yourself to have passed a long stretch of objective time without having realized "to have had a good time conversing."

There are impediments to getting in the flow. For example, especially when preoccupied with something, the chatter in the mind might go on and I will not at all experience being-in-the-flow of weeding. I am holding on to the different thought contents that emerge. During many of the long hiking trips I did during my twenties, the mental chatter initially kept on for several hours, and sometimes it continued into the second or third day of hiking. But eventually, being-in-the-flow arrived, which, as described before, I discovered and became consciously aware of only upon awakening from that form of being-in-the-world. I will not fall into the state of being-in-the-flow if something else is awaiting me, for example, if I know that I have to leave within an hour or two to do some business. In fact, I may not start the activity at all, such as academic writing, the successes of which largely depend on the productivity of being accomplished while being-in-the-flow.

Being-in-the-flow may be ended when whatever obstacle arises in activity is too great, exceeding the capacities of absorbed coping. If my spatula breaks or it is not ready to hand – because it is hidden or has been left behind – the tool will have demanded conscious attention and thereby will have broken the flow of weeding. My wife enters my office to tell me that she urgently needs the copy and printout of a document, bringing the flow to a halt. The (rare) ring of the telephone intrudes and thereby stops being-in-the-flow. That is, whenever something else calls strongly enough to be attended to, the flow of the current activity stops.

3.4 *Affect versus Emotion*

Being-in-the-flow while weeding, I do not make present the present. There is weeding. But there is no "I," "spatula tool," "to weed," or any particular emotion. This does not mean, however, that affect is absent. Indeed, affect is a condition for action, a condition for any form of life as we know it (Leont'ev, 1981). The point is that only in hindsight, after snapping back into a state where the present is present to consciousness, that I might say, "I feel good" or "This was a satisfying morning in the garden." That is, it is only after the fact that I can say that now I am feeling relaxed, or feeling well though I might have started out the morning feeling a bit tired. I experience the same in cycling, where I might feel tired, but then, after a period of riding in the state of being-in-the-flow, I feel reinvigorated. But all of these descriptions are descriptions of *emotions*. When they occur at all, it always is after the fact and after coming out of the flow. There is therefore a difference between the affectivity characterizing flow and the emotion discourse that I may use to describe what and how I felt before and after the event. In being-in-the-flow, there is a pre-objective affectivity. When it becomes the object of the description, it turns into something from the emotional repertoire. It is the same as with pain. If I say I feel pain here or there in my body, then there is something more fundamental than "pain." There are bodily events, which, when externalized, I name pain.

The essence of the phenomenon of flow comes to be falsely represented when the necessary distinction between affect and emotion is not made. From a phenomenological perspective, emotion is a social phenomenon. It requires taking the perspective of another on oneself. I would not be able to recognize anger in the expressions of another unless I knew how others can see me when I am flooded by a sense that I come to know as feeling angry (Franck, 1981; Husserl, 1973). For example, when a gamer writes, "I feel the euphoria of mastery" (Beyer, 2020, para. 2), she already needs to know how "euphoria" relates to the feelings of the living body. When I write about a feeling of wellbeing that I experience after an extensive period of weeding or cycling, then I already have to know how "wellbeing" relates to the silent affections flooding the body. I have to take an outside perspective on myself. This outside perspective on oneself, however, is antithetical to the phenomenon of flow with which I am concerned here. If in meditation you were to try to focus on your emotions, you would immediately snap out of the meditative state. The problem I see arises from the fact that emotions are states of the body viewed from the outside, and my emotions – as in "I feel euphoria" – are two external perspectives on the same phenomenon (Henry, 2000). The classical bipartite division of a feeling body and a body felt, as it appears in the works of Husserl, requires a third form: the original flesh, which is the condition for the feeling and felt body. That third form refers us to affect, which includes all the pre-thematic valuations on which feeling and talking about emotions are based. It is that originary flesh [Fr. chair], the non-objective and non-objectified body, that is characterized by affectivity. It is that body that remembers and knows to act without the intervention of the conscious mind.

3.5 *Time and Temporality*

Time and temporality are different during experiences of being-in-the-flow. I know to have been experiencing flow when I realize that I just passed three or four hours reading, gardening, thinking, writing, conversing, cycling, hiking, or meditating without consciously having noted the passage of chronological time and without having made what I have done the topic of my reflective thinking. That is, in absorbed coping reflective consciousness – when the present is the object of thinking or experience – has come to a halt. Temporality and time then are experienced differently. In fact, there no longer is a passage of time in the mundane sense. Time no longer stands out as the Kantian precondition of experience. In absorbed activity, it is as if objective time has been put at bay: it no longer is a measure of what we are doing at the moment. There is no time in moments that are denoted by *flow*; and there is no (objective, clock) time during meditation. In both instances, there is but being-in-the-flow, weeding, cycling, academic writing, and so on. Although thinking related to the activity continues to occur, it is not concerned with making anything present and thus becoming consciously aware of it by means of beings (conceptions, mental structures). I thus emerge from being-in-the-flow into consciousness without any awareness of how much clock time has passed.

4 Ways of Thinking about Being-in-the-Flow

The preceding descriptions exhibit being-in-the-flow as a phenomenon of flux, where the subject is absorbed in a continuously unfolding world, does not experience itself as subject separate from the world, and therefore does not experience itself in an entitative way. To appropriately capture the evental form of flow requires forms of thought that differ from the classical (Western) conceptions of the entitative individuum operating in and on a world separate from itself. Over the course of many years of trying to come to grips with the phenomenon of being-in-the-flow, two related forms of thought have turned out to be more promising than others that I have investigated in the course of my scholarly career. The first allows us to think about the phenomenon in terms of a continuous stream of experiencing; and the second encourages us to move from viewing the world in entitative terms (including subject, object, and actions) to thinking about it in evental terms.

4.1 *Experiencing versus an Experience*

> To be conscious of one's experiences is nothing other than to have them as object (stimulus) for other experiences. Consciousness is the experience of experiences just like experiences are simply experiences of objects. (Vygotsky, 1997, pp. 71–72)

The preceding phenomenology of being-in-the-flow characterized by absorbed coping highlights the important difference between that state and other forms of human experience where the self–other distinction is predominant. While being-in-the-flow, thinking is but one of the many forms of events that together constitute the whole flux of the current activity while it endures. My (agential) self, the tools I use, the objects "I" am oriented to, and so on do not stand out as entitative things. Instead, there is but a continued happening and a dimmest of sense of feeling well. Importantly, my (immediate past) experience no longer is the objects of the current experience: there no longer is a world of separate entitative things, including the self, as everything including experiencing is in continuous flux.

One of my early dissatisfactions with the constructivist metaphor to understand individual and social life has been the intellectualization of human affairs. Teachers and students are said to "construct" knowledge, identities, beliefs, and so on. In an extended study of knowing and learning about static electricity – which analyzed both what students did activities in their hands-on activities and my own reproduction thereof – this metaphor of construction turned out to be unhelpful (Roth, 2008). There were too many aspects of the objective and subjective data that the metaphor could not explain. Among others, my study includes a chapter in which I describe the experience of being-in-the-flow which had arisen while I was trying to reproduce with the students' curriculum materials what they had been asked to achieve. Even though I had previously obtained a Master's degree in physics, I found myself having spent an entire night doing experiments over and over again, keeping records of what I was doing and finding, trying to figure out how to understand something that ought to have been simple enough for a tenth-grade student to understand. Since then, I have tried to find ways to describe the experience of being-in-the-flow that more scientifically oriented individuals might accept rather than rejecting the phenomenon as esoteric.

An important concept developed at the beginning of the 20th century is that of experience. However, it never has had much traction in the field of psychology, increasingly orienting toward becoming more scientific and thus removed from the pursuit of understanding real people in real situations. The development makes sense given that the concept of experience, generally imprecise and double-barreled, is the best one to use when "a name is wanted to emphasize the *interconnectedness of all concerns, affairs, pursuits, etc.*" (Dewey & Bentley, 1949/1999, p. 187, emphasis added). The consequence of such a position is that it abandons reductionist approaches to understanding the essence of humans and nature, including any body–mind or mind–matter dichotomy. The concept emphasizes that "mind and external things are co-ordinate members of the world" (Alexander, 1920, p. 29). That is, the concept of experience fits into a holistic conception of humans and their lifeworld that stand in an organismic part-whole relation. Being-in-the-flow while cycling, hammering, pulling weeds, or writing academic works no longer belongs to the individual but needs to be understood from the perspective of the whole event in which person, thing, or environment are but abstractions. The concept of experience was introduced precisely in the pursuit of a non-reductionist approach to understanding human affairs.

One of the problems with the general use of the term experience arises from the fact that there are different phenomena that the term refers to but that are not normally distinguished in English (as other languages). These different phenomena are denoted in German as *Erleben* or *Erlebnis*, which may be translated as "ongoing experiencing" equivalent to Vygotsky's simple experiences, and *Erfahrung*, which refers to the experiences one has had and what one has learned. When asking people about their experiences, we generally are provided with *accounts of* experiences including everything that a person recalls and which therefore has entered consciousness. The result is something corresponding to the German *Erfahrung* and to Vygotsky's notion of the experience of experience, as defined in the opening quotation of this section. This quotation does indeed make the distinction between the two phenomena: simply experiencing – because of the evental nature of the phenomenon, the gerund form experienc*ing* may actually be more useful than the noun form experience – and the experience of experience. The latter is consciousness or conscious awareness, whereas simply experiencing does not involve conscious awareness of what is involved as such, including experiencing. However, as the preceding phenomenology shows, being-in-the-flow is a form of experiencing that does not make the different aspects of the ongoing event stand out in any entitative way. The experience of experience, on the other hand, refers to what we tend to understand as mind or intellect. The experience that is the focus of another, necessarily subsequent experience inherently is a completed (compositional) whole (Dewey, 1934/2008). Dewey thus proposes a distinction equivalent to that Vygotsky was making: between a general stream of experience and *an* experience, with the latter being equivalent to the experience of experience.

An experience is a whole, having a beginning and an end. Because the event has run its course, the narrative plot of *an* experience is oriented toward the already-given end. It is this orientation that gives *an* experience its compositional character, giving agents and things their specific place and self-identity. Readers familiar with the history of science will have encountered the same form of relation in the difference between science as practice and science as it appears in scientific publication. Although Dewey (1934/2008) uses the word verb flow, comparing *an* experience to a river, his example is inconsistent with an evental perspective. This is so because one can only after the fact talk about "that meal in a Paris restaurant of which one says 'that *was* an experience.' It stands out as an enduring memorial of what food may be" (p. 43). For example, we may think about those who had dinner in Le Petit Cambodge restaurant in the evening of November 13, 2015 did not know what kind of *an* experience they will have had until the eruption of gun fire that eventually left 15 people dead. It is unlikely that any of the survivors talked about the evening like Dewey, though they might have done so under different circumstances.

My phenomenology of being-in-the-flow provided above makes it apparent that the term experience is inappropriate for the phenomenon of being-in-the-flow when used in the sense of *an* experience. But the gerund form *experiencing,* emphasizes the ongoing and open-ended nature of what is currently happening. But that experiencing concerns the activity, weeding, cycling, academic writing, or building a garden shed. It is not an experiencing of the self – e.g., concerned with how others might think about what I am doing. Instead, the current happening is singularly organized by the event: weeding, cycling, academic writing, building a garden shed, or whatever it might be. As a result, experiencing, as being-in-the-flow, is best thought from the perspective of events. This new perspective replaces the previously critiqued predominant one of the entitative and agential subject who acts upon entitative things, or entitative subjects thinking about (constructing) entitative ideas and concepts. Being-in-the-flow, there are no things apart from subjects. There are only events overlapping – if they relate at all to one another – in ways that give rise to space and time.

4.2 *From Things to Events*

> I let my avatar fly through this level – and find myself flying high. With somnambulistic certainty, I unwind the movement sequences. There are moments when the game and I seem to be one. I feel the euphoria of mastery, the self-forgetfulness of the virtuoso: I am playing the game and not the other way around. In short: I am in the so-called flow. (Beyer, 2020, para. 2)

The introductory quotation derives from an article on the experience of flow in (computer) gaming. Although there are aspects in the description that appear consistent with the phenomenology provided above – e.g., the experience of unity with the game – it is an essentially agent-centered account. The agent is in control, playing the game, rather than the converse – or, as I would describe it, rather than being caught up and being an integral part of something larger that has its own dynamic. The account also articulates emotion, rather than hinting at the affects that predominate in experiencing. Indeed, the very experience of an emotion such as euphoria would express an orientation to the entitative self rather than to the game, which, if it really happened, would break the flow.

The description thus is based on classical Platonian ontology, which assumes that there are actors (subjects) and actions and things acted upon (predicates). Events come about when actors act. In this perspective, there is a primacy to entitative subjects, with the capacity to act, and things. The entire logic of classical (Western) philosophy is built on this framework, and, with it, the logic of technology and modern philosophy. This includes cause and effect reasoning.

The description of flow in the quotation opening this section is antithetical to my phenomenology of being-in-the-flow. My descriptions of being-in-the-flow while weeding or doing other mundane activities shows that in this state, tools and objects do not stand out in the way as they do in a theoretical gaze. The more we gaze at and consider the thing (tool), the less we actually understand its essence during the event. The less it is gazed at and the more it dissolves into the event, the more it reveals itself and we encounter it in its essence. To think about being-in-the-flow and absorbed coping, we therefore must not begin by positing the subject, who is engaged in some form of activity using some tools (gardening, cycle, computer) to produce ("construct") some entitative thing with whatever is at hand. If we did so, we would have already committed to a cinematographic approach, which assumes that movement can be reconstituted from still images and stable things (Bergson, 1908). The description of experience then is concerned with identifying permanences in past events (e.g. the spatula-tool) that "are recognised as self-identical amid different circumstances" (Whitehead, 1919, p. 63). The cinematographer reconstitutes past movement on the basis of recurrences across different stills, each representing the featured matters through a lens of immobility. But the movement is not that inherent in the things. Instead, the movement is an illusion created when an outside mechanism presents the stills in rapid succession.

To deal with the phenomenon of being-in-the-flow, as something with endogenous movement, we are better off thinking it from the perspective of the event, a perspective in which still things are but abstractions from a world considered forever in flux (Roth, 2012). The smallest part of flux still is flux rather than stable entities acting upon and relating to one another. The smallest part of being-in-the-flow therefore still is being-in-the-flow. And the subject, with emotions, feelings, thoughts, using tools oriented toward objects all are parts of still images.

Being-in-the-flow is an evental phenomenon. When we change to a viewpoint that places primacy on events, everything changes. It should be apparent that this is so because an event (flow) includes change. I am no longer the same – biologically, experientially, affectively, etc. – at the end of an event, however brief, as I was at the beginning. I cannot therefore attribute identity (or thinghood) before taking an external, retrospective view on the phenomenon of being-in-the-flow. It is only after an event that those permanences attributed to the individual can be identified despite the changes it has undergone. It is thus only after the fact that I can emphasize the role of this or that thing within an overall narrative that relates earlier parts of an event to later parts. This is so because events do not cause other events, not in the least because even the most basic event comes with novelty (Whitehead, 1919). Thus, any thinking concurrent with weeding cannot *grasp* the latter, for it is not complete and therefore not yet an act, just as my thinking concurrent with my speaking can grasp my thought until after my speaking has ended. Grasping a thought is different from thinking, just as is being-in-the-flow and the associated account of having had *an* experience.

I previously noted that the self-moving event of being-in-the-flow implies an inherent change of the subject of activity. Rather than a subject of activity, we are dealing with a subject that has changed in the course and as a result of the event – Whitehead (1929/1978) therefore proposes the notion of the subject-superject. The change may be understood in terms of the concurrent and intersecting events of the *person-becoming-thing* and the *thing-becoming-person* (Roth, 2019). We cannot usefully attribute the origin of actions in the thing or the subject: in weeding, the gardener and the weeds are but organic parts.

In an evental (as opposed to an entitative) ontology, two events only relate when they have something in common (Whitehead, 1919). They may be contemporaneous (e.g., thinking and the associated acting), give rise to another (e.g., intending), or arise from an earlier one (e.g., acting from intending). If they do not have something in common, they are external to each other and thus do not relate at all. No third thing can get them to relate, for example, by means of mediation because this approach only introduces further gaps with each additional theoretical entity (e.g., James, 1909). But if they overlap, then they are constitutive and organic (thus non-additive) parts of larger events. In weeding, weeds and gardener are events that intersect in weeding.

To clarify the relation between two events (e.g., gardener and weeds), consider the analogy of two individuals in conversation. The attentive listening and hearing on the part of the recipient is contemporaneous with the saying of the speaker. The words resonating in the mouth of the speaker and in the ear of the listener, constitute the events that intersect with the evental families corresponding to the participants. Conversations do not have a predetermined end. One turn at speaking arises out of the preceding one and leads into (gives rise to) the succeeding one. This is why succeeding turns cannot be in causal relation, for the earlier turn is an integral constituent of the later (cf. Dewey, 1938). The terrain covered by the contributions of the participants, the said, can then be referred to as the content of the conversation.

In evental terms, my weeding can be thought of as a family of events, including those of the most basic biological and physiological nature (exchanging oxygen, producing carbon dioxide, beating heart) and the basic and more advanced psychological ones (thinking, doing). Consciousness then is a form of experiencing, where the event of thinking deals with the contents of remembering what stands out from previous experiencing. The world, as intimated above, also is thought of in terms of a family of events. In the relation between the two classes of events, one related to the senses, the other to the world sensed, the former constitute "active" and the latter "passive" conditions (Whitehead, 1919). In the case of weeding, thinking, sensing, acting, and the world co-evolve, corresponding with one another as persons correspond in a conversation (cf. Roth, 2019). Co-evolution means that weeding, thinking, sensing, and acting are not separate from the world but are organic parts of and thus subject and subjected to the encompassing event.

Being-in-the-flow involves an abandonment of the self to what is happening. I think of the self a permanence recognized from a series of still photographs. Any notion of self (identity) requires a cessation of the event of experiencing typical of being-in-the-flow, and is concerned with *an* experience, with what just has ended and some conclusion. This is why I the introductory quotation uses an inappropriate description, for it privileges the human agent. Instead, while being-in-the-flow, she is playing the game as much as the game is playing her. Indeed, there is neither game nor a separable subject. And if I tried to always be in control of the game or of the weeds, then I would not fall into being-in-the-flow: I would remain external to the relation with the unfolding world.

Even though in being-in-the-flow there are no objects, subjects, actions or time in the objective sense (i.e., as standing out), this does not mean that no thinking is taking place. Indeed, for weeding to occur in the ways it does and for the bicycle to stay on the road without accidents involving other vehicles or pedestrians, thinking does occur. But it is a thinking event concurrent with other events, among which are those that get the weeds out of the ground. It is not thinking that tries to fix what is happening in theoretical terms, but one that is part of the happening as a whole. Being-in-the-flow means that what Nietzsche (1922) called the *will to power* has gone, and with it the associated reduction of the world into subject-predicate relations and the entitative ontology it presupposes. I have allowed myself to become integral and constitutive part of a larger evental whole, which also determines the nature of role.

5 Coda

In this chapter, I describe and theorize being-in-the-flow, a form of experience often described to be associated with exceptional performances and non-work-related activities. Being-in-the-flow is taken here to be a form of total involvement with life and absorbed coping with the challenges at hand without concurrently making this involvement present in conscious awareness. The predominant quality of the experience is that of an evental whole, a unity in which the separate subject and its lifeworld are but abstractions (as in "the game and I are one"). The transitive relations between an acting subject and its object that typically appear in descriptions of the phenomenon are antithetical to the phenomenon of being-in-the-flow because the agential subject ("I") does not experience itself as separate from the world. Some of the concepts typically found in the social science literature – including identity, notions of self, conceptions, emotions, and tools – are shown to be irrelevant, for they fail to describe (theorize) and categorize essential features of being-in-the-flow. Using weeding as the predominant example, my descriptions exhibit essential features of the phenomenon that are inconsistent with the (social) constructivist metaphors that are commonly used across the social sciences.

I propose understanding being-in-the-flow in terms of the concept of experiencing, contrasting it with that of *an* experience, a term that refers us to a completed event through the lens of its end. It is only through such a lens that (a) early parts of an event can be said to have caused later parts and (b) an agential subject can be constructed as having acted according to preconceived intentions. Both aspects are related to what have been called self-actional and interactional views, where "presumptively independent 'actors,' 'souls,' 'minds,' 'selves,' 'powers' or 'forces,' [are] taken as activating events" and where "particles or other objects [are] organized as operating upon one another" (Dewey & Bentley, 1949/1999, p. 122). I liken these supposedly independent entities to recognizable aspects of still photographs, which inherently are abstractions from events.

The description I provide instead is a transactional one, in which behavior and its sources cannot be located within (as in a constructivist view) or outside of the organism (as in a behaviorist). In the transactional perspective, descriptions "are employed to deal with aspects and phases of action, without final attribution to 'elements' or other presumptively detachable or independent 'entities,' 'essences,' or 'realities,' and without isolation of presumptively detachable 'relations' from such detachable 'elements'" (Dewey & Bentley, 1949/1999, p. 133). That is, the view I present here is one that takes the individual-acting-in-the-environment as an irreducible evental unit (as in "Michael-weeding-the-garden"). An evental unit can be further analyzed by investigating part events that stand in an organic relation with the whole. As outlined above, in an organic perspective, weeding then is understood as a family of events, where the person and the lifeworld are taken as constitutive families of events.

In my long academic and personal search for coherence, this is the only way in which I was able to get at the very essence of being-in-the-flow: by using evental categories to investigate evental phenomena.

References

Alexander, S. (1920). *Space time and deity: The Gifford lectures at Glasgow 1916–1918.* Macmillan.

Ambrose, G., Das, K., Fan, Y., & Ramaswami, A. (2020). Is gardening associated with greater happiness of urban residents? A multi-activity, dynamic assessment in the Twin-Cities region, USA. *Landscape and Urban Planning, 198,* Article 103776. https://doi.org/10.1016/j.landurbplan.2020.103776

Bergson, H. (1908). *L'évolution créatrice* (Creative evolution, 4th ed.). Félix Alcan.

Beyer, N. (2020, June 7). Das Geheimnis des Flow [The secret of flow]. *Spiegel Netzwelt* [Online magazine]. https://www.spiegel.de/netzwelt/games/flow-in-videospielen-wenn-alles-fliesst-a-89135cf0-b7e2-4e5b-8299-2a75cba8c0e1

Csikszentmihalyi, M. (1990). *Flow* (E-book). HarperCollins.

Dewey, J. (1938). *Logic: The theory of inquiry.* Henry Holt.

Dewey, J., & Bentley, A. F. (1999). Knowing and the known. In R. Handy & E. E. Hardwood, *Useful procedures of inquiry* (pp. 97–209). Behavioral Research Council. (Original work published 1949)

Findlay, H. (2019, February 28). How to find your flow. *Climbing.* https://www.climbing.com/skills/hazel-findlay-how-to-find-your-flow/

Franck, D. (1981). *Chair et corps: Sur la phénoménologie de Husserl* [*Flesh and body: On the phenomenology of Husserl*]. Les Éditions de Minuit.

Heidegger, M. (1977). *Sein und Zeit* [*Being and time*]. Max Niemeyer.

Henry, M. (2000). *Incarnation: Une philosophie de la chair* [*Incarnation: A philosophy of the flesh*]. Éditions du Seuil.

Husserl, E. (1973). *Husserliana Band I. Cartesianische Meditationen und Pariser Vorträge* [*Husserliana Vol. 1: Cartesian mediations and Parisian presentations*]. Martinus Nijhoff.

James, H. (1909). *A pluralistic universe.* Longmans, Green.

Leont'ev, A. N. (1981). *Problems of the development of the mind.* Progress.

Masciotra, D., Roth, W.-M., & Morel, D. (2007). *Enaction: Toward a Zen mind in learning and teaching.* Sense.

Nietzsche, F. (1922). *Nachgelassene Werke: Zweite Abteilung Band XVI* [*Unpublished works: Part 2 Vol. 16*]. Alfred Kröner Verlag.

Roth, W.-M. (2003). Competent workplace mathematics: How signs become transparent in use. *International Journal of Computers for Mathematical Learning, 8*(3), 161–189.

Roth, W.-M. (2007a). *In search of meaning and coherence: A life in research*. Sense.

Roth, W.-M. (2007b). On mediation: Toward a cultural-historical understanding of the concept. *Theory & Psychology, 15*, 655–680.

Roth, W.-M. (2011). *Passibility: At the limits of the constructivist metaphor*. Springer.

Roth, W.-M. (2012). *First-person methods: Toward an empirical phenomenology of experience*. Sense.

Roth, W.-M. (2019). *Transactional psychology of education: Toward the social in a strong sense*. Springer.

Roth, W.-M., & Jornet, A. (2017). *Understanding educational psychology. A late Vygotskian, Spinozist approach*. Springer.

Roth, W.-M., & Jornet, A. (2019). Theorizing with/out "mediators." *Integrative Psychological and Behavioral Science, 53*, 323–343.

Vygotsky, L. S. (1987). *The collected works of L. S. Vygotsky, Vol. 1: Problems of general psychology*. Springer.

Whitehead, A. N. (1919). *An enquiry concerning the principles of natural knowledge*. Cambridge University Press.

Whitehead, A. N. (1978). *Process and reality: An essay in cosmology*. The Free Press. (Original work published 1929)

Index